Breastfeeding A-Z

Terminology and Telephone Triage

Karin Cadwell, PhD, RN, FAAN, IBCLC
The Healthy Children Project
The Center for Breastfeeding
East Sandwich, MA

Cindy Turner-Maffei, MA, IBCLC
The Healthy Children Project
The Center for Breastfeeding
East Sandwich, MA

EQNK4

JONES AND BARTLETT PUBLISHERS
Sudbury, Massachusetts
BOSTON   TORONTO   LONDON   SINGAPORE

GSTM   (EQNK4)

World Headquarters
Jones and Bartlett Publishers
40 Tall Pine Drive
Sudbury, MA 01776
978-443-5000
info@jbpub.com
www.jbpub.com

Jones and Bartlett Publishers
Canada
6339 Ormindale Way
Mississauga, Ontario L5V 1J2
CANADA

Jones and Bartlett Publishers
International
Barb House, Barb Mews
London W6 7PA
UK

Jones and Bartlett's books and products are available through most bookstores and online booksellers. To contact Jones and Bartlett Publishers directly, call 800-832-0034, fax 978-443-8000, or visit our website, www.jbpub.com.

Substantial discounts on bulk quantities of Jones and Bartlett's publications are available to corporations, professional associations, and other qualified organizations. For details and specific discount information, contact the special sales department at Jones and Bartlett via the above contact information or send an email to specialsales@jbpub.com.

The authors, editor, and publisher have made every effort to provide accurate information. However, they are not responsible for errors, omissions, or for any outcomes related to the use of the contents of this book and take no responsibility for the use of the products described. Treatments and side effects described in this book may not be applicable to all patients; likewise, some patients may require a dose or experience a side effect that is not described herein. The reader should confer with his or her own physician regarding specific treatments and side effects. Drugs and medical devices are discussed that may have limited availability controlled by the Food and Drug Administration (FDA) for use only in a research study or clinical trial. The drug information presented has been derived from reference sources, recently published data, and pharmaceutical research data. Research, clinical practice, and government regulations often change the accepted standard in this field. When consideration is being given to use of any drug in the clinical setting, the healthcare provider or reader is responsible for determining FDA status of the drug, reading the package insert, reviewing prescribing information for the most up-to-date recommendations on dose, precautions, and contraindications, and determining the appropriate usage for the product. This is especially important in the case of drugs that are new or seldom used.

Production Credits
Acquisitions Editor: Kevin Sullivan
Production Director: Amy Rose
Associate Editor: Amy Sibley
Production Editor: Carolyn F. Rogers
Marketing Manager: Emily Ekle
Manufacturing and Inventory Coordinator: Amy Bacus
Composition: Auburn Associates, Inc.
Cover Design: Kristin E. Ohlin
Printing and Binding: Malloy, Inc.
Cover Printing: Malloy, Inc.

Library of Congress Cataloging-in-Publication Data
Cadwell, Karin.
    Breastfeeding A-Z : terminology and telephone triage / Karin Cadwell,
Cindy Turner-Maffei.
        p. ; cm.
    Includes bibliographical references.
    ISBN 0-7637-3533-7 (pbk. : alk. paper)
    1. Breastfeeding—Terminology.   I. Turner-Maffei, Cindy.   II. Title.
    [DNLM: 1. Breast Feeding—Terminology—English.   2. Lactation
—Terminology—English.   WS 15 C147b 2006]
    RJ216.C226 2006
    649′.33—dc22
                                                                                          2005033209

ISBN-13: 978-0-7637-3533-3
ISBN-10: 0-7637-3533-7
6048

Printed in the United States of America
10 09 08 07 06   10 9 8 7 6 5 4 3 2 1

Dedication

This book is dedicated to the volunteer and professional telephone helpers with whom we have worked over the past several decades, who have opened our eyes to the intricate skill of eliciting the mother's and baby's story.

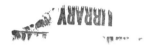

Table of Contents

Introduction

This book was developed to provide nurses, physicians, nutritionists, breastfeeding peer counselors, lactation consultants, and counselors with an evidenced-based reference about common breastfeeding terms and issues that may present as telephone calls. The need for such a tool emerged as a result of our experiences answering calls on *The Cape and Islands Breastfeeding Warmline,* and counseling mothers in person at The Center for Breastfeeding, which serves Barnstable, Dukes, and Nantucket counties in Massachusetts, USA. In addition, this book is based on collected data related to our calls.[1] We have also spoken[2] and published[3,4] information about our experiences.

One of the questions we are often asked about our warmline is "what is the difference between a helpline that is called a 'warmline' and one that is a 'hotline?'" For us, a warmline is a breastfeeding support telephone line answered in person during office hours, usually five days a week, with an opportunity for the caller to leave a voice mail message after hours and on weekends. The voice mail queries are answered the next business day. A hotline is answered in person 24 hours a day, 7 days a week.

Helping women with their breastfeeding concerns is a complex process. That complexity is amplified when the telephone answerer cannot see the mother or the baby, and the mother's description of the situation may be inadequate. The focus of the telephone interaction should be to decide the *urgency* and the *best disposition* of the case. In other words, the person answering the telephone must determine

- Do **the mother or baby need to be seen in person**, or is this telephone interaction sufficient?
- If the mother or the baby need to be seen in person, **how urgently**? Immediately? Later today? Tomorrow? Next week? Communities and health plans may have a variety of resources and options. The telephone answerer should be familiar with available community services. "Seek emergency care now" could mean a call to emergency services in one community or urgent care in another. "Seek medical care in 2 to 4 hours" means call the medical care provider now or, if the caller or baby don't have a provider, go to urgent care or an emergency care setting quickly. Agencies should give phone answerers explicit instructions regarding services in the communities they serve.

- **What** is the best disposition of the case? **Who** should be the next person to see or talk to the mother?

This book will help breastfeeding support workers to triage problems and to appropriately answer breastfeeding questions on the telephone. Key words direct further questions and provide the support person with the information needed to clarify the situation and decide the appropriate urgency and disposition of the case.

Problems may be addressed under several headings to facilitate quick reference. For example, pain in the breast is addressed under "Breast pain" and "Painful breastfeeding."

Telephone evaluation requires asking simple questions in plain language. Therefore, the keywords section contains simple keywords such as "breast pain" as well as medical terms such as "galactocele." The mother's tone of voice, sense of urgency, and concern must be considered, as well as the history of the mother and the baby. Referring to the mother or baby's chart or records is ideal, but not always possible.

It is important to always keep in mind the limitations of telephone support interactions. The telephone interaction cannot take the place of in-person assessment, evaluation, or teaching. However, for many mothers, especially those who are breastfeeding for the first time, the telephone can offer an opportunity to "check out" whether what they are experiencing is common, normal, or abnormal, and to ask questions as they arise.

Mothers may call the telephone help line when they have a specific question or problem. In some cases, the mother articulates her situation clearly, such as in the following examples:

"I called because my neighbor told me my 6-week-old baby is ready for solid foods."
"I think I have the flu. Can I still breastfeed?"
"I'm going back to work. Where can I get a breast pump?"
"I think that my baby has diarrhea. Did he get it from my milk?"

Other mothers' calls are less clear about their issues and require open-ended questions so that the telephone answerer can work with her to clarify her concerns. For example, the mother may say, "My baby isn't feeding right." We can never assume that our ideas of "feeding right" are the same as the mother's. We must work to try to gain a better understanding of what the mother means.

Breastfeeding supporters also need to be aware that mothers may construct a "door-opener" question or complaint that overlies a real concern that they are afraid is unworthy of attention. The mother may not have articulated her real concern to a point at which it can be easily communicated. For example, the mother may be worried about the quality of her milk, but ask for help with her "inverted" nipple. Upon further discussion, the telephone answerer learns from the mother's own description that her nipples are indeed nicely everted. In this case, the mother does not need false reassurance, but a thoughtful exploration of other concerns or questions she may have.

Not all questions that come to a breastfeeding support telephone line are about breastfeeding. For example, a mother may be the victim of domestic abuse. She may want to know about government programs or housing. She may call the breastfeeding support telephone line because it is a number she has handy or she has called before. How will these calls be handled? At our call center, we keep information about accessing community resources and refer mothers to specified non-breastfeeding resources. Your agency will need to make its own policy regarding appropriate referrals.

This book constitutes a first attempt to provide a quick reference and triage tool. We welcome you to give us feedback and input to enrich future editions of this book. Please send us your suggestions, so that together we may build a rich reference for telephone helpers.

Karin Cadwell and Cindy Turner-Maffei
info@healthychildren.cc

REFERENCES

[1]Philipp, B. (2001). Every call is an opportunity: Supporting breastfeeding mothers over the telephone. *Pediatric Clinics of North America, 48*(2), 525–532.

[2]Cadwell, K., & Turner-Maffei, C. (2002). *From concept to reality: Building a breastfeeding warmline.* Poster, Healthy Mothers Healthy Babies Coalition Biennial Conference, Tampa, Florida, July 22, 2002.

Turner-Maffei, C., & Cadwell, K. (1999). *From Reality to Evaluation: Documenting and Improving the Work of a Breastfeeding Warmline.* Breastfeeding: The Odds-On Best, The 1999 National Conference on the Theory and Practice of Human Lactation and Breastfeeding Management; April 11, 1999.

Philipp, B., & Cadwell, K. (1998). *Calls to a Breastfeeding Warmline: Using the Data to Shape Teaching Curriculum.* Academy of Breastfeeding Medicine Third Annual Meeting; Kansas City, November 5–8, 1998.

[3]Philipp, B.L., & Cadwell, K. (1999). Fielding questions about breastfeeding. *Contemporary Pediatrics, 16*(4).

[4]Cadwell, K., & Turner-Maffei, C. (2004). *Case studies in breastfeeding: Problem-solving skills & strategies.* Sudbury, MA: Jones & Bartlett Publishers.

How to Use This Book

This book is meant to be a quick reference for anyone who uses the phone to help support breastfeeding women. The following key features have been added throughout the text to draw attention to information that will be important to consider while on the phone. Please remember to watch for these items while you are using the book.

▶ Terms

Common breastfeeding problems, concerns, and events are listed alphabetically. Note that many items (e.g., breast pain and painful breastfeeding) repeat for ease of quick reference during telephone calls. Remember that callers may report more than one concern.

DEFINITION

If the caller gives a technical or medical name to their problem (e.g., engorgement), review the definition to ensure that the caller and the telephone helper agree on the nature of the problem and are using the appropriate definitions to describe the problem.

Ask about

Ask descriptive, simple questions in lay language about the items in this section to explore the severity of the mother's concern and possible contributing or complicating factors.

ASSESSMENT

This section presents questions designed to help the telephone answerer triage the need for referral to emergency, prompt, or routine care. Use the questions to determine the appropriate disposition of the case at hand.

SELF CARE INFORMATION

Self care information may be suggested for use until the mother receives a medical or lactation evaluation.

Notes

This section may contain information about the relevance of certain symptoms, as well as contact information for various support agencies and organizations.

See also

This section suggests other related topics that may be appropriate to review with the caller.

General Recommendations for Telephone Triage

- Maintain a welcoming tone on the telephone. Many callers may be concerned about having "silly" questions or wasting your time. Tell callers that all questions are welcome and important.
- Make sure that you write down the caller's name and telephone number before beginning to discuss the presenting concern. This will allow you to call back if further information or discussion is needed, or if you lose connection with the caller.
- When possible, pull the caller's records or chart during the call. This may help provide important history or details to the case (e.g., this mother has already experienced mastitis, or this baby was born prematurely).
- Ask open-ended questions whenever possible. Callers will provide more information when asked questions that cannot be answered with a "Yes" or "No."
- Encourage callers to talk about the history of the problem or concern, when it was first noticed, and what they think caused the problem.
- If you do not know the answer to a question the caller asks, say so, and tell the caller you will find out the answer and call them back. Do not forget to follow through on this promise.
- At the end of the call, review the triage plan. Make sure the caller has your name and telephone number in case she requires further assistance.
- Remember that callers may have more than one concern. Before ending the call, ask the caller what other concerns or problems she has.
- Document the call while you are speaking to the caller or immediately after the call. Develop a form that works for your needs and the needs of your program (see Appendix A of this book for a sample intake form).

About the Authors

Karin Cadwell, PhD, RN, FAAN, IBCLC is a nationally and internationally recognized speaker, researcher, and educator. She convened Baby-Friendly USA, implementing the WHO/UNICEF Baby-Friendly Hospital Initiative in the United States, is a delegate to the U.S. Breastfeeding Committee, was visiting professor and chair of the Health Communications Masters Degree program at Emerson College, and is an adjunct professor at the Union Institute and University. Dr. Cadwell served on the International Board of Lactation Consultant Examiners (IBLCE) Panel of Experts to develop the first lactation consultant certification exam. Her extensive clinical experience includes hospital and community practice, and she continues to counsel nursing mothers on Cape Cod in Massachusetts. Dr. Cadwell is the author of numerous publications, including *Maternal and Infant Assessment for Breastfeeding and Human Lactation: A Guide for the Practitioner* and *Reclaiming Breastfeeding for the U.S.: Protection, Promotion, and Support.* She was awarded the designation International Board Certified Lactation Consultant (IBCLC) in 1985 for "significant contribution to the field" and has since recertified.

Cindy Turner-Maffei, MA, IBCLC is the national coordinator of Baby-Friendly USA, implementing the WHO/UNICEF Baby-Friendly Hospital Initiative in the United States. She has extensive experience as a breastfeeding educator in The Special Supplemental Nutrition Program for Women, Infants, and Children (WIC) and other maternal child health programs, and she continues to counsel nursing mothers on Cape Cod in Massachusetts. Ms. Turner-Maffei is a delegate to breastfeeding coalitions on the local, state, and national level, including the U.S. Breastfeeding Committee. A faculty member of the Healthy Children Project and adjunct faculty of the Union Institute and University, Ms. Turner-Maffei is also an author of numerous publications, including *Case Studies in Breastfeeding: Problem-Solving Skills and Strategies* and *Ten Steps to Successful Breastfeeding: An 18-Hour Interdisclipinary Breastfeeding Management Course for the United States.*

Acknowledgments

We are eternally grateful to Kimberly G. Lee, MD, MS, IBCLC, Assistant Professor of Pediatrics, Harvard Medical School, and Assistant Director, Newborn Nursery, Beth Israel Deaconess Medical Center, Boston, MA, for her thoughtful, insightful review of this book.

We also gratefully acknowledge the support of our colleagues at the Center for Breastfeeding and our wonderful families.

The information contained in this book is intended for use in understanding and triaging client's concerns in order to direct them to the most appropriate route of care. Medical information obtained from this publication is not intended as a substitute for professional care. If you have or suspect you have a problem, please consult your health care provider immediately. Health care is an ever-changing science; as new research and clinical experience broaden our knowledge, changes in treatment are required.

The authors have checked with sources believed to be reliable in their efforts to provide information that is complete and generally in accord with the standards accepted at the time of publication.

▶ AA

DEFINITION Arachidonic acid. A long-chain polyunsaturated fatty acid (LCPUFA) found naturally in human milk. These fatty acids assist in the development of nerve and brain tissue, and may account for some of the differences between formula and breastfed children in terms of IQ, test scores, and visual acuity.

> **Notes**
>
> While LCPUFAs have been added to formula in recent years, there is little evidence of beneficial outcomes for children who have consumed them.

▶ AABA

See also African-American Breastfeeding Alliance (AABA)

▶ AAFP

See also American Academy of Family Physicians (AAFP)

▶ AAN

See also American Academy of Nursing (AAN)

▶ AAP

See also American Academy of Pediatrics (AAP)

▶ ABI

See also American Breastfeeding Institute (ABI)

▶ ABM

See also The Academy of Breastfeeding Medicine (ABM)

▶ Abrupt weaning

DEFINITION Sudden cessation of breastfeeding. May be initiated by either mother or baby.

Ask about

Onset.
Age of baby.
Reason for abrupt weaning.
Whether initiated by mother or baby.

ASSESSMENT

EMERGENT CARE NEEDED?

Are any of the following present?

Extreme lethargy in baby.
Extreme irritability in baby.
Sudden change in baby's muscle tone (extremely floppy or stiff).
Sudden disinterest in feeding.
Unable to wake baby.
Baby does not calm, even with cuddles.

IF YES, *Seek emergency care now.*

PROMPT MEDICAL CARE NEEDED?

Are any of the following present?

For mothers or for babies older than 3 months, fever higher than 101° F (38.5° C). In a baby under 3 months, fever higher than 100.4° F (38° C).
In mother, extreme breast discomfort or redness.
In mother, flu-like aching throughout body.

IF YES, *Seek medical care within 2 to 4 hours.*

Are any of the following present?

Unexplained **breast refusal** of baby.
Lack of appetite in baby lasting one day.

IF YES, *Call pediatric care provider today.*

PROMPT LACTATION CARE NEEDED?

Are any of the following present?

Breast discomfort.

Difficulty relieving pressure in the breast.

Concern about effects of weaning on baby.

Sadness about weaning.

Nursing strike.

Mother has taken a drug which negatively affects milk supply (e.g., pseudoephedrine).

IF YES, *Call lactation care provider today.*

ROUTINE CARE NEEDED?

Are any of the following present?

Mild breast swelling.

Mild breast discomfort.

Ongoing adjustment difficulty.

IF YES, *Give self care information.*

Report to lactation care provider if no improvement in 2 days.

SELF CARE INFORMATION

Consider supportive bra.

Nonprescription pain relief.

Expect some emotional response to abrupt weaning.

Talk out your feelings with a trusted friend, family member, or counselor.

Baby requires an appropriate substitute for breastmilk (formula if younger than 12 months, other foods if older than 12 months).

Ensure that baby receives emotional and physical comfort during adjustment to weaning.

IMPORTANT CONDITIONS TO REPORT

Fever.

Signs of infection.

Ongoing discomfort.

Unresolved symptoms after 48 hours.

Weaning is best accomplished in a gradual manner. Slow weaning allows time for mother and baby to adjust physically and emotionally to this change. Rarely, **abrupt weaning** may be necessary for mothers to take one of the rare **contraindicated medications**, undergo surgery, or be separated from their babies for an extended period (e.g., women in the military who are deployed overseas).

Babies may abruptly refuse feeding. In this case, it is important to distinguish medical from developmental reasons for the infant's disinterest in breastfeeding. Rarely, babies can experience life threatening infections or events that cause extreme lethargy and disinterest in feeding. They may be suddenly floppy or stiff. These symptoms indicate a medical emergency, as they may reflect botulism, meningitis or other life threatening infection.

More commonly, babies may refuse to nurse for developmental or other reasons. For babies four to six months old, this may be due to distractibility. Refusal to nurse is often considered a **nursing strike**, rather than weaning. Typically it is an indication that something is troubling the baby. Troubles can range from teething and ear infection to a negative reaction to mother-baby separation or family stress. When nursing strike persists, the baby should be examined to rule out ear infection or other contributing factors.

Strategies for overcoming nursing strike include not forcing nursing, offering lots of contact and holding, having mom lie down beside a sleepy baby and offering the breast, having mom and baby take a bath together, and applying "peer pressure" by bringing an older baby in contact with other nursing babies.

Mother may need assistance with expressing milk to continue her milk supply during this phase. She may wish to discuss her reaction to the baby's refusal to feed.

While weaning abruptly, women usually need to remove some milk to relieve the pressure in their breasts. Women who are weaning permanently should remove as little milk as possible, as milk removal continues milk synthesis. Other women may be weaning temporarily due to short term separation from baby, or short term use of a contraindicated medication. In this situation, mothers should be encouraged to hand express or pump milk as many times daily as their baby would nurse.

See also Nursing strike; Relactation; Weaning

▶ Abscess, breast

DEFINITION A localized collection of pus resulting from the breakdown of breast tissue. Inflammation often occurs around the abscess. Breast abscess is often the outcome of unresolved breast infection.

Abscess may or may not be visible on the surface of the breast. Breast abscess is often the outcome of unresolved mastitis.

Abscesses are typically drained through aspiration or by surgical incision and drainage. Antibiotic treatment will be prescribed based on suspected pathogen.

Ask about

Onset.
Prior breast infection.
Known drug allergies.

ASSESSMENT

EMERGENT CARE NEEDED?

Are any of the following present?

Visible or palpable breast abscess.
Maternal fever higher than 100° F (37.7° C).
Extreme breast discomfort.
Flu-like aching throughout body.
Chills.
Continuing fever after abscess drainage.
Reaction to antibiotic prescribed postdrainage.
Green or odorous change to fluid seeping from site after drainage.

IF YES, *Seek medical care within 2 to 4 hours.*

PROMPT CARE NEEDED?

Are any of the following present?

Continuation of pain, swelling, or redness after drainage.
Difficulty with breastfeeding following abscess drainage.

IF YES, *Seek medical care within 24 hours and call lactation care provider today.*

ROUTINE CARE NEEDED?

Are any of the following present?

Questions about resumption of breastfeeding on affected breast.

IF YES, *Call obstetric or surgical care provider today.*

SELF CARE INFORMATION

Finish full course of antibiotics prescribed (unless told to stop by a physician).

Continue nonprescription pain relief as recommended.

Continue to monitor breasts for symptoms of recurring breast infection (redness, heat, fever, blockage, pain).

IMPORTANT CONDITIONS TO REPORT

Symptoms worsen or persist.

Signs of infection.

> ### Notes
>
> Abscess indicates a need for urgent medical treatment. Symptoms include reddened areas of the breast, occasionally with a visible fluid filled sac protruding through the surface of the breast, and overall body sensation of **malaise**, aching, fever, or fatigue. Abscess may follow **mastitis**. Typical treatment includes appropriate antibiotic administration and drainage by lancing or aspiration. Presence of one identified abscess may indicate presence of multiple other abscesses, some of which may be deep in the breast, visible only by imaging technology. When symptoms do not resolve after treatment, presence of additional abscesses must be considered.
>
> Breastfeeding is not contraindicated on the noninvolved breast. Breastfeeding may continue on the affected breast if determined safe. Drainage may cause leaking of milk from severed ducts. Women may feel very ill and need practical and emotional support.

See also Acute infection; Breast infection

▶ Abuse

DEFINITION Improper treatment, misuse, or physical, emotional or sexual maltreatment.

Ask about

Location.

Physical safety at this moment.

EMERGENT CARE NEEDED?

Are any of the following present?

Physical safety of baby and caller in danger at this moment.

IF YES, *Seek emergency protection now.*

PROMPT CARE NEEDED?

Are any of the following present?

Caller or baby endangered, but not at the current moment.

IF YES, *Contact social services immediately.*

SELF CARE INFORMATION

Contact local abuse resources.

Know local emergency assistance numbers.

Know the location of area police stations.

Notes

Physical and emotional abuse are disturbingly common in families. When individuals reach out for help with abuse, appropriate response is crucial.

Follow your office protocol for abuse referrals. Protocols should be based on existing state or territorial laws and resources. Know the rules regarding mandated reporting. Have the emergency social service numbers on hand for easy reference.

Careful response to the abuser is critical; otherwise the caller and her family may be further endangered. Refer abusive situations to the appropriate authorities.

▶ Academy of Breastfeeding Medicine (ABM)

DEFINITION "The Academy of Breastfeeding Medicine is a worldwide organization of physicians dedicated to the promotion, protection and support of breastfeeding and human lactation. Its mission is to unite into one association members of the various medical specialties with this common purpose."[1]

Footnotes

[1]The Academy of Breastfeeding Medicine. (n.d.). Untitled. Retrieved June 19, 2005 from http://www.bfmed.org.

▶ Academy for Educational Development (AED)

DEFINITION "Founded in 1961, AED is an independent, nonprofit organization committed to solving critical social problems and building the capacity of individuals, communities, and institutions to become more self-sufficient. AED works in all the major areas of human development, with a focus on improving education, health, and economic opportunities for the least advantaged in the United States and developing countries throughout the world."[2]

Footnotes

[2]Academy for Educational Development. (2005). *What We Do.* Retrieved June 19, 2005 from http://www.aed.org/WhatWeDo/.

▶ ## Academy of Lactation Policy & Practice (ALPP)

DEFINITION "The Academy of Lactation Policy and Practice strives to promote interdisciplinary, professional knowledge about breastfeeding and human lactation, and thereby to promote, protect and support breastfeeding for individuals and the society of the United States at large.

Founded in 1999, ALPP is dedicated to improving the foundation of breastfeeding comprehension and understanding throughout the United States by providing certificates of added qualification in breastfeeding."[3,4]

Notes
The Academy of Lactation Policy and Practice
Post Office Box 1288
Forestdale, MA 02644
Phone: 508-833-1500
Web: www.talpp.org

Footnotes

[3]Academy of Lactation Policy and Practice. (n.d.). *Mission.* Retrieved August 11, 2005, from http://www.talpp.org.

[4]Academy of Lactation Policy and Practice. (n.d.). *What is ALPP?* Retrieved August 11, 2005, from http://www.talpp.org.

▶ ## Accessory breast tissue

DEFINITION Extra breast and nipple tissue. Women may have extra "accessory" breast or nipple tissue anywhere on the ventral surface of their trunk, as well as in the axillary, groin, and upper thigh areas.

▶ ACNM

See also American College of Nurse-Midwives (ACNM)

▶ ACOG

See also The American College of Obstetricians and Gynecologists (ACOG)

▶ Acquired immunodeficiency syndrome (AIDS)

DEFINITION A life threatening disease of the immune system caused by the human immunodeficiency virus (HIV). People with AIDS have increased susceptibility to infections and rare cancers including Kaposi's sarcoma. HIV is transmitted primarily by exposure to contaminated body fluids, especially blood, semen, and potentially breastmilk.

Ask about

Onset of illness.
Age of baby.

ASSESSMENT

EMERGENT CARE NEEDED?
Are any of the following present?

Breastfeeding mother with concern about possibility of recently contracting HIV.
Breastfeeding mother diagnosed with HIV.

IF YES, *Seek medical care within 2 to 4 hours.*

PROMPT CARE NEEDED?

Are any of the following present?

Pregnant mother with concerns about possibility of recently contracting HIV.

Pregnant mother diagnosed with HIV.

IF YES, *Call obstetric care provider today.*

ROUTINE CARE NEEDED?

Are any of the following present?

General questions about HIV.

IF YES, *Call pediatric or obstetric care provider today.*

SELF CARE INFORMATION

Know your HIV status.

Know your treatment options.

Know the HIV status of all sexual partners.

Practice safe sex.

Avoid intravenous drug use.

IMPORTANT CONDITIONS TO REPORT

Need for testing.

Notes

In the United States, breastfeeding is contraindicated in women diagnosed as HIV positive or with AIDS. Women at high risk for **HIV** (e.g., women who are sex workers, women with an HIV positive sexual partner, women using intravenous drugs, women whose sexual partners use intravenous drugs, and women who are raped or coerced to have sex) should receive testing and ongoing counseling regarding infant feeding.

See also Contraindicated conditions

▶ Acrocyanosis

DEFINITION Blue color of the hands and feet. This condition is caused by constriction of the tiny arterioles (small arteries) and results in mottled blue or red discoloration of the wrists, hands, ankles and toes.

▶ Acute infection

DEFINITION Invasion and reproduction of microorganisms in the cells or tissues of the body. Infectious microorganisms include bacteria, viruses, fungi, and others. Symptoms of infection may include fever and malaise. Lack of desire to feed can be an additional symptom of infection in the baby.

Ask about

Onset.
Age of baby.
Medications taken.
Known drug allergies.

ASSESSMENT

EMERGENT CARE NEEDED?
Are any of the following present?
Extreme **lethargy or irritability** in baby.
Sudden change in baby's muscle tone (extremely floppy or stiff) or repetitive jerking movements (e.g., seizure activity).
Baby shows sudden disinterest in feeding.
Unable to wake baby.

IF YES, *Call pediatrician now.*

PROMPT CARE NEEDED?
Are any of the following present?
About mother
Fever higher than 100° F (37.7° C).

Extreme breast discomfort.

Flu-like aching throughout body.

Extreme exhaustion.

Visible or palpable breast **abscess**.

About baby

Extreme discomfort.

Any fever in a baby younger than 3 to 4 months of age.

Fever higher than 100° F (37.7° C) in an older baby or child.

Vomiting and diarrhea that last for more than a few hours in a child of any age.

Rash, especially if there is also a fever.

Any cough or cold that does not improve within several days, or a cold that worsens and includes a fever.

Drainage from an ear.

Problems swallowing.

Sharp or persistent pains as described by older baby in the throat, ear, abdomen or stomach.

Fever and vomiting at the same time.

Not eating for more than a day.

IF YES, *Seek medical care within 2 to 4 hours.*

SELF CARE INFORMATION

Feed baby at least 10–24 times per 24 hours.

Soften breasts between feedings with gentle hand expression.

Finish full course of antibiotics prescribed (unless told to stop by a prescriber).

Continue nonprescription pain relief as recommended.

Continue to monitor for symptoms of recurring breast infection (redness, heat, fever, chills, pain).

IMPORTANT CONDITIONS TO REPORT

Symptoms worsen or persist.

Signs of infection.

Rarely, babies experience life threatening infections or events that cause extreme lethargy and disinterest in feeding. They may be suddenly floppy or stiff. These symptoms indicate a medical emergency, as they may reflect botulism, meningitis or other life threatening infection.

Many mothers experiencing **mastitis** may mistake symptoms of mastitis for flu. When a mother calls to ask for recommendations of safe flu medications, remember to ask her if she has any red, painful, hot spots on her breasts. See **Mastitis** and **Flu, maternal** for more information.

Few infections are incompatible with breastfeeding. Infections in the breastfeeding mother that are not compatible with breastfeeding include **HIV**, **HTLV-1**, and active **Herpes** lesion on the nipple or other area that will be in contact with baby's mouth.[5]

Mothers with certain infections may breastfeed once a period of treatment is initiated. These infections include tuberculosis, hepatitis, and Lyme disease. The Centers for Disease Control & Prevention and health departments can provide further information.

See also Breast infection; Flu, maternal

Footnotes

[5]American Academy of Pediatrics Section on Breastfeeding. (2005). Breastfeeding and the use of human milk. *Pediatrics, 115,* 496–506.

▶ ADA

See also American Dietetic Association (ADA)

▶ Adolescent breastfeeding

DEFINITION Adolescent mothers (ages 13–19) should be encouraged to breastfeed. Like all mothers, teens also need breastfeeding support.

Ask about

Age of baby.

PROMPT CARE NEEDED?

Are any of the following present?

Difficulty with breastfeeding.

Breast or nipple discomfort or trauma.

Misshapen nipple after feedings.

Visible fissures on nipples.

Concern about adequate milk production.

IF YES, *Call lactation care provider today.*

ROUTINE CARE NEEDED?

Are any of the following present?

Mother has questions or concerns about breastfeeding.

IF YES, *Call lactation care provider today.*

SELF CARE INFORMATION

Practice skin-to-skin contact frequently.

Feed baby at first sign of hunger cues (signs that say "feed me" include hand-to-face or hand-to-mouth movements, lip smacking, seeking with lips, rooting, and head bobbing).

Feed baby at least 10–12 times per 24 hours.

Listen for signs of baby swallowing.

Allow baby to end feedings.

Expect at least 3–4 infant stools per 24 hours after the first 4 days of life.

Good positioning and attachment are crucial to reduce nipple pain.

If baby is fed away from the breast, hand express or pump milk to maintain supply.

Eat well to preserve your energy.

IMPORTANT CONDITIONS TO REPORT

Discomfort with nursing.

Feeding or stooling expectations are not met.

There is no reason to suspect that adolescent women will have difficulty making milk.

The Dietary Reference Intake for breastfeeding teens call for an additional 500 calories over the amount required to maintain prepregnant weight.[6] 1300 mg of **calcium** is suggested for teens younger than 18 in order to protect bone density. Recent research indicates that breastfeeding was not detrimental to bone density in adolescent mothers, and may have been protective.[7] Eating more healthful foods is important to maintain mothers' energy level and nutrient stores. Eating more or less healthfully will *not* change milk composition or affect infant growth.

See also Teenaged mothers

Footnotes

[6]Food and Nutrition Information Center, Food and Nutrition Board. (2002). *Dietary Reference Intake: Recommended Intakes for Individuals.* Retrieved August 25, 2005, from http://www.nal.usda.gov/fnic/etext/000105.html

[7]Chantry, C.J., Auinger, P., & Byrd, R.S. (2004). Lactation among adolescent mothers and subsequent bone mineral density. *Archives of Pediatric & Adolescent Medicine, 158*(7), 650–656.

▶ Adoption and induced lactation

DEFINITION Induced lactation is the process of establishing a milk supply in a woman who has not given birth.

Ask about

Age of baby.

ASSESSMENT

ROUTINE CARE NEEDED?
Are any of the following present?
Mother wishes to induce lactation for an adopted infant.

IF YES, *Call lactation care provider.*

SELF CARE INFORMATION

Frequent stimulation may enable milk production.

Practice skin-to-skin contact frequently.

Feed baby at first sign of hunger cues (Signs that say "feed me" include hand-to-face or hand-to-mouth mouth movements, lip smacking, seeking with lips, rooting, and head bobbing).

Work with pediatric care provider to determine need for supplementation of the adopted baby.

Listen for signs of baby swallowing.

Allow baby to end feedings.

Expect at least 3–4 infant stools per 24 hours after the first 4 days of life.

Good positioning and attachment are crucial to reduce nipple pain.

If baby is not yet with you, or is fed away from the breast, hand express or pump milk to maintain supply.

IMPORTANT CONDITIONS TO REPORT

Arrival of baby.

First visible milk produced.

Lack of milk production after weeks of attempt.

Notes

Feeding adopted babies at the breast can be a wonderful bonding experience for mothers and babies. Adoptive mothers can produce milk with frequent breast stimulation (from a baby or a pump). It may take weeks of stimulation for a partial supply to develop. There is a wide range of volume of milk produced. Women need much practical guidance and support during this time and should consult with a lactation care provider early and often while awaiting the arrival of their adopted child.

Adopted babies may take right to the breast, or may take longer to learn to feed. Devices may be used to deliver supplements to the baby at the breast in the event that mother does not have a full milk supply.

See also At-breast supplementation; Increasing milk supply; Induced lactation; Relactation

---

► **AED**

See also Academy for Educational Development (AED)

▶ African-American Breastfeeding Alliance (AABA)

DEFINITION "AABA's overall purpose is to raise the numbers of African-American women (and women of African descent) who breastfeed; educate African-American women about the infant and maternal benefits of breastfeeding; provide valuable resources about breastfeeding; offer on-going support to women who decide to breastfeed; and collaborate with other organizations that have an interest in the health and well-being of African-American women and infants."[8]

Notes

African-American Breastfeeding Alliance
940 Madison Avenue
Baltimore, MD 21201
Phone: 410-225-2006
Web: www.aabaonline.com

Footnotes

[8]African-American Breastfeeding Alliance. (n.d). *Our Purpose.* Retrieved June 19, 2005, from http://www.aabaonline.com.

▶ AGA

DEFINITION Appropriate for gestational age. Babies who are classified **appropriate for gestational age** are of weight, length, and development considered appropriate for their gestational age at birth.

▶ AIDS

DEFINITION Acquired immunodeficiency syndrome. A life threatening disease of the immune system caused by the human immunodeficiency virus (HIV). People with AIDS have increased susceptibility to infections and rare cancers including Kaposi's sarcoma. HIV is transmitted primarily by exposure to contaminated body fluids, especially blood, semen, and potentially breastmilk.

Onset of illness.

Age of baby.

ASSESSMENT

EMERGENT CARE NEEDED?

Are any of the following present?

   Breastfeeding mother with concern about possibility of recently contracting HIV.

   Breastfeeding mother diagnosed with HIV.

IF YES, *Seek medical care now.*

PROMPT CARE NEEDED?

Are any of the following present?

   Pregnant mother with concerns about possibility of recently contracting HIV.

   Pregnant mother diagnosed with HIV.

IF YES, *Call obstetric care provider today.*

ROUTINE CARE NEEDED?

Are any of the following present?

   General questions about HIV.

IF YES, *Call pediatric or obstetric care provider today.*

SELF CARE INFORMATION

Know your HIV status.

Know your treatment options.

Know the HIV status of all sexual partners.

Practice safe sex.

Avoid intravenous drug use.

IMPORTANT CONDITIONS TO REPORT

Need for testing.

See also Contraindicated conditions

▶ Alcohol

DEFINITION An intoxicating chemical component of fermented and distilled beverages.

Ask about

Age of baby.
Status of alcohol consumption.

ASSESSMENT

EMERGENT CARE NEEDED?
Are any of the following present?
   Symptoms of alcohol poisoning (confusion, vomiting, seizures, slow or
      irregular breathing, pale or blue-tinged skin, unconsciousness).
   Symptoms of alcohol withdrawal [Delirium tremens (confusion and
      hallucinations), fever, agitation, convulsions, blacking out].

IF YES,   *Seek emergency care now.*

PROMPT CARE NEEDED?
Are any of the following present?
   Admits chronic dependence on alcohol.

IF YES,   *Seek medical care within 2 to 4 hours.*

ROUTINE CARE NEEDED?

> *Are any of the following present?*
>> Occasional social use of alcohol.
>> Plans to use alcohol occasionally.

IF YES,	*Call lactation care provider today.*

SELF CARE INFORMATION

Avoid or limit alcohol consumption.

Avoid consuming alcohol with an empty stomach.

It takes about two hours for the body to metabolize the alcohol in one drink.

Alcohol is not trapped in breastmilk. When you have had an occasional drink of alcohol and you no longer feel the effects of alcohol, it is safe to breastfeed.

Do not give alcohol to a baby or child.

IMPORTANT CONDITIONS TO REPORT

Sleepiness in baby.

Difficulty waking baby.

Notes

Alcohol passes quickly and easily into the mother's bloodstream and into her milk. As alcohol levels fall in her blood, alcohol is reabsorbed from her milk and metabolized by her body. Alcohol from a single drink (one drink is considered to be one 12-oz beer, one 4- to 5-oz glass of wine, or one shot of 80-proof alcohol) may be removed from her milk in approximately two hours. Mothers are best encouraged to avoid alcohol during the breastfeeding period. The American Academy of Pediatrics states, "Breastfeeding mothers should avoid the use of alcoholic beverages, because alcohol is concentrated in breastmilk and its use can inhibit milk production. An occasional celebratory single, small alcoholic drink is acceptable, but breastfeeding should be avoided for 2 hours after the drink."[9]

Other lines of inquiry and counseling surround the safety of the baby during the time mother is drinking. Who will care for the baby? Mother and other caregivers should be advised not to sleep in the same bed as baby when under the influence of alcohol and other medications that may alter awareness and sleep states.

Footnotes

[9]American Academy of Pediatrics Section on Breastfeeding. (2005). Breastfeeding and the use of human milk. *Pediatrics, 115*, 496–506.

▶ Allergen

DEFINITION A protein perceived as foreign by the body, thus triggering an allergic response.

See also Allergy in the breastfed infant

▶ Allergy in the breastfed infant

DEFINITION An abnormal immune reaction to substances consumed, breathed, touched, or injected.

Ask about

Onset.
Age of baby.
Known allergies.

ASSESSMENT
EMERGENT CARE NEEDED?
Are any of the following present?
Difficulty breathing.
Difficulty swallowing.
Swelling of tongue.
IF YES, Seek emergency care now.
PROMPT CARE NEEDED?
Are any of the following present?
Swelling of the face, hands, or feet.
Persistent rash, headache, or fever.
Persistent diarrhea, nausea, or vomiting.
Bloody stool.
IF YES, Seek medical care within 2 to 4 hours.

SELF CARE INFORMATION

Monitor symptoms.

Possibility of developing allergy to other proteins.

Comfort techniques for irritable baby (rocking, singing, skin-to-skin contact, bathing, seeking quiet, calm environment, etc.).

IMPORTANT CONDITIONS TO REPORT

Family history of allergy.

Symptoms worsen, persist, or reoccur.

Notes

If breathing difficulty or other extreme symptoms are reported, refer the caller to emergency care immediately.

Babies born into allergic families are more likely to develop allergy, particularly those with two allergic parents or one allergic parent and an allergic sibling. Exclusive breastfeeding is the optimal feeding choice for these babies in particular. Should the baby develop allergy symptoms, mother may be counseled to avoid consuming offending allergens such as cow's milk, fish, eggs, peanuts, and tree nuts.

Mothers who have not chosen breastfeeding may **relactate** for their allergic infant. Babies whose mothers do not choose to relactate may be fed hypoallergenic formula.

In the event that the allergic response is to a solid food, that food should not be fed to the baby. The breastfeeding mother should avoid the food until directed by a medical care provider to reintroduce allergen.

Rarely, babies develop allergies to fragments of foreign proteins consumed by their breastfeeding mother. The most potent allergens in the United States' diet include cow's milk, fish, eggs, peanuts, and tree nuts. Infantile symptoms of an allergic reaction include hives, facial swelling, runny nose, wheezing, eczema, vomiting, irritability (colic), blood in the stool, and **anaphylaxis**. Treatment centers on identification and avoidance of the proteins that are triggering the allergic reaction.

If supplementation is required, babies with documented allergy should be fed protein hydrolysate formula identified by a medical care provider. Soy protein may also be allergenic.[10]

Concern about infant allergy is much more predominant than actual allergy. The American Academy of Pediatrics reports that the prevalence of infant cow's milk allergy is two to three percent.[11] The overall prevalence of childhood food allergy is four to six percent.[12]

Counseling and education should include comfort techniques for the irritable baby and coping methods for parents.

See also Atopic eczema

Footnotes

[10]American Academy of Pediatrics Committee on Nutrition. (2000). Hypoallergenic infant formulas. *Pediatrics, 106*, 346–349.

[11]American Academy of Pediatrics Committee on Nutrition. (2000). Hypoallergenic infant formulas. *Pediatrics, 106*, 346.

[12]Ziegler, R.S. (2003). Food allergen avoidance in prevention of food allergy in infants and children. *Pediatrics, 111*, 1662–1671.

▶ **ALPP**

See also Academy of Lactation Policy & Practice

▶ **Alternate breast massage**

DEFINITION A technique used to encourage milk to flow from the breast. When the suckling baby pauses, the mother gently but firmly massages and compresses the breast to which the baby is attached, thereby increasing the flow of milk and starting the suckling again.

▶ Aluminum in breastmilk and formula

DEFINITION Aluminum is a toxic metal that is present in the environment. It affects the nervous system and other tissues.

Notes

Aluminum levels are higher in formula than in human milk. Levels are highest in soy-based formulae.[13]
   Infants born prematurely or with kidney disease are at greater risk for aluminum toxicity.

Footnotes
   [13]American Academy of Pediatrics Committee on Nutrition. (1996). Aluminum Toxicity in Infants and Children. *Pediatrics, 97*, 413–416.

▶ Alveoli

DEFINITION Tiny sacs containing milk producing cells within the breast.

Notes

These cells produce droplets of milk in response to suckling and the resulting rise in maternal blood levels of the hormone prolactin. Milk produced passes through the cell membrane into the center of the alveolar cluster, causing it to fill. The hormone oxytocin (which is created by nipple stretching, breast massage, and other stimuli) causes the myoepithelial bands around the alveoli to contract, squeezing the milk into the ductules and ducts, propelling it toward the nipple.

When the breast is very full, alveolar lobes and clusters may be palpable through the skin of the breast. Encouraging frequent feeding, good positioning, and using techniques such as **alternate breast massage** may assist mothers through this period.

If lumps or fullness do not resolve within a day or two, the mother should be seen by a physician to rule out other pathology in the breast.

▶ Amenorrhea

DEFINITION A period of cessation of menses (monthly flow of blood from the uterus).

Ask about

Age of baby.

ASSESSMENT

ROUTINE CARE NEEDED?

Are any of the following present?

Concern about prolonged lack of menses.

Concern about contraceptive usage.

Desire to conceive again.

IF YES, *Schedule routine obstetric visit.*

Are any of the following present?

Desire to extend amenorrhea.

IF YES, *Call lactation care provider today.*

SELF CARE INFORMATION

Characteristics of breastfeeding thought to increase the chances of amenorrhea include baby older than 6 months, **exclusive breastfeeding,** unrestricted feeding (10–12 or more feeds per day), avoidance of pacifiers, and **co-sleeping.**

Once any of these criteria no longer apply, secure another family planning method (unless pregnancy is desired at this time).

IMPORTANT CONDITIONS TO REPORT
Past fertility problems.
Resumption of menses.

Notes

A woman who breastfeeds exclusively during the first six months of her baby's life is likely to experience amenorrhea (that is, no menstrual period). Many breastfeeding women experience amenorrhea of a year or more, as long as they continue to breast-feed frequently.

Lactational Amenorrhea Method (LAM) is a form of natural family planning which is 98% effective in the first six months of the baby's life, so long as the mother's menses have not returned, her baby is exclusively breastfed, and there are no long periods of time between feedings, day and night. Once the baby is older than 6 months, or any of the above criteria no longer apply, LAM is no longer effective, and mothers should utilize other forms of birth control.

See also Bellagio Consensus; Lactational Amenorrhea Method (LAM); Menstrual cycle; Natural family planning

---

▶ American Academy of Family Physicians (AAFP)

DEFINITION "The Academy was founded in 1947 to promote and maintain high quality standards for family doctors who are providing continuing comprehensive health care to the public."[14]

Notes

American Academy of Family Physicians
P.O. Box 11210
Shawnee Mission, KS 66207-1210
Phone: 913-906-6000
Web: www.aafp.org

The AAFP publishes articles regarding breastfeeding in its journal, *American Family Physician®*. A breastfeeding position paper is available on its Web site.

Footnotes

[14]American Academy of Family Physicians. (2005). *Facts About AAFP*. Retrieved June 19, 2005, from http://www.aafp.org/x7637.xml.

▶ ## American Academy of Nursing (AAN)

DEFINITION "The mission of the AAN is to serve the public and nursing profession by advancing health policy and practice through the generation, synthesis, and dissemination of nursing knowledge."[15]

> **Notes**
>
> American Academy of Nursing
> 555 East Wells Street
> Suite 1100
> Milwaukee, WI 53202-3823
> Phone: 414-287-0289
> Web: www.aannet.org
>   AAN convenes an expert panel on breastfeeding.

Footnotes

[15]American Academy of Nursing. (2005). *Mission Statement*. Retrieved June 19, 2005 from http://www.aannet.org.

▶ ## American Academy of Pediatrics (AAP)

DEFINITION "The mission of the American Academy of Pediatrics is to attain optimal physical, mental, and social health and well-being for all infants, children, adolescents, and young adults."[16]

> **Notes**
>
> American Academy of Pediatrics
> 141 Northwest Point Boulevard
> Elk Grove Village, IL 60007-1098
> Phone: 847-434-4000

Fax: 847-434-8000
Web: www.aap.org
    The AAP publishes several articles, as well as policies and protocols covering breast-feeding, on its Web site and in its journal, *Pediatrics*.

Footnotes

[16]American Academy of Pediatrics. (n.d.). *Mission Statement.* Retrieved June 19, 2005 from http://www.aap.org/visit/facts.htm.

► American Breastfeeding Institute (ABI)

DEFINITION "The purpose of the American Breastfeeding Institute shall be to promote, protect and support breastfeeding in the United States through research and education."[17]

Notes

American Breastfeeding Institute
327 Quaker Meeting House Road
East Sandwich, MA 02537
Phone: 508-888-9366
    The American Breastfeeding Institute was incorporated in 2000 as a non-profit corporation.

Footnotes

[17]Articles of Incorporation, American Breastfeeding Institute.

► American College of Nurse-Midwives (ACNM)

DEFINITION "With roots dating to 1929, the American College of Nurse-Midwives (ACNM) is the oldest women's health care organization in the U.S. ACNM provides research, accredits midwifery education programs, administers and promotes continuing education programs, establishes clinical practice standards, creates liaisons with state and federal agencies and members of Congress."[18]

American College of Nurse-Midwives
8403 Colesville Rd
Suite 1550
Silver Spring, MD 20910
Phone: 240-485-1800
Web: www.midwife.org
The ACNM publishes policy papers on breastfeeding on its Web site and in the *Journal of Midwifery and Women's Health.*

Footnotes

[18]American College of Nurse-Midwives. (2005). *About the American College of Nurse-Midwives.* Retrieved June 19, 2005 from http://www.midwife.org/about.cfm.

▶ # The American College of Obstetricians and Gynecologists (ACOG)

DEFINITION "2001 marked the 50th Anniversary of The American College of Obstetricians and Gynecologists (ACOG). Founded in 1951 in Chicago, Illinois, ACOG today has over 46,000 members and is the nation's leading group of professionals providing health care for women. Now based in Washington, DC, it is a private, voluntary, nonprofit membership organization."[19]

Notes

The American College of Obstetricians and Gynecologists
409 12th Street, SW
P.O. Box 96920
Washington, DC 20090-6920
Phone: 202-638-5577
Web: www.acog.org
ACOG publishes several documents addressing breastfeeding on its Web site and in its journal, *Obstetrics & Gynecology.*

Footnotes

[19]American College of Obstetricians and Gynecologists. (2005). Untitled. Retrieved June 19, 2005 from http://www.acog.org/from_home/acoginfo.cfm.

▶ American Dietetic Association (ADA)

DEFINITION "With nearly 70,000 members, the American Dietetic Association is the nation's largest organization of food and nutrition professionals. ADA serves the public by promoting optimal nutrition, health and well-being."[20]

> **Notes**
>
> American Dietetic Association
> 120 South Riverside Plaza
> Suite 2000
> Chicago, IL 60606-6995
> Phone: 800-877-1600
> Web: www.eatright.org
>   The ADA publishes articles and policy statements about breastfeeding on its Web site and in the *Journal of the American Dietetic Association*.

Footnotes

[20]American Dietetic Association. (2005). *Welcome*. Retrieved June 19, 2005 from http://www.eatright.org/Public.

▶ American Public Health Association (APHA)

DEFINITION The American Public Health Association (APHA) is the oldest and largest organization of public health professionals in the world, representing more than 50,000 members from over 50 occupations of public health.

▶ ## Amoxicillin

DEFINITION A commonly used oral form of the antibiotic penicillin.

Notes

Amoxicillin is considered "usually compatible with breastfeeding" by the American Academy of Pediatrics (Table 6),[21] and L1 (safest) by Hale.[22]

See also Lactation risk category; Medications

Footnotes

[21]American Academy of Pediatrics Committee on Drugs. (2001). Transfer of drugs and other chemicals into human milk. *Pediatrics, 108,* 776–789.

[22]Hale, T.W. (2004). *Medications and mothers milk* (pp. 53–54). Amarillo, TX: Pharmasoft Publishing.

Drug References

Briggs, G.G., Freeman, R.K., & Yaffee, S.J. (Eds.). (2002). *Drugs in pregnancy and lactation* (6th ed.). Philadelphia: Lippincott, Williams, and Wilkins.

Lawrence, R.A., & Lawrence, R.M. (2005). *Breastfeeding: A guide for the medical profession* (6th ed.). St. Louis: Mosby.

Amphetamines

DEFINITION A category of drugs that stimulate the central nervous system.

> **Notes**
>
> Amphetamines and methamphetamines are considered "drugs of abuse for which adverse effects on the infant during breastfeeding have been reported" by the American Academy of Pediatrics (Table 2)[23] and L5 (contraindicated) by Hale.[24] Specific concerns mentioned include irritability and sleep problems in the infant.
>
> Street names for these drugs include *speed, crank, crystal, crystal meth, ecstasy,* and *"x."* Women reporting use of these drugs should receive substance abuse counseling.

See also Illegal drugs and breastfeeding; Lactation risk category; Medications

Footnotes

[23]American Academy of Pediatrics Committee on Drugs. (2001). Transfer of drugs and other chemicals into human milk. *Pediatrics, 108,* 776–789.

[24]Hale, T.W. (2004). *Medications and mothers milk* (pp. 55–56). Amarillo, TX: Pharmasoft Publishing.

Drug References

Briggs, G.G., Freeman, R.K., & Yaffee, S.J. (Eds.). (2002). *Drugs in pregnancy and lactation* (6th ed.). Philadelphia: Lippincott, Williams, and Wilkins.

Lawrence, R.A., & Lawrence, R.M. (2005). *Breastfeeding: A guide for the medical profession* (6th ed.). St. Louis: Mosby.

Analgesia

DEFINITION A category of drugs used for pain relief.

SELF CARE INFORMATION

When mothers receive pain medications during the birth process, extended skin-to-skin contact should be practiced until the infant shows feeding cues.

Feeding difficulties after labor pain medication.

> ### Notes
>
> A wide range of drugs are used to relieve pain. An up-to-date drug reference should be consulted to determine the safety and possible side effects of individual drugs.
>
> Breastfeeding and skin-to-skin contact have been demonstrated to be analgesic for infants, and may be recommended for babies while undergoing painful procedures, e.g., immunization, blood draw, etc.[25]
>
> Newborn and premature babies are at greater risk of side effects due to limited ability to clear drugs from their systems.[26]

Footnotes

[25]Gray, L., Watt, L., Blass, E.M. (2000). Skin-to-skin contact is analgesic in healthy newborns. *Pediatrics, 105*(1), e14.

[26]Carbajal, R., Veerapen, S., Couderc, S., Jugie, M., & Ville, Y. (2003). Analgesic effect of breast feeding in term neonates: Randomised controlled trial. *The British Medical Journal, 326*(7379), 13.

Drug References

American Academy of Pediatrics Committee on Drugs. (2001). Transfer of drugs and other chemicals into human milk. *Pediatrics, 108,* 776–789.

Briggs, G.G., Freeman, R.K., & Yaffee, S.J. (Eds.). (2002). *Drugs in pregnancy and lactation* (6th ed.). Philadelphia: Lippincott, Williams, and Wilkins.

Hale, T.W. (2004). *Medications and mothers milk.* Amarillo, TX: Pharmasoft Publishing.

Lawrence, R.A., & Lawrence, R.M. (2005). *Breastfeeding: A guide for the medical profession* (6th ed.). St. Louis: Mosby.

▶ Anaphylaxis

DEFINITION A potentially life threatening, full body response to an allergen consumed, touched, or breathed.

Anaphylactic reactions are serious medical conditions. Symptoms may involve the skin and respiratory, digestive, circulatory and nervous systems. Common symptoms include swelling, itching, and burning of the face (especially the lips, tongue, and inside of the mouth), nausea, vomiting, abdominal pain, diarrhea, difficulty breathing, coughing, constriction of the throat, wheezing, itching of the skin, hives, swelling of the eyelids, hands, and feet, rapid or irregular heartbeat, dizziness, low blood pressure (leading to loss of consciousness), confusion, and panic.

According to the Canadian Paediatric Society, "Children with a history of anaphylaxis are at risk for subsequent episodes and death. All children who have had one or more episodes of anaphylaxis should have injectable epinephrine with them or with their parent or caregiver at all times, and should wear some form of Medic-Alert identification."[27]

See also Allergy in the breastfed infant

Footnotes

[27]Simons, F.E.R., Chad, Z.H., & Gold, M. (2001). *Anaphylaxis* (Canadian Paediatric Surveillance Project). Retrieved March 5, 2005, from http://www.cps.ca/english/CPSP/Resources/Ranaphylaxis.htm.

▶ Anemia

DEFINITION A deficiency in the oxygen-carrying capacity of blood cells, typically caused by iron deficiency (although other nutrient deficiencies and medical conditions can cause anemia).

Iron deficiency anemia is a common problem in childbearing women. In a nonpregnant woman older than 18 years, hemoglobin levels below 12.0 g/dL and hematocrit levels lower than 35.7 are considered anemia. In children between 6 months and 2 years of age, hemoglobin levels of less than 11.0 g/dL and hematocrit of less than 32.9% are considered anemia.[28]

Preterm infants are at risk for anemia due to decreased transfer of iron prenatally. The American Academy of Pediatrics and the Academy of Breastfeeding Medicine recommend supplementation of 2 mg/kg/day in exclusively breastfeeding premature infants for the first year of life.

More commonly, anemia may influence energy levels and coping behaviors. Anemic women may not initiate an adequate number of feedings daily, and may be more likely to use formula or pacifiers due to their exhaustion.

Rarely, women who have experienced a severe blood loss during childbirth may be at risk for **Sheehan's syndrome**, a failure of the pituitary gland caused by altered blood flow to the brain. Symptoms of this syndrome include sudden onset of hypothyroidism, diabetes insipidus, and hair loss along with menstrual irregularities. Medical evaluation should include measurement of prolactin levels before and after sucklings. The extent to which women recover from Sheehan's is variable with the degree of infarct.[29]

Anemic children should be evaluated for developmental delays, behavioral disturbances, and lead poisoning.

Several other conditions and nutrient deficiencies can contribute to anemia. Anemia should be treated and monitored in an ongoing manner.

See also Iron; Retained placental fragments; Sheehan's syndrome

Footnotes

[28]Centers for Disease Control and Prevention. (1998). Recommendations to prevent and control iron deficiency in the United States. *Morbidity and Mortality Weekly Report, 47*(RR-3).

[29]Lawrence, R.A., & Lawrence, R.M. (2005). *Breastfeeding: A guide for the medical profession* (6th ed., p. 573). St. Louis: Mosby.

▶ Anesthesia

DEFINITION Administration of drugs used to cause total or partial loss of sensation for surgical or other medical purposes.

SELF CARE INFORMATION

When mothers receive pain medications during the birth process, extended skin-to-skin contact should be practiced until the infant shows feeding cues.

IMPORTANT CONDITIONS TO REPORT

Feeding difficulties after anesthesia.

Drug References

American Academy of Pediatrics Committee on Drugs. (2001). Transfer of drugs and other chemicals into human milk. *Pediatrics, 108*, 776–789.

Briggs, G.G., Freeman, R.K., & Yaffee, S.J. (Eds.). (2002). *Drugs in pregnancy and lactation* (6th ed.). Philadelphia: Lippincott, Williams, and Wilkins.

Hale, T.W. (2004). *Medications and mothers milk.* Amarillo, TX: Pharmasoft Publishing.

Lawrence, R.A., & Lawrence, R.M. (2005). *Breastfeeding: A guide for the medical profession* (6th ed.). St. Louis: Mosby.

▶ Angle of the dangle

DEFINITION A colloquial expression describing the way the breasts naturally hang. Just as there are multiple variations on normal breast shape, size, where the nipples point, etc., there is variation on the angle of the dangle. There is no right or wrong angle.

> **Notes**
>
> In order to allow milk to flow easily from the alveoli through the ducts and to the nipples, it is important that the mother's clothing and hands do not alter the "angle of the dangle."
>
> The baby's mouth should be angled to allow the milk to flow through the nipple without impediment.

▶ Animal milks

DEFINITION Referring to the nutritive mammary secretions of mammals.

▶ Ankyloglossia

DEFINITION A tight lingual frenulum (the membrane attaching the tongue to the bottom of the mouth).

When the frenulum is tight, it can restrict the movement of the tongue, resulting in breastfeeding problems for some mothers and babies.

Ask about

Age of baby.
Appearance of tongue.

ASSESSMENT

PROMPT MEDICAL CARE NEEDED?

Are any of the following present?

Inadequate urine or stool output.

Baby not back to birthweight by 2 weeks of age.

Poor growth of breastfed infant.

IF YES, *Seek medical care within 2 to 4 hours.*

Are any of the following present?

Presence of tight lingual frenulum in baby in conjunction with feeding or breast/nipple problems in breastfeeding mother.

IF YES, *Call pediatric care provider today.*

SELF CARE INFORMATION

Practice skin-to-skin contact frequently.

Watch for hunger cues (signs that say "feed me" include hand-to-face or hand-to-mouth movements, lip smacking, seeking with lips, rooting, and head bobbing).

Feed baby at first sign of hunger cues.

Practice good attachment:

Offer the breast as soon as it is seen.

Wait for baby to open mouth wide (greater than a 100° angle).

Pull baby in so that chin touches the breast first, and nipple enters the mouth along the top of the tongue; this should result in a wide open mouth on breast. Baby may need to be in a semi-upright position to assist in attaining the widest mouth angle.

Lips should be flanged outward.

Baby's lips should look off center when compared with the areola; the bottom lip should be farther away from the nipple than the top lip.

IMPORTANT CONDITIONS TO REPORT

Unresolved symptoms.

Ongoing concerns.

Notes

Babies with ankyloglossia may have difficulty performing the tongue motions required to strip a breast or bottle of milk. On visual assessment, the tongue may appear to be heart-shaped at the tip. The infant may be unable to extend the tongue beyond the lower gum ridge.

Breastfeeding mothers of babies with tongue-tie may experience sore nipples, mastitis, and milk supply problems.

Babies with ankyloglossia should be evaluated for their tongue mobility, and possibly for frenotomy.[30,31] Mothers should receive lactation assistance to improve positioning and milk removal. Occupational therapists and/or speech language pathologists have specialized skills for assisting babies with ankyloglossia.

See also Nipple pain

Footnotes

[30]Ballard, J.L., Auer, C.E., Khoury, J.C. (2002). Ankyloglossia: assessment, incidence, and effect of frenuloplasty on the breastfeeding dyad. *Pediatrics, 110*(5), e63.

[31]Lalakea, M.L., & Messner, A.H. (2003). Ankyloglossia: does it matter? *Pediatric Clinics of North America, 50,* 381–397.

▶ ## Antibacterial agents in breastmilk

DEFINITION Referring to immunologically active components found in human milk.

Notes

Human milk is a rich source of active immune factors. Breastfeeding children receive several different types of immunoglobulins as well as live immune cells and factors from their mother's milk.

With very few exceptions (e.g., maternal infection with **HIV** or **HTLV-1, herpes** vesicles on the nipple or other area that would be in contact with baby's mouth), mothers may continue to breastfeed their babies through illness.[32]

See also Antibodies

Footnotes

[32]American Academy of Pediatrics Section on Breastfeeding. (2005). Breastfeeding and the use of human milk. *Pediatrics, 115,* 496–506.

▶ Antibiotics

DEFINITION A group of drugs that fight infection.

See also Antibacterial agents in breastmilk

Drug References

American Academy of Pediatrics Committee on Drugs. (2001). Transfer of drugs and other chemicals into human milk. *Pediatrics, 108*, 776–789.

Briggs, G.G., Freeman, R.K., & Yaffee, S.J. (Eds.). (2002). *Drugs in pregnancy and lactation* (6th ed.). Philadelphia: Lippincott, Williams, and Wilkins.

Hale, T.W. (2004). *Medications and mothers milk.* Amarillo, TX: Pharmasoft Publishing.

Lawrence, R.A., & Lawrence, R.M. (2005). *Breastfeeding: A guide for the medical profession* (6th ed.). St. Louis: Mosby.

▶ Antibodies

DEFINITION Referring to specific proteins on the surface of immune cells that are secreted in response to the presence of a specific antigen (bacteria, viruses, or other invader) in the body. An antibody attacks and neutralizes the specific antigen to which it is sensitized.

Notes

Human milk is a rich source of active immune factors, including antibodies. Breastfeeding children receive several different types of immunoglobulins as well as live immune cells and factors from their mother's milk.

With very few exceptions (e.g., maternal infection with **HIV** or **HTLV-1, herpes** vesicles on the nipple or other area that would be in contact with baby's mouth), mothers should continue to breastfeed their babies through illness.[33] Mothers are usually exposed to the same illnesses as their babies and are producing specific antibodies which help the baby to mount an immune response.

See also Acute infection; Antigen; Immunoglobulin; Secretory IgA

Footnotes

[33]American Academy of Pediatrics Section on Breastfeeding. (2005). Breastfeeding and the use of human milk. *Pediatrics, 115*, 496–506.

▶ Antidepressants

DEFINITION A category of drugs used to treat clinical depression. Depression is a state of extreme sadness, feelings of hopelessness, difficulty concentrating, difficulty sleeping, and often decreased appetite.

Ask about

Onset.
Age of baby.
Past history of depression.

ASSESSMENT

EMERGENT CARE NEEDED?
  Are any of the following present?
      Suicidal thoughts.
      Thoughts of harming baby.

IF YES,   *Seek emergency medical and protective care now.*

SELF CARE INFORMATION

Mood swings are normal in the postpartum period, but may become more severe. Report symptoms and any worsening of symptoms to health care provider immediately.

Seek support.

IMPORTANT CONDITIONS TO REPORT

Worsening of depression.

Failure of treatment in alleviating symptoms.

Reoccurrence of depression.

Past history of depression, mood disorders, premenstrual syndrome, or thyroid disorders.

Notes

Postpartum mood disorders affect most new mothers. Mood disorders cover a broad spectrum from "baby blues" to postpartum psychosis. While mood disorders are common, they are not to be ignored. Avoid giving false reassurance. Depression can be life threatening for mother and baby.

Women who experienced depression during pregnancy and those with a prior history of depression, mood disorders, or premenstrual syndrome are at greater risk for postpartum depression.

Hypothyroidism, anemia, and other physical disorders share many symptoms with postpartum depression.

A wide range of drugs are used as antidepressants. An up-to-date drug reference should be consulted to determine the safety and possible side effects of individual drugs. Many antidepressants are compatible with breastfeeding.

Newborn and premature babies are at greater risk of side effects due to limited ability to clear drugs from their systems.

See also Baby blues; Postpartum depression

Drug References

American Academy of Pediatrics Committee on Drugs. (2001). Transfer of drugs and other chemicals into human milk. *Pediatrics, 108,* 776–789.

Briggs, G.G., Freeman, R.K., & Yaffee, S.J. (Eds.). (2002). *Drugs in pregnancy and lactation* (6th ed.). Philadelphia: Lippincott, Williams, and Wilkins.

Hale, T.W. (2004). *Medications and mothers milk.* Amarillo, TX: Pharmasoft Publishing.

Lawrence, R.A., & Lawrence, R.M. (2005). *Breastfeeding: A guide for the medical profession* (6th ed.). St. Louis: Mosby.

▶ Antigen

DEFINITION A foreign substance that stimulates the production of an antibody when introduced into the body.

▶ Antihistamines

DEFINITION A category of drugs that reduce the histamine response in allergic reactions and upper respiratory infections. Histamine response includes vasodilation, constriction of the bronchial muscles, and increased gastric secretion.

Notes

A wide range of drugs are used as antihistamines. An up-to-date drug reference should be consulted to determine the safety and possible side effects of individual drugs.

Some antihistamines have been noted to suppress lactation.

Newborn and premature babies are at greater risk of drug side effects due to limited ability to clear drugs from their systems.

See also Allergen; Allergy in the breastfed infant; Medications

Drug References

American Academy of Pediatrics Committee on Drugs. (2001). Transfer of drugs and other chemicals into human milk. *Pediatrics, 108,* 776–789.

Briggs, G.G., Freeman, R.K., & Yaffee, S.J. (Eds.). (2002). *Drugs in pregnancy and lactation* (6th ed.). Philadelphia: Lippincott, Williams, and Wilkins.

Hale, T.W. (2004). *Medications and mothers milk.* Amarillo, TX: Pharmasoft Publishing.

Lawrence, R.A., & Lawrence, R.M. (2005). *Breastfeeding: A guide for the medical profession* (6th ed.). St. Louis: Mosby.

▶ Anti-infective agents in breastmilk

DEFINITION Referring to immunologically active components found in human milk. This includes antimicrobial, antiviral, antibacterial, and anti-inflammatory properties.

Notes

Human milk is a rich source of active immune factors. Breastfeeding children receive several different types of immunoglobulins as well as live immune cells and factors from their mother's milk.

With very few exceptions (e.g., maternal infection with **HIV** or **HTLV-1**, **herpes** vesicles on the nipple or other area that would be in contact with baby's mouth), mothers may continue to breastfeed their babies through illness.[34]

See also Antibodies, Anti-inflammatory agents in breastmilk

Footnotes

[34]American Academy of Pediatrics Section on Breastfeeding. (2005). Breastfeeding and the use of human milk. *Pediatrics, 115*, 496–506.

▶ Anti-inflammatory agents in breastmilk

DEFINITION Substances that reduce the body's inflammatory response (a reaction of the immune system to injury or infection that results in pain, redness, swelling, and sometimes impaired function of the affected area).

See also Allergy in the breastfed infant; Bioactive components of breastmilk

▶ APHA

See also American Public Health Association (APHA)

▶ Appropriate for gestational age (AGA)

DEFINITION Babies who are classified **appropriate for gestational age** are of weight, length, and development considered appropriate for their gestational age at birth.

▶ Arachidonic acid (AA)

DEFINITION A long-chain polyunsaturated fatty acid (LCPUFA) found naturally in human milk. These fatty acids assist in the development of nerve and brain tissue, and may account for some of the differences between formula and breastfed children in terms of IQ, test scores, and visual acuity.

▶ Areola

DEFINITION The area of darkened pigmentation around the nipple. The size and color of the areola varies among women.

> **Notes**
>
> It is normal for the areola to become much darker during pregnancy and lactation. **Montgomery's glands** or tubercules are mixed sebaceous and milk glands that look like "goose bumps" on the surface of the areola. These glands become more prominent during pregnancy and lactation.
>
> It is normal for the areolar area to be slightly enlarged and darkened. Any reddening or lumpiness in this area should be examined by a medical care provider to rule out anomalies.

▶ Aspirin

DEFINITION A drug used to reduce fever and inflammation.

> **Notes**
>
> Aspirin is listed on AAP Table 5, "Drugs that have been associated with significant effects on some nursing infants and should be given to nursing mothers with caution."[35] Hale rates aspirin as "moderately safe."[36]
>
> Medical evaluation should determine what analgesic is appropriate for mother's and baby's situation.
>
> Aspirin should never be given to infants or children due to concern about Reye's Syndrome.

See also Medications; Over-the-counter (OTC) drugs

Footnotes

[35]American Academy of Pediatrics Committee on Drugs. (2001). Transfer of drugs and other chemicals into human milk. *Pediatrics, 108,* 776–789.

[36]Hale, T.W. (2004). *Medications and mothers milk* (pp. 69–70). Amarillo, TX: Pharmasoft Publishing.

Drug References

American Academy of Pediatrics Committee on Drugs. (2001). Transfer of drugs and other chemicals into human milk. *Pediatrics, 108,* 776–789.

Briggs, G.G., Freeman, R.K., & Yaffee, S.J. (Eds.). (2002). *Drugs in pregnancy and lactation* (6th ed.). Philadelphia: Lippincott, Williams, and Wilkins.

Hale, T.W. (2004). *Medications and mothers milk.* Amarillo, TX: Pharmasoft Publishing.

Lawrence, R.A., & Lawrence, R.M. (2005). *Breastfeeding: A guide for the medical profession* (6th ed.). St. Louis: Mosby.

Association of Women's Health, Obstetric, and Neonatal Nurses (AWHONN)

DEFINITION "AWHONN is the leading professional association for nurses who specialize in the care of women and newborns. Our members include neonatal nurses, APRNs, women's health nurses, OB/GYN and labor and delivery nurses, nurse scientists, nurse executives and managers, childbirth educators and nurse practitioners."[37]

> **Notes**
>
> Association of Women's Health, Obstetric, and Neonatal Nurses
> 2000 L Street, NW
> Suite 740
> Washington, DC 20036
> Phone: 202-261-2400
> Web: www.awhonn.org
>   Articles and policy statements about breastfeeding can be found in the *Journal of Obstetric, Gynecologic, and Neonatal Nursing,* and on the AWHONN's Web site.

Footnotes

[37]Association of Women's Health, Obstetric and Neonatal Nurses. (2002). *Welcome.* Retrieved June 19, 2005, from http://www.awhonn.org.

Asthma and lactation

DEFINITION Asthma is a chronic respiratory disease characterized by difficulty breathing, constriction of the airways, and coughing attacks often triggered by allergens.

> **Notes**
>
> Research has indicated that breastfeeding may reduce the risk and severity of asthma in susceptible children.
>   Mothers with asthma may breastfeed their babies. Any medications used by a mother with asthma should be reviewed. Consult an up-to-date drug reference to determine the safety and possible side effects of individual drugs.

Asthmatic women who take theophylline may need to be monitored for cumulative effects of this drug in combination with any dietary caffeine.

Newborn and premature babies are at greater risk of side effects due to limited ability to clear drugs from their systems.

Drug References

American Academy of Pediatrics Committee on Drugs. (2001). Transfer of drugs and other chemicals into human milk. *Pediatrics, 108*, 776–789.

Briggs, G.G., Freeman, R.K., & Yaffee, S.J. (Eds.). (2002). *Drugs in pregnancy and lactation* (6th ed.). Philadelphia: Lippincott, Williams, and Wilkins.

Hale, T.W. (2004). *Medications and mothers milk.* Amarillo, TX: Pharmasoft Publishing.

Lawrence, R.A., & Lawrence, R.M. (2005). *Breastfeeding: A guide for the medical profession* (6th ed.). St. Louis: Mosby.

▶ Asymmetric breasts

DEFINITION Lack of similarity of appearance, size, or other characteristic of one breast as compared with the other.

Ask about

Onset.
Age of baby.

ASSESSMENT

PROMPT CARE NEEDED?

Are any of the following present?

Reported breast asymmetry coupled with concern about milk supply or infant's weight gain.

IF YES, *Call pediatric care provider and lactation care provider today.*

ROUTINE CARE NEEDED?

Are any of the following present?

Reported asymmetry with no concerns about milk supply or infant's growth.

IF YES, *Call lactation care provider today.*

SELF CARE INFORMATION

Practice skin-to-skin contact frequently.

Feed baby at first sign of hunger cues (signs that say "feed me" include hand-to-face or hand-to-mouth movements, lip smacking, seeking with lips, rooting, and head bobbing).

Feed baby at least 10–12 times per 24 hours.

Listen for signs of baby swallowing.

Allow baby to end feedings.

Expect at least 3–4 infant stools per 24 hours after the first 4 days of life.

Good positioning and attachment are crucial to reduce nipple pain.

If baby is fed away from the breast, hand express or pump milk to maintain supply.

IMPORTANT CONDITIONS TO REPORT

Feeding or stooling expectations are not met.

> **Notes**
>
> Most women have some discrepancy between their breasts in terms of size, shape, position, **"angle of the dangle,"** etc. The hormones of pregnancy may alter the discrepancy, either exacerbating or equalizing it. Minor asymmetry is common and normal.
>
> When a lactating woman's breasts are markedly different, particularly with one or both breasts appearing underdeveloped, insufficient glandular tissue may exist in one or both breasts.
>
> Marked asymmetry indicates the need for careful medical and lactation evaluation and monitoring. The baby's weight gain should be closely followed to ensure that adequate milk-making potential exists.

See also Breast, insufficient glandular tissue; Insufficient milk supply; Milk transfer, estimating

▶ Asymmetric latch

DEFINITION An ideal way for baby to remove maximal milk from the breast, referring to the position of the mother's nipple in the baby's mouth.

Notes

In order to allow the baby to get as much breast tissue into the mouth as possible, an asymmetric latch position is recommended. In this position, baby's mouth is open to a 100° or larger angle, and baby grasps more of the underside of the breast than the tissue above the nipple. Baby's lips will appear to be off-center on the nipple, with the upper lips closer to the nipple than the lower.

Because nipple and breast pain is a major reason for discontinuing breastfeeding, any woman reporting such pain should be seen within 24 hours by a skilled breastfeeding helper. Baby's growth should also be evaluated, as painful breastfeeding is associated with poor growth.

See also Latch-on; Taking the baby off the breast

▶ At-breast supplementation

DEFINITION Administration of extra fluids (expressed breastmilk or formula) to the baby through a tube device attached to the breast.

Notes

At-breast supplementation is useful when a baby is not receiving an adequate amount of milk from the breast. This may be due to a temporary or permanent problem with milk supply on the part of the mother. It may also result from weak or inefficient suckling on the part of the baby, due to temporary or permanent conditions (e.g., prematurity, undernourishment, Down syndrome, cardiac problems).

See also Adoption and induced lactation; Supplemental feeding

▶ Atopic eczema

DEFINITION An allergic inflammation of the skin characterized by itching, redness, and scaling.

Ask about

Onset.
Age of baby.
Medications used.

ASSESSMENT

PROMPT CARE NEEDED?
Are any of the following present?
Eczema on the breast.
Eczema in the baby.
Concerns about medications to treat eczema.

IF YES, *Seek medical care today.*

SELF CARE INFORMATION

Follow instructions from the health care provider and report problems as directed.

IMPORTANT CONDITIONS TO REPORT

Allergy and eczema in parents and siblings.
Infant symptoms of blood in stool, wheezing, hives, facial swelling, runny nose, vomiting, or irritability.

Notes

Research has identified that exclusive breastfeeding reduces the risk of atopic eczema in susceptible children.

In adults, atopic eczema is typically treated with topical steroid creams. The specific cream indicated should be examined in an up-to-date drug reference to ensure that it is safe for use by the breastfeeding mother.

Steroid cream use is of greater concern when the affected area is on the breast where the baby's mouth will be placed, as the baby could then absorb the steroid both through direct contact and through the milk.

> *In the breastfed baby,* atopic eczema may be a symptom of food allergy, or related to an allergen in food that the mother or baby is consuming. Mother and baby should avoid consuming offending allergens such as cow's milk, fish, eggs, peanuts, and tree nuts.
>
> Infantile symptoms of an allergic reaction include hives, facial swelling, runny nose, wheezing, eczema, vomiting, irritability (colic), blood in the stool, and **anaphylaxis**. Treatment centers on identification and avoidance of the proteins that are triggering the allergic reaction.
>
> Babies born into allergic families are more likely to develop allergy, particularly those with two allergic parents or one allergic parent and an allergic sibling. Exclusive breast-feeding is the optimal feeding choice for these babies in particular.
>
> If babies with documented allergy are supplemented, a protein hydrolysate formula should be considered.

See also Allergy in the breastfed infant

Drug References

American Academy of Pediatrics Committee on Drugs. (2001). Transfer of drugs and other chemicals into human milk. *Pediatrics, 108,* 776–789.

Briggs, G.G., Freeman, R.K., & Yaffee, S.J. (Eds.). (2002). *Drugs in pregnancy and lactation* (6th ed.). Philadelphia: Lippincott, Williams, and Wilkins.

Hale, T.W. (2004). *Medications and mothers milk.* Amarillo, TX: Pharmasoft Publishing.

Lawrence, R.A., & Lawrence, R.M. (2005). *Breastfeeding: A guide for the medical profession* (6th ed.). St. Louis: Mosby.

▶ Attachment

DEFINITION Refers to the way in which the nursing baby latches on to the breast.

Notes

Correct attachment of the baby to the breast is crucial to comfortable breastfeeding, to adequate milk manufacture and transfer, and ultimately to infant growth. When a baby is attached well, mother should feel no pain or discomfort and should hear sounds of swallowing on the part of the baby.

Since concerns about pain and inadequate milk are major reasons mothers stop breastfeeding, mothers should be seen for a feeding evaluation within 24–48 hours of expressing breastfeeding concerns.

See also Asymmetric latch

▶ Attachment parenting

DEFINITION A phrase used to describe a parenting style that includes continuous, nurturing contact between a baby and its parents. The goal of attachment parenting is to develop a secure emotional bond between the baby and its primary caregivers.

> **Notes**
>
> Attachment parenting typically includes carrying babies in a sling, breastfeeding exclusively, co-sleeping, and avoiding prolonged parent–baby separation.

See also Co-sleeping

▶ Augmentation surgery

DEFINITION A procedure that increases the size of the breast, typically by inserting a saline or silicone implant in the breast.

Ask about

Date of surgery.
Age of baby.
Location of surgical incision.

ASSESSMENT

PROMPT CARE NEEDED?

Are any of the following present?

History of augmentation surgery.
Concerns about milk supply.
Poor stool output in breastfed baby.
Poor weight gain in breastfed baby.

IF YES, *Call pediatric care provider and lactation care provider today.*

SELF CARE INFORMATION

Practice skin-to-skin contact frequently.

Feed baby at first sign of hunger cues (signs that say "feed me" include hand-to-face or hand-to-mouth movements, lip smacking, seeking with lips, rooting, and head bobbing).

Feed baby at least 10–12 times per 24 hours.

Listen for signs of baby swallowing.

Allow baby to end feedings.

Expect at least 3–4 infant stools per 24 hours after the first 4 days of life.

Good positioning and attachment are crucial to reduce nipple pain.

If baby is fed away from the breast, hand express or pump milk to maintain supply.

IMPORTANT CONDITIONS TO REPORT

Fewer than four bowel movements daily in newborn time period after the fourth day.

Ongoing problems with baby's weight gain.

Ongoing concerns or problems with milk supply.

Notes

The location and extent of the incision may impact the sensation of the nerves in the nipple area. Loss of or decreased sensation may decrease milk-making potential. Trauma to the nerves may hinder the stimulation of the brain to release prolactin (the milk-making hormone) in response to suckling. Periareolar incisions suggest more potential injury than do incisions underneath the breast.

Babies of women who have had breast augmentation surgery should be followed closely to ensure milk transfer and growth.

If the mother reports that she had an implant in one breast only, inquire about the reason for this surgery. If augmentation corrected breast asymmetry, there may be increased concern regarding the mother's ability to make a full milk supply. Marked asymmetry may indicate insufficient glandular tissue in both breasts. Baby and mother should be closely followed. (Breasts are rarely identical in shape and size. Minor asymmetry is common and normal.)

See also Breast surgery

▶ Australian posture

DEFINITION A breastfeeding position where the baby is above the mother (or the mother is "down-under" the baby—the reason for the name of the posture).

This posture is suggested to deal with fast milk flow, which may cause the baby to pull away from the breast gasping.

Some mothers are successful managing the flow by nursing while lying on their back with the baby positioned flat on top. The baby has more head control in this position.

▶ Autoimmune diseases

DEFINITION Chronic illnesses caused by a person's immune cells acting on the body's own cells and tissues. Crohn's disease, lupus, and type 1 diabetes are examples of autoimmune diseases.

> **Notes**
>
> A reduction in development of autoimmune diseases such as diabetes, some thyroid diseases, and multiple sclerosis, has been documented in breastfed infants.
>
> Autoimmune diseases are more common in women. A wide range of drugs are used to treat autoimmune disorders. An up-to-date drug reference should be consulted to determine the safety and possible side effects of individual drugs.
>
> Newborn and premature babies are at greater risk of drug side effects due to limited ability to clear drugs from their systems.

See also Diabetes and breastfeeding; Lupus; Thyroid disease

▶ Automatic electric breast pumps

DEFINITION These fully automated devices are designed to remove milk from the lactating breast with minimal work on the part of the woman.

SELF CARE INFORMATION

A breast pump cannot tell you how much milk you are making.

If you have concerns about milk supply, please call or see a lactation specialist.

> **Notes**
>
> Automatic electric breast pumps are ideally suited for women who are pumping for a baby from whom they are separated many hours daily. This includes women pumping for babies who are hospitalized in special care, as well as women who are separated from their babies due to work or school.
>
> Automatic electric pumps can be rented or purchased from representatives of various companies.
>
> There is no one pump that works best for all women. Please note that it is never appropriate to recommend mixing one manufacturer's pump kits with another manufacturer's pump.
>
> Women will sometimes request a breast pump when they have doubts about their milk supply. Pumps should not be used to quantify a woman's milk supply. Refer women to a lactation specialist regarding this concern.

See also Breast pump

▶ AWHONN

See also Association of Women's Health, Obstetric, and Neonatal Nurses (AWHONN)

▶ Azidothymidine (AZT)

DEFINITION An antiretroviral drug used to treat infection with human immunodeficiency virus (HIV). Trade name *Retrovir®*.

> **Notes**
>
> In the United States, breastfeeding is **contraindicated** for women who have tested positive for HIV/AIDS, due to the risk of transmission of the HIV virus to the baby via breastmilk.
>
> Women at risk for HIV infection (those who have used intravenous drugs, or who have HIV positive sexual partners or partners who are intravenous drug users should be tested for HIV before a recommendation is made regarding breastfeeding.

See also Acquired immunodeficiency syndrome (AIDS); Contraindicated conditions; Human immunodeficiency virus (HIV)

▶ **AZT**

See also Azidothymidine (AZT)

▶ **Baby**

DEFINITION A child younger than 12 months of age.

▶ **Baby blues**

DEFINITION Transient mood swings experienced by more than 50% of women during the early days postpartum. Women may feel alternately giddy, sad, tearful, and anxious.

Ask about

Onset.
Age of baby.
Past history of depression.

ASSESSMENT

EMERGENT CARE NEEDED?
Are any of the following present?
　　Suicidal thoughts.
　　Thoughts of harming baby.

IF YES, *Seek emergency care and protective services now.*

PROMPT CARE NEEDED?
Are any of the following present?
　　Persistent sadness.
　　Inability to function.

IF YES, *Seek medical care within 2 to 4 hours and seek psychological counseling today.*

SELF CARE INFORMATION

Mood swings are normal in the postpartum period, but may become more severe.

Seek support from friends and family members.

Practice skin-to-skin contact frequently.

Feed baby at least 10–12 times per 24 hours.

IMPORTANT CONDITIONS TO REPORT

Continuation of baby blues.

Worsening of symptoms.

Past history of depression, mood disorders, premenstrual syndrome, or thyroid disorders.

Notes

While the "baby blues" are a common postpartum experience, women can progress to postpartum depression among other postpartum mood disorders. It is important to encourage mothers to report any worsening of symptoms.

Women who experienced depression during pregnancy and those with a prior history of depression, mood disorders, or premenstrual syndrome are at greater risk for postpartum depression.

Hypothyroidism, anemia, and other physical disorders share many symptoms with postpartum depression.

See also Antidepressants; Postpartum depression

▶ Baby food

DEFINITION Refers to ground, mashed, or blended foods intended for use by babies between the ages of 6 and 12 months. Baby foods may be made at home or purchased.

Ask about

Age of baby.

Foods already introduced.

EMERGENT CARE NEEDED?

Are any of the following present in the baby?

Difficulty breathing or swallowing.

Swelling of tongue.

IF YES, *Seek emergency care now.*

PROMPT CARE NEEDED?

Are any of the following present in the baby?

Swelling of the face, hands, or feet.

Persistent rash, headache, or fever.

Persistent diarrhea, nausea, or vomiting.

Bloody stool.

Wheezing.

IF YES, *Seek medical care within 2 to 4 hours.*

ROUTINE CARE NEEDED?

Are any of the following present in the baby?

Suspected reaction to food or medication.

Occasional nausea, vomiting, or diarrhea.

Persistent runny nose.

Rash and itching.

IF YES, *Schedule a pediatric appointment.*

SELF CARE INFORMATION

Monitor baby's symptoms.

Be aware of the possibility of developing allergy to other proteins.

IMPORTANT CONDITIONS TO REPORT

Family history of allergy.

Symptoms occur, worsen, persist, or reoccur.

Exclusive breastfeeding is the ideal food for infants younger than 6 months. Around 6 months of age, babies may be introduced to solid foods as advised by their pediatric care provider. Around 12 months of age, whole cow's milk and other dairy foods may be introduced. There is limited need for commercial baby foods—homemade foods are often fresher and tastier. Cooked fruits and vegetables and ripe bananas and avocados can be mashed with a fork or pureed until babies are able to handle lumpier foods.

In children of allergic families, potent allergenic foods such as cow's milk, egg whites, peanuts, and other tree nuts, should be introduced per medical advice.

Care should be taken to avoid introducing foods that present choking hazards to babies and young children, including peanut butter, popcorn, hot dogs, and other sticky, hard, and rigid foods that can become lodged in the throat.

Mothers should be encouraged to continue breastfeeding as they wish throughout and beyond the first year of life.

See also **Allergy in the breastfed infant; Mixed feeds; Solid foods for breastfed babies**

▶ Baby Food Action Network (IBFAN)

DEFINITION The International Baby Food Action Network (IBFAN) is a network of public interest groups working around the world to reduce infant and young child morbidity and mortality.

Notes

International Baby Food Action Network
North American Office
INFACT Canada
P.O. Box 781
10 Trinity Square
Toronto, Ontario M5G 1B1
Canada
Phone: 416-595-9819
Fax: 416-591-9355
E-mail: infact@ftn.net
Web: www.ibfan.org

▶ Baby-Friendly Hospital Initiative (BFHI)

DEFINITION The Baby-Friendly Hospital Initiative (BFHI) is an international project of the United Nations Children's Fund (UNICEF) and the World Health Organization (WHO). The BFHI seeks to encourage hospitals and birth centers to implement the *Ten Steps to Successful Breastfeeding*, a set of best practices to ensure positive breastfeeding outcomes.

▶ Baby-Friendly USA

DEFINITION Baby-Friendly USA is the national organization responsible for the implementation of the United Nations Children's Fund (UNICEF) and World Health Organization (WHO) Baby-Friendly Hospital Initiative (BFHI) in the United States.

Notes

Baby-Friendly USA
327 Quaker Meeting House Road
East Sandwich, MA 02537
Phone: 508-888-8092
Fax: 508-888-8050
E-mail: info@babyfriendlyusa.org
Web: www.babyfriendlyusa.org

▶ Bacteria in mother's milk

DEFINITION Bacteria are single celled microorganisms. Of concern in this context are those bacteria that are pathogenic.

Notes

Bacteria are typically of concern only in milk expressed for a premature or ill baby, or in milk collected for a donor milk bank. To avoid bacterial contamination of expressed milk, it is important to employ careful handwashing techniques and careful cleaning of any equipment used to collect, store, and feed milk. Breast pumps are more likely to introduce bacteria than manual expression.[38]

> In the event of infant infection, it may be necessary to test mother's milk to identify if the pathogen originates with the mother or a contaminant in the expression, collection, or feeding process.

See also Antibacterial agents in breastmilk

Footnotes

[38]Lawrence, R.A., & Lawrence, R.M. (2005). *Breastfeeding: A guide for the medical profession* (6th ed., p. 768). St. Louis: Mosby.

▶ BALT

DEFINITION Bronchus-associated lymphoid tissue. Immunologically active tissue found within the lungs.

Notes

The breast is thought to act as an extension of bronchus-associated lymphoid tissue (BALT). When a pathogen is breathed into the lung, BALT tissue responds by triggering the production of an immunoglobulin to attach the pathogen. The breast may also respond to the BALT trigger by manufacturing and releasing appropriate immunoglobulins to fight the organism through the milk.

See also Bioactive components of breastmilk

▶ Battery operated breast pump

DEFINITION A motorized device designed to remove milk from the lactating breast using battery power.

SELF CARE INFORMATION

A breast pump cannot tell you how much milk you are making.
If you have concerns about milk supply, please call or see a lactation specialist.

See also **Automatic electric breast pumps; Breast pump**

▶ Bellagio Consensus

DEFINITION A statement made in 1998 by a group of experts about the efficacy of the Lactational Amenorrhea Method of family planning.

> **Notes**
>
> In 1998, a group of specialists met in Bellagio, Italy to review what was known about the cessation of menses, or lactational amennorhea, experienced by exclusively breast-feeding women. This group produced the Bellagio Consensus, which set forth what has been named the Lactational Amenorrhea Method (LAM) of family planning.
>
> Research suggests that LAM is 98% effective in the first six months following the birth of a baby, so long as the mother's menses have not returned ("**amenorrhea**"), her baby is exclusively breastfed, receiving no other foods or drinks, nursing at least 8–10 times daily and there are no long periods of time (6 hours or greater) between feedings, day and night. Once the baby is older than 6 months, or any of the other criteria above is no longer true, LAM is no longer effective and women should utilize other family planning methods.

See also **Amenorrhea; Lactational Amenorrhea Method (LAM)**

▶ Benadryl

DEFINITION A commonly used antihistamine (also known as Diphenhydramine).

> **Notes**
>
> This drug is not reviewed by the American Academy of Pediatrics, but Hale has determined it to be a lactation risk category 2 "safer" drug.[39]
>
> An up-to-date drug reference should be consulted to determine the safety and possible side effects of individual drugs.
>
> Newborn and premature babies are at greater risk of drug side effects due to limited ability to clear drugs from their systems.

Footnotes

[39]Hale, T.W. (2004). *Medications and mothers milk* (pp. 248–249). Amarillo, TX: Pharmasoft Publishing.

Drug References

American Academy of Pediatrics Committee on Drugs. (2001). Transfer of drugs and other chemicals into human milk. *Pediatrics, 108,* 776–789.

Briggs, G.G., Freeman, R.K., & Yaffee, S.J. (Eds.). (2002). *Drugs in pregnancy and lactation* (6th ed.). Philadelphia: Lippincott, Williams, and Wilkins.

Hale, T.W. (2004). *Medications and mothers milk.* Amarillo, TX: Pharmasoft Publishing.

Lawrence, R.A., & Lawrence, R.M. (2005). *Breastfeeding: A guide for the medical profession* (6th ed.). St. Louis: Mosby.

See also Lactation risk category; Medications, Over-the-counter (OTC) drugs

▶ Benefits of breastfeeding

DEFINITION Advantages of human milk over artificial replacement foods.

> **Notes**
>
> Breastfeeding has innumerable positive effects for children, mothers, and society in general.

Benefits include (but are not limited to):
> *Child*: Optimal growth and development as well as protection against chronic and acute diseases.
> *Mother*: Respite to recover physically from childbirth as well as protection against some chronic diseases.
> *Society*: Less health care expenditure on acute and chronic illness for mothers and children; less environmental waste; far-reaching advantages from optimally healthy and bonded families.

When clients have questions about advantages of breastfeeding, refer them to a lactation care provider or medical care provider. Fathers may be particularly receptive to messages about the benefits of breastfeeding.

▶ Best Start Social Marketing

DEFINITION "Best Start Social Marketing is a not-for-profit, 501(c)(3) corporation that provides social marketing services to public health, education, social service and other organizations that serve economically disadvantaged families."[40]

Notes

Best Start Social Marketing
4809 E. Busch Boulevard
Suite 104
Tampa, FL 33617
Phone: 813-971-2119
Fax: 813-971-2280
E-mail: beststart@beststartinc.org
Web: www.beststartinc.org

Best Start has conducted several social marketing programs addressing breastfeeding, including the USDA's *Loving Support Makes Breastfeeding Work* campaign.

Footnotes

[40]Best Start Social Marketing. (2005). *Who We Are*. Retrieved June 19, 2005, from http://www.beststartinc.org/who_we_are.asp.

Beta-agonists

DEFINITION A category of drugs that mimic the effects of adrenaline on the body's beta receptors. These drugs are often used to relax the muscles of the airway, making breathing easier and reducing bronchial spasms.

> **Notes**
>
> There are several different beta-agonists in use. An up-to-date drug reference should be consulted to determine the safety and possible side effects of individual drugs.
>   Newborn and premature babies are at greater risk of side effects due to limited ability to clear drugs from their systems.

See also Medications

Drug References

American Academy of Pediatrics Committee on Drugs. (2001). Transfer of drugs and other chemicals into human milk. *Pediatrics, 108,* 776–789.

Briggs, G.G., Freeman, R.K., & Yaffee, S.J. (Eds.). (2002). *Drugs in pregnancy and lactation* (6th ed.). Philadelphia: Lippincott, Williams, and Wilkins.

Hale, T.W. (2004). *Medications and mothers milk.* Amarillo, TX: Pharmasoft Publishing.

Lawrence, R.A., & Lawrence, R.M. (2005). *Breastfeeding: A guide for the medical profession* (6th ed.). St. Louis: Mosby.

Beta-blockers

DEFINITION A category of drugs that block the effects of adrenaline on the body's beta receptors. These drugs are often used to reduce high blood pressure.

> **Notes**
>
> There are several different beta-blockers in use. An up-to-date drug reference should be consulted to determine the safety and possible side effects of individual drugs.
>   Newborn and premature babies are at greater risk of side effects due to limited ability to clear drugs from their systems.

See also Medications

Drug References

American Academy of Pediatrics Committee on Drugs. (2001). Transfer of drugs and other chemicals into human milk. *Pediatrics, 108,* 776–789.

Briggs, G.G., Freeman, R.K., & Yaffee, S.J. (Eds.). (2002). *Drugs in pregnancy and lactation* (6th ed.). Philadelphia: Lippincott, Williams, and Wilkins.

Hale, T.W. (2004). *Medications and mothers milk.* Amarillo, TX: Pharmasoft Publishing.

Lawrence, R.A., & Lawrence, R.M. (2005). *Breastfeeding: A guide for the medical profession* (6th ed.). St. Louis: Mosby.

▶ **BFHI**

See also Baby-Friendly Hospital Initiative (BFHI)

▶ **Bicycle-horn breast pump**

DEFINITION A manually operated device designed to remove milk from the lactating breast. This particular manual pump employs a rubber bulb syringe which is compressed to generate pressure.

SELF CARE INFORMATION

A breast pump cannot tell you how much milk you are making.

If you have concerns about milk supply, please call or see a lactation specialist.

> **Notes**
>
> These inexpensive hand pumps are named for a rubber bulb syringe that the mother compresses to withdraw milk. These pumps are not recommended, due to two problems: (1) compression of the bulb can generate very high pressure, possibly injuring the breast and nipple, and (2) milk can flow backward into the bulb of most pumps of this type, creating a potential contamination problem (as the interior of the bulb cannot be cleaned thoroughly).

There is no one pump that works best for all mothers. It is never appropriate to recommend mixing one manufacturer's pump kits with another manufacturer's pump. Pumps in this category are not intended to be used by more than one woman. It is possible for the interior of the pump to be contaminated with pathogens.

Women will sometimes request a breast pump when they have doubts about their milk supply. Pumps should not be used to quantify a woman's milk supply.

See also Breast pump

▶ Bifidus factor

DEFINITION A group of components of human milk that stimulate the growth of *Lactobacillus bifidus,* a "friendly" bacterium, in the gut of the breastfed baby.

Notes

Lactobacillus bifidus is the predominant bacterium present in the gut of the breastfed baby. This friendly microbe helps to protect the baby's gut from infection.

Infant formula does not contain bifidus factor.

▶ Bilateral

DEFINITION Meaning two sides. In this context, the term refers to something occurring in or on both breasts or nipples.

▶ Bilateral mastitis

DEFINITION The presence of mastitis (breast inflammation) in both breasts at the same time. Mastitis can be infective or noninfective.

Onset.
Prior breast inflammation.
Sore nipples.
Known drug allergies.

ASSESSMENT

EMERGENT CARE NEEDED?

Are any of the following present?

Visible red areas on the breast(s).
Maternal fever higher than 101° F (38.5° C).
Extreme breast discomfort.
Flu-like aching throughout body.
Continuing fever after treatment.
Reaction to antibiotic prescribed.

IF YES, *Seek emergency care now.*

PROMPT CARE NEEDED?

Are any of the following present?

Continuing symptoms after treatment.
Difficulty breastfeeding.

IF YES, *Call obstetric care provider today and call lactation care provider today.*

ROUTINE CARE NEEDED?

Are any of the following present?

Questions about treatment.
Questions about breastfeeding.

IF YES, *Call obstetric care provider today and call lactation care provider today.*

SELF CARE INFORMATION

Breastfeed on both breasts, keeping them as soft as possible.
Take care of yourself as though you have the flu (rest in bed, drink plenty of fluids, and request help for other children and household chores).

Take medications as they have been prescribed, even after you feel better.

Call your health care provider or lactation care provider if you have questions.

IMPORTANT CONDITIONS TO REPORT

Symptoms that worsen or do not resolve.

> **Notes**
>
> Bilateral presentation may indicate infection with *Streptococcus*. Lawrence and Lawrence state "bilateral mastitis should always be treated as *Streptococcus* unless cultures disprove it. The infant needs to be treated as well."[41]

See also Breast infection; Breast inflammation

Footnotes

[41]Lawrence, R.A., & Lawrence, R.M. (2005). *Breastfeeding: A guide for the medical profession* (6th ed., p. 570). St. Louis: Mosby.

▶ Bilirubin

DEFINITION A breakdown product of red blood cells. When bilirubin accumulates in the blood stream, a yellow discoloration of the skin and the whites of the eyes called **jaundice** can occur.

> **Notes**
>
> Jaundice is the most common condition requiring medical treatment in the newborn period.
>
> Bilirubin is removed from the blood by the liver.
>
> Although jaundice may be benign, it may be a symptom of other more serious conditions, e.g., **kernicterus**.

See also Jaundice; Late onset jaundice

► Bioactive components of breastmilk

DEFINITION Referring to living cells and other active components in human milk that stimulate growth, build the baby's immune response, and promote health.

> **Notes**
>
> Human milk is a rich source of bioactive factors, including antibodies, antiviral factors, white blood cells, enzymes, immune-active proteins, fats, sugars, and numerous growth and immune factors.

See also Antibacterial agents in breastmilk; Antibodies; Anti-infective agents in breastmilk; Anti-inflammatory agents in breastmilk; Bifidus factor; Bronchus-associated lymphoid tissue (BALT); Cytokine; Epidermal growth factor; Enzymes in breastmilk; Fat-soluble vitamins in breastmilk; Gut-associated lymphoid tissue (GALT); Hormones; IgA; IgE; IGF-I; Immunoglobulin; Lactoferrin; Lymphocytes; Macrophages; Mucosa-associated lymphoid tissue (MALT); Oligosaccharides in breastmilk; Secretory IgA

► Biopsy, breast

DEFINITION A surgical procedure performed to remove a sample of breast tissue for diagnostic purposes.

Ask about

Reason for biopsy.
Date of biopsy.
Age of baby.

PROMPT CARE NEEDED?

Are any of the following present?

Biopsy scheduled in a lactating woman.

Breast or feeding problems post biopsy.

IF YES, *Call lactation care provider today.*

ROUTINE CARE NEEDED?

Are any of the following present?

Concern about effect of past biopsy on breastfeeding.

IF YES, *Call lactation care provider.*

SELF CARE INFORMATION

Follow instructions about caring for biopsy site.

IMPORTANT CONDITIONS TO REPORT

Excessive leakage from biopsy site.

Increased pain.

Fever.

Notes

Breast biopsy may be performed during lactation due to concern about masses in the breast. While many masses in the lactating breast are often associated with plugged milk ducts, and galactocele. Growths—including cancerous ones—are possible.

Women can continue to breastfeed after biopsy, assuming they are not taking contraindicated medications. Women often need support and assistance in breastfeeding during the healing process.

Women who have had past biopsy surgery may experience decreased milk production in the segments of the breast surgically involved.

See also **Abrupt weaning; Breast surgery**

▶ Birth, Cesarean

DEFINITION Delivery of baby through surgical incision made through the abdomen and uterus.

Ask about

Date of Cesarean.
Age of baby.
Feeding status.

ASSESSMENT

EMERGENT CARE NEEDED?

Are any of the following present?

Baby refuses to feed for more than six hours.

Exclusively breastfed baby stools less than one time daily after the first day of the newborn period.

Extreme **lethargy or irritability** in baby.

Sudden change in baby's muscle tone (extremely floppy or stiff) or repetitive jerking movements (e.g., seizure activity).

Baby shows sudden disinterest in feeding.

Unable to wake baby.

Baby does not calm, even with cuddles.

IF YES, *Call pediatric care provider now.*

PROMPT MEDICAL CARE NEEDED?

Are any of the following present?

Maternal temperature higher than 100.4° F.

Foul smelling drainage or fluid from the incision.

Increased tenderness or soreness at the incision.

Incision edges are no longer together.

Redness or swelling at the incision site.

Exclusively breastfed baby stools less than 3–4 times daily in the newborn period (after fourth day).

IF YES, *Call medical care provider today.*

PROMPT LACTATION CARE NEEDED?

Are any of the following present?

Breast engorgement.

Difficulty latching baby onto breast.

Difficulty finding comfortable feeding positions post surgery.

Concerns about adequacy of milk supply.

Concerns about adequacy of infant growth.

IF YES,   *Call lactation care provider today.*

SELF CARE INFORMATION

Practice skin-to-skin contact frequently.

Feed baby at first sign of hunger cues (signs that say "feed me" include hand-to-face or hand-to-mouth movements, lip smacking, seeking with lips, rooting, and head bobbing).

Feed baby at least 10–12 times per 24 hours.

Listen for signs of baby swallowing.

Allow baby to end feedings.

Expect at least 3–4 infant stools per 24 hours after the first 4 days of life.

Good positioning and attachment are crucial to reduce nipple pain.

If baby is being fed away from the breast, hand express or pump milk to maintain supply.

IMPORTANT CONDITIONS TO REPORT

Maternal fever.

Ongoing discomfort at incision site.

Ongoing difficulty with breastfeeding.

Ongoing concerns about infant growth.

Lethargy or irritability in baby.

Notes

Mothers and babies who experience Cesarean birth have greater risk of mother–baby separation, delayed breastfeeding initiation, delayed development of mature milk, and early supplementation. Mothers should be monitored to ensure that they are healing well after surgery and receiving appropriate post-operative pain relief.

A wide range of drugs are used to relieve pain. An up-to-date drug reference should be consulted to determine the safety and possible side effects of individual drugs.

Newborn and premature babies are at greater risk of side effects due to limited ability to clear drugs from their systems.

Face-to-face lactation counseling can assist mothers in finding comfortable breastfeeding positions and learning their baby's feeding cues.

See also Analgesia; Anesthesia; Childbirth

Drug References

American Academy of Pediatrics Committee on Drugs. (2001). Transfer of drugs and other chemicals into human milk. *Pediatrics, 108,* 776–789.

Briggs, G.G., Freeman, R.K., & Yaffee, S.J. (Eds.). (2002). *Drugs in pregnancy and lactation* (6th ed.). Philadelphia: Lippincott, Williams, and Wilkins.

Hale, T.W. (2004). *Medications and mothers milk.* Amarillo, TX: Pharmasoft Publishing.

Lawrence, R.A., & Lawrence, R.M. (2005). *Breastfeeding: A guide for the medical profession* (6th ed.). St. Louis: Mosby.

▶ Birth control

DEFINITION Devices and drugs used to reduce fertility.

Many contraceptive methods are compatible with breastfeeding, including all barrier methods (condoms, foam, diaphragms, and cervical caps), intrauterine devices (IUDs), and progestin-only hormonal methods.[*] Combined estrogen/progestin methods are generally not recommended as they may reduce milk supply and affect infant growth.

The **Lactational Amenorrhea Method (LAM)** is a form of natural family planning which is 98% effective in the first 6 months following the birth of a baby, so long as the mother's menses have not returned, her baby is exclusively breastfed, and there are no long periods of time between feedings, day and night. Once the baby is older than 6 months, or any of the above criteria is no longer true, LAM is no longer effective and mothers should utilize other forms of family planning.

See also Amenorrhea; Birth interval and breastfeeding; Lactational Amenorrhea Method (LAM); Medications; Progestin-only contraceptives

▶ Birth injury

DEFINITION Damage to the infant's body sustained during delivery.

Ask about

Type, degree, and effects of injury.

ASSESSMENT

EMERGENT CARE NEEDED?
Are any of the following present?
      Baby refuses to feed for more than six hours.
      Extreme **lethargy or irritability** in baby.
      Sudden change in baby's muscle tone (extremely floppy or stiff) or repetitive jerking movements (e.g., seizure activity).
      Baby shows sudden disinterest in feeding.
      Unable to wake baby.
      Baby does not calm, even with cuddles.

IF YES,   *Seek emergency care now.*

PROMPT MEDICAL CARE NEEDED?
Are any of the following present?
      Inadequate urine/stool output.
      Infant discomfort during feeding.

IF YES,   *Seek medical care within 2 to 4 hours.*

PROMPT LACTATION CARE NEEDED?

Are any of the following present?

Baby has difficulty latching on to the breast.

Baby has difficulty sustaining feeding.

Difficulty finding comfortable feeding positioning on one breast or both.

Milk leaking from baby's mouth during feeding.

IF YES,   *Call lactation care provider today.*

SELF CARE INFORMATION

Practice skin-to-skin contact frequently.

Feed baby at first sign of hunger cues (signs that say "feed me" include hand-to-face or hand-to-mouth movements, lip smacking, seeking with lips, rooting, and head bobbing).

Feed baby at least 10–12 times per 24 hours.

Listen for signs of baby swallowing.

Allow baby to end feedings.

Expect at least 3–4 infant stools per 24 hours after the first 4 days of life.

Good positioning and attachment are crucial to reduce nipple pain.

If baby is fed away from the breast, hand express or pump milk to maintain supply.

IMPORTANT CONDITIONS TO REPORT

Persistent unresolved symptoms.

Notes

Birth injuries are sometimes identified because of feeding problems. Birth injuries (e.g., fractured clavicle) may affect baby's ability to feed well temporarily or permanently. Babies with birth injuries should be closely monitored for healing, development, and growth. Feeding positions may need adjustment to accommodate baby's comfort.

Mothers may also experience injuries to soft tissue and coccyx that affect her comfort level.

A wide range of drugs are used to relieve pain. An up-to-date drug reference should be consulted to determine the safety and possible side effects of individual drugs.

Newborn and premature babies are at greater risk of side effects due to limited ability to clear drugs from their systems.

See also Breast refusal

Drug References

American Academy of Pediatrics Committee on Drugs. (2001). Transfer of drugs and other chemicals into human milk. *Pediatrics, 108*, 776–789.

Briggs, G.G., Freeman, R.K., & Yaffee, S.J. (Eds.). (2002). *Drugs in pregnancy and lactation* (6th ed.). Philadelphia: Lippincott, Williams, and Wilkins.

Hale, T.W. (2004). *Medications and mothers milk.* Amarillo, TX: Pharmasoft Publishing.

Lawrence, R.A., & Lawrence, R.M. (2005). *Breastfeeding: A guide for the medical profession* (6th ed.). St. Louis: Mosby.

▶ Birth interval and breastfeeding

DEFINITION Birth interval refers to the length of time from one birth date to the next birth date.

Notes

Women who are exclusively breastfeeding a young baby are likely to experience a lack of menses (**amenorrhea**). Women may be amenorrheic for more than one year while breastfeeding.

Birth intervals of two years or more (international health agencies recommend three years or more[42]) are recommended to allow time for the mother's body to recover and replenish nutrient stores.

Women who wish to become pregnant again may consider breastfeeding less intensively to trigger resumption of their menses. Nutritionally appropriate foods should be offered to the baby when mother begins to **wean**.

See also Amenorrhea; Lactational Amenorrhea Method (LAM); Birth control; Natural family planning

Footnotes

[42]Rutstein, S. (2003, June). *Effect of Birth Intervals on Mortality and Health: Multivariate Cross Country Analyses.* Presentation to the USAID-sponsored Conference on Optimal Birth Spacing for Central America, Antigua.

▶ Birthweight

DEFINITION The weight of the baby at the time of birth. Full term babies are expected to weigh more than 5 lb, 8 oz (2500 g). The average full term baby born in the United States weighs more than 7 lb at birth.

Low birthweight babies weigh less than 2500 g (5 lb, 8 oz) at birth. **Very low birthweight** babies weigh between 1000 and 1500 g (2 lb, 3 oz to 3 lb, 5 oz) at birth. Many low birthweight babies are born prematurely. Others are full term babies who have experienced slow growth in the uterus—these babies are also considered small for gestational age (**SGA**).

Babies born above the 90th percentile for gestational age are considered large for gestational age (**LGA**).

Notes

Low birthweight babies may be more challenging to feed, as they are usually premature and thus may be sleepier and more lethargic. Even if not premature, their smaller size and lower muscle mass may make it more difficult for them to latch well. Ongoing lactation support and attention to stool output, feeding frequency, and weight is indicated.

Babies of diabetic mothers are at increased risk of hypoglycemia and concommitant LGA status. Due to screening procedures and possibly treatment, these babies may experience more separation from their mother and a more difficult start to breastfeeding than appropriate gestational age (**AGA**) babies. Ongoing lactation support can assist in overcoming early difficulties

▶ Biting

DEFINITION This action occurs when the baby closes its teeth or jaw on the nipple and breast.

Age of baby.

ASSESSMENT

ROUTINE CARE NEEDED?

Are any of the following present?

Runny or stuffy nose in baby.

Difficulty nursing.

IF YES, *Call pediatric care provider today and call lactation care provider today.*

Are any of the following present?

New onset of sore nipples.

Biting at the breast.

Questions about soothing the teething baby.

IF YES, *Call lactation care provider today.*

SELF CARE INFORMATION

Teething is a temporary (but reoccurring) stage. Teething can be difficult for some babies and families. Allowing the baby to bite down on a cool, textured teething toy prior to feeding may make feeding more comfortable.

IMPORTANT CONDITIONS TO REPORT

Difficulty breathing.

Wheezing.

Fever.

Notes

Babies do not need to be weaned because they are teething or because they have teeth, although mothers may be told this by friends or family.

Because their gums are uncomfortable, teething babies may try chewing at the breast.

Mothers may have sore nipples when the baby is teething.

Babies often have stuffy noses at the teething ages.

See also Clenching or clamping onto the nipple/areola; Sore nipples; Teething

▶ Bleb

DEFINITION A tiny white, milky blockage of a single duct opening on the surface of the nipple. Mothers often describe excruciating, pinpoint pain at the site of the blockage. Blebs may need to be lanced by a medical care provider.

Ask about

Onset.
Age of baby.
History of herpes lesions or other skin conditions on breast or nipple.

ASSESSMENT

EMERGENT CARE NEEDED?
Are any of the following present?
History of herpes lesions on the nipple.
History of herpes lesions elsewhere on mother or partner's body with current bleb or lesion on nipple or breast.

IF YES, *Seek medical care within 2 to 4 hours.*

PROMPT CARE NEEDED?
Are any of the following present?
Painful, protruberant bleb on nipple.

IF YES, *Call obstetric care provider today and call lactation care provider today.*

SELF CARE INFORMATION
Follow directions for post lancing care.
Breastfeeding can usually resume right away.

IMPORTANT CONDITIONS TO REPORT
Symptoms of infection (fever, aching, chills, redness at site).

Because of the serious nature of some infectious conditions, including *Herpes,* women reporting rashes or lesions on the breast and nipple should be seen immediately by medical personnel to rule out contraindicated infections.

Emergency differential diagnosis is crucial in women with breast or nipple lesions who have a history of herpes lesions or a partner with a history of herpes. As herpes can be fatal to the newborn, breastfeeding should be discontinued on the affected nipple until differential diagnosis is obtained.

A bleb "may be 'cured' or disappear when the health professional opens it with a sterile needle. It may reappear and have to be opened again."[43]

See also Blisters on nipple or breast; Nipple pain

Footnotes

[43]Lawrence, R.A., & Lawrence, R.M. (2005). *Breastfeeding: A guide for the medical profession* (6th ed., p. 300). St. Louis: Mosby.

▶ Bleeding, breast

DEFINITION Visible evidence of blood flow from the breast.

Ask about

Onset.
Age of baby.
History of trauma or surgery to breast.

ASSESSMENT

EMERGENT CARE NEEDED?

Are any of the following present?

Persistent bleeding from breast between feedings.
Symptoms of infection (redness or pus at the site of bleeding, fever, chills, achiness, malaise).
Mass or lump in the breast (**intraductal papilloma**).

IF YES, *Seek medical care within 2 to 4 hours.*

SELF CARE INFORMATION

Watch for feeding cues and offer the breast as soon as it is seen.

Wait for baby to open mouth wide (greater than a 100° angle).

Pull baby in so that chin touches the breast first, and nipple enters the mouth along the top of the tongue; this should result in a wide open mouth full of breast tissue.

Lips should be flanged outward.

Baby's lips should look off center when compared with the areola; the bottom lip should be farther away from the nipple than the top lip.

IMPORTANT CONDITIONS TO REPORT

Any substance or item being used to decrease pain.

Worsening symptoms.

Persistent symptoms.

Notes

Due to its highly vascular nature, the lactating breast may be more prone to bleeding. Blood may be seen in pumped milk. It may also appear on injured nipples. The nursing baby may spit up blood-tinged milk. Blood in the milk or coming from the breast indicates need for medical evaluation. Breast trauma, intraductal **papilloma,** and other findings are possible.

Mothers may be concerned about the safety of nursing the baby when they are bleeding. There is no reason for concern about the infant consuming small amounts of blood.

See also Bleeding, nipple; Papilloma, intraductal

▶ Bleeding, nipple

DEFINITION Visible evidence of blood flow from the nipple.

Ask about

Onset.
Age of baby.
History of trauma or surgery to breast.

ASSESSMENT

EMERGENT CARE NEEDED?

Are any of the following present?

Persistent bleeding from nipple between feedings.

Symptoms of infection (redness or pus at the site of bleeding, fever, chills, achiness, malaise).

Mass or lump in the breast (**intraductal papilloma**).

IF YES, *Seek medical care within 2 to 4 hours.*

PROMPT CARE NEEDED?

Are any of the following present?

Bleeding during feedings.

Pain on latch.

IF YES, *Seek lactation care within 2 to 4 hours.*

SELF CARE INFORMATION

Practice good attachment:

Watch for feeding cues and offer the breast as soon as they are seen.

Wait for baby to open mouth wide (greater than a 100° angle).

Pull baby in so that chin touches the breast first, and nipple enters the mouth along the top of the tongue; this should result in a wide open mouth full of breast tissue.

Lips should be flanged outward.

Baby's lips should look off center when compared with the areola; the bottom lip should be farther away from the nipple than the top lip.

IMPORTANT CONDITIONS TO REPORT

Any substance or item being used to decrease pain.

Worsening symptoms.

Persistent symptoms.

> **Notes**
>
> Bleeding nipples are most often due to nipple trauma from poor breastfeeding positioning and attachment. The degree of pain women express varies widely.
>
> Nipple pain is one of the main reasons women stop breastfeeding before they intended to do so. Nipple pain indicates need for a consultation with the lactation care provider.
>
> Mothers may be concerned about the safety of nursing the baby when they are bleeding. There is no reason for concern about the infant consuming small amounts of blood.

See also Bleeding, breast; Nipple pain

▶ Bleeding, postpartum hemorrhage

DEFINITION An abnormally high amount (generally more than 500 ml) of blood loss during or after delivery.

> **Notes**
>
> Postpartum hemorrhage is of concern related to breastfeeding because extreme blood loss can cause **Sheehan's syndrome,** an insult to the **pituitary gland,** where the hormones of lactation (**prolactin** and **oxytocin**) are manufactured. Women affected by Sheehan's syndrome may be unable to make an adequate amount of milk.
>
> Other symptoms of this syndrome include sudden onset of hypothyroidism, diabetes insipidus, and hair loss along with menstrual irregularities. Medical evaluation should include measurement of prolactin levels before and after sucklings. The extent to which women recover from Sheehan's is variable with the degree of infarct.[44]
>
> Babies of mothers who suffered postpartum hemorrhage should be closely monitored for signs of adequate milk intake (e.g., swallowing, milk transfer, stool output) and growth.

See also Sheehan's syndrome

Footnotes

[44]Lawrence, R.A., & Lawrence, R.M. (2005). *Breastfeeding: A guide for the medical profession* (6th ed., pp. 573–574). St. Louis: Mosby.

▶ Bleeding, postpartum vaginal

DEFINITION Vaginal blood flow is expected after delivery. This is also called "lochia." Three types of lochia are recognized, including Lochia rubra (red), Lochia serosa (pink), and Lochia alba (white).

Lochia rubra, a red discharge, begins after delivery and continues for two to three days.

Lochia serosa, a paler, pinkish discharge continues for the next week or so. Lochia alba, a whitish discharge, starts around the tenth day postpartum and should be resolved within a month.[45]

Ask about

Onset.
Date of delivery.

ASSESSMENT

EMERGENT CARE NEEDED?
Are any of the following present?

Soaking more than one pad per hour.
Offensive odor to lochia.
Green color to lochia.

IF YES, *Seek medical care now.*

PROMPT CARE NEEDED?

Are any of the following present?

Sudden resumption of lochia rubra (bright red blood flow).

Lack of cessation of lochia rubra after four days postpartum.

Lack of cessation of lochia serosa.

Signs of infection (fever, chills, pain, malaise, overall aching).

Milk supply problems coupled with ongoing lochia rubra or serosa.

IF YES, *Seek medical care within 2 to 4 hours.*

SELF CARE INFORMATION

Monitor blood flow.

IMPORTANT CONDITIONS TO REPORT

Continuation of symptoms.

Sudden gushing of blood.

Multiple blood clots passed.

Concerns about milk supply.

Notes

As time progresses, the volume of lochia should also decrease. Sudden return of bright red bleeding is of concern and should be evaluated medically. Retained placental fragments can be indicated by ongoing lochia rubra. In this event, mature milk production may not occur until placental fragments are expelled or removed.

See also Lochia; Retained placental fragments

Footnotes

[45]Varney, H., Kriebs, J.M., Gegor, C.L. (Eds.). (2004). *Varney's midwifery* (4th ed., p. 1043). Sudbury, MA: Jones & Bartlett Publishers.

▶ Blisters on nipple or breast

DEFINITION A local swelling of the skin of the nipple or breast that contains fluid. May be caused by pressure of baby's mouth or device, or by infectious or inflammatory process.

Because of the serious nature of some infectious conditions, including *Herpes*, women reporting rashes or lesions on the breast or nipple should be seen immediately by medical personnel to rule out contraindicated infections.

Ask about

Onset.
Age of baby.
Known history of herpes lesions or other skin conditions.

ASSESSMENT

PROMPT MEDICAL CARE NEEDED?
Are any of the following present?
   History of herpes lesions on the nipple or breast.
   Blisters plus fever, aching, and systemic symptoms in mother or baby.
   History of herpes lesions elsewhere on mother or partner's body with
      current bleb or lesion on nipple or breast.

IF YES, *Seek medical care within 2 to 4 hours.*

PROMPT LACTATION CARE NEEDED?
Are any of the following present?
   Pain during breast pumping or feeding.
   Trauma to nipple or breast from pumping or feeding.
   Concerns about adequacy of supply.

IF YES, *Call lactation care provider today.*

SELF CARE INFORMATION
   Practice good attachment:
      Watch baby for hunger cues, and offer the breast as soon as it is seen.
      Place baby so that nose is opposite nipple.

Wait for baby to open mouth wide (greater than a 100° angle).

Pull baby in so that chin touches the breast first, and nipple enters the mouth along the top of the tongue; this should result in a wide open mouth full of breast tissue.

Lips should be flanged outward.

Baby's lips should look off center when compared with the areola; the bottom lip should be farther away from the nipple than the top lip.

IMPORTANT CONDITIONS TO REPORT

History of other skin conditions.

Known skin reaction.

Notes

Blisters may appear on the nipple and breast for several reasons, including poor latch, trauma, damage from **nipple shields**, **abscess**, and **blebs**.

Emergency differential diagnosis is crucial in women with history of herpes lesions on the nipple or elsewhere on mother or partner's body. As herpes can be fatal to the newborn, breastfeeding should be discontinued on the affected nipple until differential diagnosis is obtained. *Active herpes or chicken pox lesions on the nipple and breast are potentially life threatening for the baby.* Herpes lesions elsewhere on the body do not contraindicate breastfeeding. However, parents should practice very careful handwashing techniques to avoid touching lesions and then touching the baby.

Other conditions to consider include poison ivy, allergic response to surface antigens ("contact dermatitis"), and eczema.

A **bleb** is a tiny white, milky blockage of a single duct opening on the surface of the nipple. Mothers often describe excruciating, pinpoint pain at the site of the blockage. Counseling and visual inspection may be required to assure correct diagnosis. A bleb "may be 'cured' or disappear when the health professional opens it with a sterile needle. It may reappear and have to be opened again."[46]

See also Bleb; Nipple pain; Milk blister, bleb

Footnotes

[46]Lawrence, R.A., & Lawrence, R.M. (2005). *Breastfeeding: A guide for the medical profession* (6th ed., p. 300). St. Louis: Mosby.

▶ Blood in milk

DEFINITION Visible blood in expressed or dripped milk.

Ask about

Onset.
Age of baby.
Trauma or injury to the breast.

ASSESSMENT

EMERGENT CARE NEEDED?
   Are any of the following present?
      Persistent bleeding from breast between feedings.
      Symptoms of infection (redness or pus at the site of bleeding, fever, chills, achiness, malaise).
      Breast lump or mass (**intraductal papilloma**)

IF YES, *Seek medical care within 2 to 4 hours.*

PROMPT CARE NEEDED?
   Are any of the following present?
      Bleeding during feedings.
      Pain on latch.

IF YES, *Call lactation care provider today.*

ROUTINE CARE NEEDED?
   Are any of the following present?
      Bloody tinge to pumped milk with no other symptoms.

IF YES, *Call lactation care provider.*

SELF CARE INFORMATION
   Practice good attachment:
      Watch for feeding cues and offer the breast as soon as it is seen.
      Hold baby so that nose is opposite nipple.
      Wait for baby to open mouth wide (greater than a 100° angle).

Pull baby in so that chin touches the breast first, and nipple enters the mouth along the top of the tongue; this should result in a wide open mouth full of breast tissue.

Lips should be flanged outward.

Baby's lips should look off center when compared with the areola; the bottom lip should be farther away from the nipple than the top lip.

IMPORTANT CONDITIONS TO REPORT

Worsening symptoms.

Persistent symptoms.

> **Notes**
>
> Due to its highly vascular nature, the lactating breast may be more prone to bleeding. Blood may be seen in pumped milk. It may also appear on injured nipples. The nursing baby may spit up blood-tinged milk. Blood in the milk or coming from the breast indicates need for medical evaluation. Breast trauma, intraductal **papilloma,** and other findings are possible.
>
> Mothers may be concerned about the safety of nursing the baby when there is blood in their milk. There is no reason for concern about the infant consuming small amounts of blood.

See also Bleeding, breast; Bleeding, nipple; Rusty-pipe syndrome

▶ Blood in stool

DEFINITION Visible evidence of blood in infant's stool. This finding needs immediate medical evaluation.

> **Notes**
>
> Blood in stool may indicate infection, reaction to protein in formula, physiologic disorder, or, in the breastfed infant, a reaction to protein in the mother's diet. If the infant is reacting to a protein in its mother's diet, the problem may be improved by an allergen avoidance diet. In this case, mother may benefit from consultation with a dietitian or nutritionist.

See also Proctocolitis

▶ BMD

See also Bone mineral density (BMD)

▶ Bonding

DEFINITION The complex process of parent–baby attachment, which develops over a period of weeks and months.

> **Notes**
>
> Mothers may feel guilty if they do not feel immediately bonded to their infant.
>
> Several experiences can interfere with bonding, including traumatic birth experiences, childbirth trauma and pain, real or perceived problems for the baby, separation from the baby due to prematurity or illness, postpartum mood disorders, and familial or life stress.
>
> Skin-to-skin contact, breastfeeding, learning soothing techniques for baby, and receiving emotional and practical support enhance bonding.
>
> Blanket reassurance does not help mothers with perceived bonding problems—genuine listening does. Refer mothers with concerns about bonding to a lactation care provider or parent educator.

▶ Bone loss

DEFINITION Referring to the liberation of calcium from bone(s) during lactation.

> **Notes**
>
> Bone mineral density (BMD) generally peaks in young adulthood. Some BMD is lost during extended breastfeeding, as calcium is liberated to be used in milk manufacture. After weaning, BMD is regained and often increased from prenatal BMD.
>
> While eating calcium rich foods is a healthful choice, it will not prevent bone loss from occurring during extended breastfeeding.

Women who entered pregnancy with **osteoporosis** or other bone density problems need ongoing medical and dietary counseling during this time.

See also Osteoporosis

Bone mineral density (BMD)

DEFINITION A measure of the abundance of calcium phosphate, the major mineral composing bone.

Notes

Bone mineral density (BMD) generally peaks in young adulthood. Some BMD is lost during extended breastfeeding, as calcium is liberated to be used in milk manufacture. During and after weaning, BMD is regained and often increased from prenatal BMD.

While eating calcium rich foods is a healthful choice, it will not prevent bone loss from occurring during extended breastfeeding.

Women who entered pregnancy with **osteoporosis** or other bone density problems need special medical and dietary counseling during this time.

See also Osteoporosis

Bottle feeding

DEFINITION Giving a baby expressed breastmilk or formula with a feeding bottle.

Ask about

Age of baby.
Reason for bottle feeding.

PROMPT CARE NEEDED?

Are any of the following present?

Baby refuses to breastfeed after having a bottle.

Baby refuses to accept bottle.

Questions about weaning.

IF YES, *Call lactation care provider today.*

ROUTINE CARE NEEDED?

Are any of the following present?

Questions about bottle feeding methods or equipment.

IF YES, *Call lactation care provider.*

SELF CARE INFORMATION

Offer baby comfort during change (cuddling, rocking, walking, etc.).

IMPORTANT CONDITIONS TO REPORT

Persistent feeding refusal.

Notes

Mothers may have heard that offering a bottle to their newborn babies will cause **nipple confusion** or other problems. While there is no scientific evidence of nipple confusion, some babies seem to have more difficulty sensing the mother's softer, more pliable nipple in their mouth after being bottlefed. This may be particularly true of preterm babies and those with low muscle tone and/or neurological issues.

There are many different bottle and nipple shapes available on the market. However, few have been studied scientifically to support any claims that they are "most like the breast."

There are many alternative ways to supplement breastfed babies, including spoons, cups, **paladai**, droppers, and other feeding devices. The cup is one of the easiest feeding devices to clean. A lactation care provider should teach parents the safe method for cup feeding infants.

If mother does not wish to, or is unable to, express her milk as a supplement, then the baby younger than 1 year of age should receive properly prepared infant formula in the bottle.

See also Feeding methods, alternate; Formula, infant; Paladai

▶ Botulism, infantile

DEFINITION An illness caused by a nerve toxin produced by *Clostridium botulinum*, resulting in symptoms of constipation, lethargy, and lack of muscle control (e.g., sudden inability to hold up head). These findings indicate the need for emergency care.

Ask about

Onset.
Age of baby.

ASSESSMENT

EMERGENT CARE NEEDED?
Are any of the following present?
Extreme **lethargy** in baby.
Sudden change in baby's muscle tone (extremely floppy or hypertense).
Sudden disinterest in feeding.

IF YES, *Seek emergency care.*

IMPORTANT CONDITIONS TO REPORT
Administration of honey to baby.

Notes

Botulism is uncommon in exclusively breastfed infants, whose guts are less hospitable to the *C. botulinum* spores that create this illness.

Feeding honey to a baby younger than 12 months (including putting honey on the breast or bottle nipples) is not recommended, as honey may contain botulism spores. Botulism spores are also found in the environment, particularly in soil.

See also Acute infection; Constipation; Lethargy

▶ Bovine milk

DEFINITION The fluid produced by the lactating cow. Cow's milk is not recommended for children younger than 1 year of age.

Notes

Human milk and infant formula are the only appropriate milks for babies younger than 1 year of age. While cow's milk-based formula is a substitute for breastmilk, unaltered cow's milk is not, as it may lead to mineral and nutrient imbalance and bleeding in the gut. Similarly, soy and rice milks are not appropriate replacements for human milk or infant formula.

Between 1 and 2 years of age, whole cow's milk may be offered to children. Low fat milk should not be offered until children are older than 2 years.

Concern about infant allergy is much more common than actual allergy. The American Academy of Pediatrics reports that the prevalence of infant cow's milk allergy is two to three percent.[47] The overall prevalence of childhood food allergy is four to six percent.[48]

Counseling and education should include comfort techniques for the irritable baby and coping methods for parents.

See also Allergy in the breastfed infant; Colic, infantile

Footnotes

[47]American Academy of Pediatrics Committee on Nutrition. (2000). Hypoallergenic infant formulas. *Pediatrics, 106,* 346–349.

[48]Ziegler, R.S. (2003). Food allergen avoidance in prevention of food allergy in infants and children. *Pediatrics, 111,* 1662–1671.

▶ Bowel movements, infant

DEFINITION Fecal matter produced by the infant. In this context, stools passed daily are a good indicator of the adequacy of feeding. Exclusively breastfed newborn babies should pass at least three to four stools daily (fewer stools may be produced during the first four days of life). Fewer stools daily may be normal in the older breastfed baby.

Ask about

Age of baby.
Stooling pattern.
Supplements given.

ASSESSMENT

EMERGENT CARE NEEDED?

Are any of the following present?

Exclusively breastfed newborn baby with less than one stool per day.
Meconium bowel movements after day five of life.
Constipation (hard stool) in a breastfed baby.
Blood in stool.
Persistent mucous in stool.
Pain with stooling.

IF YES, *Call pediatric care provider now.*

PROMPT CARE NEEDED?

Are any of the following present?

Concern about inadequate feeding.
Concern about inadequate stooling.
Fewer than 3–4 stools daily in the excusively breastfead baby over four days old.

IF YES, *Call pediatric and lactation care provider today.*

SELF CARE INFORMATION

Practice skin-to-skin contact frequently.
Feed baby at first sign of hunger cues (signs that say "feed me" include hand-to-face or hand-to-mouth movements, lip smacking, seeking with lips, rooting, and head bobbing).

Feed baby at least 10–12 times per 24 hours.

Observe for signs of baby swallowing (sounds, pauses, etc.).

Allow baby to end feedings.

Expect at least 3–4 infant stools per 24 hours after the first 4 days of life during the newborn period.

Good positioning and attachment are crucial to reduce nipple pain.

If baby is fed away from the breast, hand express or pump milk to maintain supply.

IMPORTANT CONDITIONS TO REPORT

Worsening of symptoms.

Persistent problems with bowel movements.

Notes

Stool appearance:
All babies pass thick, black-green, tarry stool called **meconium** in the first days post-partum. In the breastfed baby, meconium gives way to transitional stool, which is brownish and very soft. After five days of life, exclusively breastfed babies pass stool that is mustard-like in color and consistency.

Until they are started on solid foods or formula, breastfed babies have very soft, liquid stools with flecks of curd. Once other foods are introduced, the color of the stool may change back to a brownish color, and be harder and more formed in shape.

Stool frequency:
Breastfed newborns pass small amounts of stool frequently during the day. They may stool during or after every feeding. *It is not normal for a breastfed newborn to go days without a bowel movement*. More than four stools daily are expected in the newborn period.

Infrequent stooling in the breastfed newborn may indicate inadequate feeding fre-quency (less than 10 feeds per 24 hours) or poor feeding dynamics. Consultation with a lactation care provider is indicated.

Rarely, constipation may be a symptom of **infantile botulism**.

See also Botulism, infantile; Constipation

▶ Bras

DEFINITION Clothing worn to support the breasts. Special bras are made for breast-feeding mothers.

> **Notes**
>
> Finding a comfortable nursing bra often takes some work. It is helpful to have referral information to a shop or service that will determine the appropriate size bra, as breast size changes during pregnancy and lactation. If breastfeeding women choose to wear a bra, one specifically designed for breastfeeding is indicated. Women have damaged their breast tissue by pulling regular or sports bras up over their breasts, or squeezing their breasts out over the top of the bra cup to feed.
>
> Bras that are too tight or constricting can cause breast problems including reduced milk supply, plugged ducts, and mastitis. Some women have been told to wear a bra day and night. This is unnecessary and may cause problems. Many nursing mothers are more comfortable wearing natural fiber camisoles, sleeveless T-shirts, or tank tops with shelf bras.
>
> There is no need for nursing mothers to wear bras around the clock. Bras are more likely to cause breast problems when worn continuously.

See also Mastitis

▶ Breast abscess

DEFINITION A localized collection of pus resulting from the breakdown of breast tissue. Inflammation often occurs around the abscess. Breast abscess is often the outcome of unresolved mastitis. Abscesses are typically drained through aspiration or by surgical incision and drainage. Antibiotic treatment will be prescribed based on suspected pathogen.

Ask about

Onset.
Prior breast infection.
Known drug allergies.

EMERGENT CARE NEEDED?

Are any of the following present?

Visible or palpable breast abscess.

Fever higher than 100° F (37.7° C).

Extreme breast discomfort.

Flu-like aching throughout body.

Chills.

Continuing fever after abscess drainage.

Reaction to antibiotic prescribed post-drainage.

Green or odorous change to fluid seeping from site after drainage.

IF YES, *Seek medical care within 2 to 4 hours.*

PROMPT CARE NEEDED?

Are any of the following present?

Continuation of symptoms after drainage.

Difficulty with breastfeeding following abscess drainage.

IF YES, *Seek medical care today and call lactation care provider today.*

ROUTINE CARE NEEDED?

Are any of the following present?

Questions about resumption of breastfeeding on affected breast.

IF YES, *Call obstetric care provider today.*

SELF CARE INFORMATION

Finish full course of antibiotics prescribed (unless told to stop by a prescriber).

Continue nonprescription pain relief as recommended.

Continue to monitor breasts for symptoms of recurring breast infection (redness, heat, fever, blockage, pain).

IMPORTANT CONDITIONS TO REPORT

Symptoms worsen or persist.

Signs of infection.

Abscess indicates a need for urgent medical treatment. Symptoms include reddened areas of the breast, occasionally with a visible fluid filled sac protruding through the surface of the breast, and overall body sensation of **malaise**, aching, fever, and fatigue. Abscess may follow **mastitis**. Typical treatment includes appropriate antibiotic administration and drainage by lancing or aspiration. Presence of one identified abscess may indicate presence of multiple other abscesses, some of which may be deep in the breast, visible only by imaging technology. When symptoms do not resolve after treatment, presence of additional abscesses must be considered.

Breastfeeding is not contraindicated on the noninvolved breast. Breastfeeding may continue on the affected breast if determined safe. Drainage may cause leaking of milk from severed ducts. Women may feel very ill and need practical and emotional support.

See also Acute infection; Breast infection

▶ **Breast augmentation**

DEFINITION A procedure that increases the size of the breast, typically by inserting a saline or silicone implant in the breast.

Ask about

Date of surgery.
Age of baby.
Location of surgical incision.

ASSESSMENT

PROMPT CARE NEEDED?
Are any of the following present?
Concerns about milk supply.
Failure of breastfed baby to grow adequately.

IF YES, *Seek medical care today and call lactation care provider today.*

SELF CARE INFORMATION

Practice skin-to-skin contact frequently.

Feed baby at first sign of hunger cues (signs that say "feed me" include hand-to-face or hand-to-mouth movements, lip smacking, seeking with lips, rooting, and head bobbing).

Feed baby at least 10–12 times per 24 hours.

Listen for signs of baby swallowing.

Allow baby to end feedings.

Expect at least 3–4 infant stools per 24 hours after the first 4 days of life.

Good positioning and attachment are crucial to reduce nipple pain.

If baby is fed away from the breast, hand express or pump milk to maintain supply.

IMPORTANT CONDITIONS TO REPORT

Fewer than four bowel movements daily in the first month of life, after the fourth day.

Ongoing concerns or problems with milk supply.

Notes

The location and extent of the incision may impact the sensation of the nerves in the nipple area. Loss of or decreased sensation may decrease milk-making potential. Trauma to the nerves may hinder the stimulation of the brain to release prolactin (the milk-making hormone) in response to suckling. Periareolar incisions suggest more potential injury than do incisions underneath the breast.

Babies of women who have had breast augmentation surgery should be followed closely to ensure proper milk transfer and growth.

If the mother reports that she had an implant in one breast only, inquire about the reason for this surgery. If augmentation corrected breast asymmetry, there may be increased concern regarding the mother's ability to make a full milk supply. Marked asymmetry may indicate insufficient glandular tissue in both breasts. Baby and mother should be closely followed.

See also Breast surgery

▶ Breast, bleeding from

DEFINITION Visible evidence of blood flow from the breast.

Ask about

Onset.
Age of baby.
History of trauma or surgery to breast.

ASSESSMENT

EMERGENT CARE NEEDED?

Are any of the following present?

Persistent bleeding from breast between feedings.

Symptoms of infection (redness or pus at the site of bleeding, fever, chills, achiness, malaise).

IF YES, *Seek medical care within 2 to 4 hours.*

PROMPT CARE NEEDED?

Are any of the following present?

Bleeding during feedings.

Pain on latch.

IF YES, *Call lactation care provider today.*

SELF CARE INFORMATION

Practice good attachment:

Watch for feeding cues and offer the breast as soon as they are seen.

Wait for baby to open mouth wide (greater than a 100° angle).

Pull baby in so that chin touches the breast first, and nipple enters the mouth along the top of the tongue; this should result in a wide open mouth full of breast tissue.

Lips should be flanged outward.

Baby's lips should look off center when compared with the areola; the bottom lip should be farther away from the nipple than the top lip.

Any substance or item being used to decrease pain.

Worsening symptoms.

Persistent symptoms.

> **Notes**
>
> Due to its highly vascular nature, the lactating breast may be more prone to bleeding. Blood may be seen in pumped milk. It may also appear on injured nipples. The nursing baby may spit up blood-tinged milk. Blood in the milk or coming from the breast indicates need for medical evaluation. Breast trauma, intraductal **papilloma,** and other findings are possible.
>
> Mothers may be concerned about the safety of nursing the baby when they are bleeding. There is no reason for concern about the infant consuming small amounts of blood.

See also Bleeding, nipple; Papilloma, intraductal; Rusty-pipe syndrome

▶ Breast cancer

DEFINITION Malignant growth within the tissues of the breast. Unexplained and unusual lumps in the lactating breast must be examined by medical personnel.

> **Notes**
>
> While many masses in the lactating breast are often associated with plugged milk ducts, other types of growths, including cancerous ones, are possible. When lumps in the breast do not resolve within 24–48 hours, complete breast evaluation should be performed.
>
> Women who have previously been diagnosed and treated for breast cancer can breastfeed. Those who have had past breast surgery may experience decreased milk production in the segments of the breast surgically involved.
>
> When cancer is identified in the lactating breast, weaning is generally indicated because of the nature of the drugs and other therapies used to treat cancer.
>
> Breastfeeding reduces the risk of developing breast cancer in the mother, and possibly the child.

See also Abrupt weaning; Biopsy, breast; Breast lumps; Breast refusal; Breast surgery; Goldsmith's sign

▶ Breast engorgement

DEFINITION Swelling in the breast associated with increase in the flow of blood and lymph to the breast, as well as the manufacture of milk. More common in the first days postpartum, engorgement may also occur whenever feedings are infrequent.

Ask about

Onset.
Age of baby.
Feeding pattern.

ASSESSMENT

EMERGENT CARE NEEDED?
> *Are any of the following present?*
>> Symptoms of infection (fever, aching, chills, malaise).
>> Red streaks on the breast.

IF YES, *Seek medical care within 2 to 4 hours.*

PROMPT CARE NEEDED?
> *Are any of the following present?*
>> Baby unable to latch on to breast.
>> Engorgement not resolving after latch-on.

IF YES, *Call lactation care provider now.*

SELF CARE INFORMATION

Consider soaking breasts in warm water before feeding and applying cool gel packs between feedings.
Gently hand express to soften breasts before feedings.
Nonprescription anti-inflammatory agents may also be helpful.

IMPORTANT CONDITIONS TO REPORT

Lack of resolution of engorgement in 24–48 hours.

Symptoms of infection (fever, chills, aching, redness, malaise).

Notes

Engorgement is best resolved by softening the breast so that baby can latch on to the breast. Nursing the baby offers more relief than does pumping.

See also Breast infection; Hand expression of breastmilk

Breastfeeding

DEFINITION Feeding a baby milk produced by the breast.

See also Exclusive breastfeeding; Full breastfeeding; Token breastfeeding

Breastfeeding assessment tools

DEFINITION Refers to documents or rubrics used to evaluate the adequacy of feeding. Documents include the IBFAT,[49] LAT,[50] LATCH,[51] MBA,[52] and SAIB[53] tools.

Footnotes

[49]Matthews, M.K. (1993). Assessment and suggested interventions to assist newborn breastfeeding behavior. *Journal of Human Lactation, 9*(4), 243–248.

[50]Blair, A., Cadwell, K., Turner-Maffei, C., & Brimdyr, K. (2003). The relationship between positioning, the breastfeeding dynamic, the latching process and pain in breastfeeding mothers with sore nipples. *Breastfeeding Review, 11*(2), 5–10.

[51]Jensen, D., Wallace, S., & Kelsay, P. (1994). LATCH: A breastfeeding charting system and documentation tool. *Journal of Obstetrics, Gynecology and Neonatal Nursing, 23*(1), 27–32.

[52]Mulford, C. (1992). The mother-baby assessment (MBA): An "APGAR" score for breastfeeding. *Journal of Human Lactation, 8*, 79–82.

[53]Shrago, L., & Bocar, D. (1990). The infant's contribution to breastfeeding. *Journal of Obstetrics, Gynecology and Neonatal Nursing, 19*(3), 209–215.

▶ Breastfeeding during pregnancy

DEFINITION If a mother becomes pregnant while she is breastfeeding a baby from a prior pregnancy, she may experience extremely sore nipples, a decrease in her milk supply, and production of colostrum. It is possible to continue breastfeeding through the pregnancy and then continue nursing the two babies together. This is called "tandem nursing."

SELF CARE INFORMATION

Nursing during pregnancy and tandem nursing are individual choices that the mother makes for herself and her family. Although there are no reported problems with nursing during pregnancy and increased risk of premature labor, mothers with a prior history of premature birth or threatened premature labor should consider the theoretical risk as they make their decision.

Mothers should seek help for sore nipples and other discomforts of breastfeeding during pregnancy.

See also Tandem nursing

▶ Breast, fibrocystic

DEFINITION A common breast condition in women that includes variable lumpiness, tenderness, and palpable cysts (pockets of fluid). Symptoms may change during the menstrual period. This benign condition is compatible with breastfeeding.

Notes
Plugged ducts respond to improving breast milk drainage by moving in 24–48 hours. Lumps that do not resolve should be medically examined to rule out **plugged ducts** and other problems.
Women who have experienced fibrocystic breasts may misdiagnose **plugged ducts** and other breastfeeding problems as fibrocystic changes.

See also Breast lumps

▶ Breast infection

DEFINITION Invasion of the breast tissue by *Staphylococcus aureus* or other common pathogens, resulting in symptoms of red, hot, painful, swollen wedges of tissue of the breast, malaise, and overall aching. This condition is usually unilateral. Bilateral presentation may indicate infection with *Streptococcus*. Breast infection is a type of *mastitis*.

Ask about

Onset.
Breast involvement.

ASSESSMENT

EMERGENT CARE NEEDED?
Are any of the following present?
Sudden bilateral red streaks with fever, aching, chills, etc.

IF YES, *Seek emergency care now.*

PROMPT CARE NEEDED?
Are any of the following present?
Unilateral red streaks.
Symptoms of infection (fever, aching, chills).

IF YES, *Call obstetric care provider now.*

SELF CARE INFORMATION
Feed baby at least 10–24 times per 24 hours.
Soften breasts between feedings with gentle hand expression.
Finish full course of antibiotics prescribed (unless told to stop by a health care provider).
Continue nonprescription pain relief as recommended.
Continue to monitor for symptoms of recurring breast infection (redness, heat, fever, chills, pain).

IMPORTANT CONDITIONS TO REPORT

Worsening of symptoms.
Persistence of symptoms.
Recurrence of symptoms.

> **Notes**
>
> The Academy of Breastfeeding Medicine states that preferred antibiotics are "penicillinase-resistant penicillins, such as dicloxacillin or flucloxacillin 500mg qid."[54]
> Mothers should continue to breastfeed through the infection. There is no reason to cease breastfeeding due to concern about infecting the infant.
> Occasionally breast infection does not respond to antibiotic treatment. In this case, clean-catch culture of the breastmilk may be taken to determine presence of infective organisms.
> The symptoms listed previously may also indicate noninfectious inflammation due to a local reaction to overfull breast tissue. Mastitis can have both inflammatory and infectious causes.

See also Acute infection; Bilateral mastitis; Breast inflammation; Mastitis

Footnotes

[54]Academy of Breastfeeding Medicine. (2002). *Clinical Protocol #4: Mastitis.* Retrieved March 10, 2005, from http://www.bfmed.org/Protocols.html.

▶ Breast inflammation

DEFINITION The body's response to injury, infection, or foreign matter that results in pain, redness, swelling, and sometimes impaired function of the affected area (in this case, the breast). This is also known as **mastitis**.

Ask about

Onset.
Extent of redness and involvement.

EMERGENT CARE NEEDED?

Are any of the following present?

Sudden bilateral red streaks with fever, aching, chills, etc.

IF YES, *Seek emergency care now.*

PROMPT CARE NEEDED?

Are any of the following present?

Unilateral red streaks.

Symptoms of infection (fever, aching, chills, etc.).

IF YES, *Seek medical care within 2 to 4 hours.*

SELF CARE INFORMATION

Feed baby at least 10–24 times per 24 hours.

Soften breasts between feedings with gentle hand expression.

Finish full course of treatment prescribed (unless told to stop by a health care provider).

Continue nonprescription pain relief as recommended.

Continue to monitor for symptoms of recurring breast infection (redness, heat, fever, chills, pain).

IMPORTANT CONDITIONS TO REPORT

Worsening of symptoms.

Persistence of symptoms.

Recurrence of symptoms.

Notes

Mothers with mastitis should continue to breastfeed. There is no reason to cease breast-feeding.

The symptoms listed previously may also indicate infection. Mastitis can have both inflammatory and infectious causes.

See also Acute infection; Bilateral mastitis; Breast infection; Mastitis

▶ Breast, insufficient glandular tissue

DEFINITION A rare condition in which women have an inadequate amount of milk-making tissue in the breasts. This may be congenital, or the result of trauma or surgery to the chest. Asymmetry between the breasts may be a hallmark of this condition.

Ask about

Onset.
Age of baby.

ASSESSMENT

PROMPT CARE NEEDED?
> *Are any of the following present?*
>> Failure of breastfed baby to grow adequately.

IF YES, *Seek medical care today and call lactation care provider today.*

ROUTINE CARE NEEDED?
> *Are any of the following present?*
>> Reported asymmetry with no concerns about milk supply or infant growth.

IF YES, *Call lactation specialist.*

SELF CARE INFORMATION
Practice skin-to-skin contact frequently.
Feed baby at first sign of hunger cues (signs that say "feed me" include hand-to-face or hand-to-mouth movements, lip smacking, seeking with lips, rooting, and head bobbing).
Feed baby at least 10–12 times per 24 hours.
Listen for signs of baby swallowing.
Allow baby to end feedings.
Expect at least 3–4 infant stools per 24 hours after the first 4 days of life.

Good positioning and attachment are crucial.

If baby is fed away from the breast, hand express or pump milk to maintain supply.

IMPORTANT CONDITIONS TO REPORT

Feeding or stooling expectations are not met.

> **Notes**
>
> Growth of baby should be closely followed by medical care provider.
>
> One sign of possible insufficient glandular tissue is marked asymmetry of the breasts. This may indicate problems with glandular tissue in both breasts. If the mother reports that she had an implant in one breast only, inquire about the reason for this surgery. If the surgery was to correct breast asymmetry, there may be increased concern regarding the mother's ability to make a full milk supply. Marked asymmetry may indicate insufficient glandular tissue in both breasts. Milk transfer and infant growth should be monitored closely.

See also Asymmetric breasts; Insufficient milk supply

▶ Breast lumps

DEFINITION Hard, knotty areas inside the breast. In the lactating breast, these are commonly due to overfull milk ducts and alveoli or exterior pressure on the milk-making cells due to restrictive clothing, bras, etc. These are called "**plugged ducts**." Lumps may also be fibroadenomas, fibrocystic changes, **abscess**, and, rarely, cancerous tumors.

Ask about

Onset.

Location of lumps.

Whether unilateral or bilateral.

PROMPT CARE NEEDED?

Are any of the following present?

Presence of lump that does not respond to changes in feeding position and frequency.

Symptoms of inflammation or infection (fever, redness, malaise, chills, achiness) in the mother.

Concerns about breastfeeding.

IF YES, *Seek medical care within 2 to 4 hours and call lactation care provider today.*

SELF CARE INFORMATION

Check for and remove any restrictive clothing.

Practice good attachment:

Watch baby for hunger cues, and offer the breast as soon as they are seen.

Place baby so that nose is opposite nipple.

Wait for baby to open mouth wide (greater than a 100° angle).

Pull baby in so that chin touches the breast first, and nipple enters the mouth along the top of the tongue; this should result in a wide open mouth full of breast tissue.

Lips should be flanged outward.

Baby's lips should look off center when compared with the areola; the bottom lip should be farther away from the nipple than the top lip.

Try nursing baby in positions where baby's chin points toward lumpy area.

Massage the affected areas gently during nursing.

Consider warm soaks before feedings and cool gel packs on affected areas between feedings.

Monitor body temperature.

Watch for signs of infection.

IMPORTANT CONDITIONS TO REPORT

Worsening of symptoms.

Persistence of symptoms—call if lumps do not resolve in 24–48 hours.

Symptoms of infection.

See also Breast abscess; Breast infection; Breast inflammation; Mastitis

▶ Breast massage

DEFINITION Gentle stroking technique used to encourage milk to flow from the breast.

See also Alternate breast massage

▶ Breastmilk, abnormal secretion

DEFINITION Production of milk from the breast that is outside normal expectations. This condition, also called **galactorrhea,** can include production of milk by women who are neither pregnant nor lactating, as well as both excessive and inadequate amounts of milk produced during lactation.

Ask about

Onset.

PROMPT MEDICAL CARE NEEDED?

Are any of the following present?

Less than 1 stool per 24 hours in a breastfed newborn.

Refusal to feed for longer than six hours in a newborn infant.

IF YES, *Seek medical care within 2 to 4 hours.*

Are any of the following present?

Production of milk in a nonlactating, nonpregnant woman.

IF YES, *Call primary care provider today.*

PROMPT LACTATION CARE NEEDED?

Are any of the following present?

Concern about inadequate milk supply.

Concern about overabundant milk supply.

Fewer than three stools daily in a breastfed newborn.

Less than 0.5 oz gain daily by breastfed newborn.

Excessively large or frequent stools in a breastfed baby.

Recurrent engorgement or mastitis.

Colic symptoms in the baby.

IF YES, *Call pediatric and lactation care providers today.*

SELF CARE INFORMATION

Frequency of feeding and amount of milk removal drives milk supply.

IMPORTANT CONDITIONS TO REPORT

Worsening of symptoms.

Continuation of symptoms.

Ongoing concerns.

Notes

Because production of milk relies on many different body systems in both mother and baby, any milk supply problem requires consideration of maternal and infant factors. Occasionally medical factors such as endocrine imbalance may require evaluation.

It is common for mothers to continue to produce milk for prolonged periods after weaning.

See also Galactorrhea; Insufficient milk supply; Milk production; Overactive let-down reflex

▶ Breastmilk, environmental contaminants

DEFINITION All foods, including breastmilk, may contain traces of chemical contaminants present in the environment. Breastmilk is one of the easiest and least painful body tissues to sample. For this reason, it is used to monitor population exposure to chemicals. According to the American Academy of Pediatrics, low level exposure to contaminants should not contraindicate breastfeeding.

Ask about

Known contaminant exposure.
Age of baby.

ASSESSMENT

EMERGENT CARE NEEDED?
Sudden exposure of mother to toxic chemical.

IF YES, *Seek emergency care now.*

PROMPT CARE NEEDED?
History of past high level exposure to toxic chemicals in a breastfeeding woman.

IF YES, *Seek medical care today.*

ROUTINE CARE NEEDED?
General questions about environmental exposure.

IF YES, *Call lactation care provider today.*

IMPORTANT CONDITIONS TO REPORT

Known history of environmental or workplace exposure to toxic chemicals. Any negative effects of past exposure.

> **Notes**
>
> Women who know they have been exposed to specific chemicals or pollutants should consult with their physician regarding analysis of the contaminant content of their milk. Several contaminants are addressed in the American Academy of Pediatrics's drug reference.[55]
>
> Researchers have looked for negative effects of toxin exposure via breastmilk, and found only benefits for breastfed babies, as compared with formula fed babies.

See also DDT in breastmilk; Pesticides and pollutants in breastmilk

Footnotes

[55]American Academy of Pediatrics Committee on Drugs. (2001). Transfer of drugs and other chemicals into human milk. *Pediatrics, 108,* 776–789.

▶ Breastmilk for preterm infants

DEFINITION A preterm infant is any infant born before 37 weeks gestation. Multiple pregnancy (e.g., twins) accounts for 15% of all premature births.

SELF CARE INFORMATION

Express milk with a double-pumping kit and hospital grade pump eight or more times daily while your baby is hospitalized.

Ask the baby's nurse for instructions for the collection and storage of milk.

Ask how soon you can hold your baby skin-to-skin.

Premature babies can learn to breastfeed. Seek skilled lactation help.

The preterm infant may require specialized care in a nursery until closer to baby's due date when his or her organ systems have developed enough to sustain life without specialized support. Depending on the extent of prematurity, this may take weeks or months.

Mothers of premature infants should begin expressing milk as soon as possible and do so regularly in order to increase the supply for the growing baby.

For about the first 30 days after she gives birth, the mother of the premature baby will produce milk that is higher in some of the components the baby needs.

See also Preterm milk

Breastmilk secretion

DEFINITION The production of a complete food for human infants within the mammary gland.

Notes

The hormonal changes of pregnancy and birth trigger milk production in the breast. The first milk, called **colostrum**, begins in mid-pregnancy. Some mothers see dried yellowish secretions on their nipples in this phase.

Following birth of the baby and complete birth of the placenta, the breasts begin to produce mature milk. Increase in breast fullness, prominence of veins, and slight fever around days two to five postpartum indicate the production of mature milk.

To facilitate milk making, babies should be breastfed in response to hunger cues, at least 10–12 times per 24 hours. Frequent nipple stimulation and milk removal stimulate the hormones **prolactin** and **oxytocin** that control the manufacture and release of milk.

There is no known limit to the amount of milk that a woman can make. Case studies of mothers producing enough milk for quadruplets have been published. This is possible due to the supply and demand nature of milk production.

Some nursing mothers produce too little or too much milk. Refer to a lactation care provider for evaluation of milk supply questions. Occasionally medical factors such as endocrine imbalance may require evaluation.

Secretion of milk may happen outside of pregnancy and lactation in response to hormonal changes, pituitary conditions, and drug side effects. This condition, called **galactorrhea**, requires medical evaluation.

See also Feeding cues; Galactorrhea; Insufficient milk supply

▶ Breast pads

DEFINITION Cloth or paper placed inside the bra to absorb leaked milk. Pads may be reusable or disposable.

SELF CARE INFORMATION

Choose soft, absorbent pads.

Replace damp pads with fresh ones frequently to avoid irritation and softening of breast tissue.

Avoid waterproof or plastic-lined pads, which can cause irritation.

Pads may be easily made by cutting appropriately sized circles out of new cloth diapers (edge stitching is recommended to hold the pad together in the wash).

> **Notes**
>
> Many baby supply, breast pump, and nursing bra companies carry pads designed for breastfeeding mothers. Caution mothers to change pads frequently and to avoid waterproof pads.

▶ Breast pain

DEFINITION Uncomfortable sensations in the breast. Pain is not an expected part of breastfeeding and indicates need for feeding evaluation.

There can be many reasons for pain in the breast including breast infection or inflammation, clogs, or cysts. Poor latch-on or positioning is a common reason for pain.

Ask about

Onset.

Location of pain.

Whether unilateral or bilateral.

PROMPT MEDICAL CARE NEEDED?

Are any of the following present?

Constant pain.

Pain combined with color change of nipple(s).

Pain with visible fissure or bleeding of the nipple.

IF YES, *Seek medical care within 2 to 4 hours.*

PROMPT LACTATION CARE NEEDED?

Are any of the following present?

Pain with feeding.

Pain between feedings.

IF YES, *Seek lactation care within 2 to 4 hours.*

ROUTINE CARE NEEDED?

Are any of the following present?

Brief pain at beginning of feeding.

Mild recurrent pain.

IF YES, *Call lactation care provider today.*

SELF CARE INFORMATION

Practice skin-to-skin contact frequently.

Feed baby at first sign of hunger cues (signs that say "feed me" include hand-to-face or hand-to-mouth movements, lip smacking, seeking with lips, rooting, and head bobbing).

Feed baby at least 10–12 times per 24 hours.

Listen for signs of baby swallowing.

Allow baby to end feedings.

Expect at least 3–4 infant stools per 24 hours after the first 4 days of life until 1 month of age.

Good positioning and attachment are crucial to reduce nipple pain.

IMPORTANT CONDITIONS TO REPORT

Symptoms worsen or persist.

Signs of infection.

Feeding or stooling expectations are not met.

> **Notes**
>
> Breastfeeding should not be painful. Advise mothers to seek medical or lactation care for breast pain.

See also Latch-on; Nipple pain

▶ Breast, preparation for breastfeeding during pregnancy

DEFINITION The best preparation for breastfeeding is reading and learning about breastfeeding, and connecting with community breastfeeding groups and resources.

> **Notes**
>
> No physical preparation is suggested for breastfeeding. Outdated practices such as "toughening up" nipples by brushing, toweling, or pulling are no longer recommended, and may actually cause damage to the skin or trigger uterine contractions.

▶ Breast pump

DEFINITION A device designed to remove milk from the lactating breast.

SELF CARE INFORMATION

A breast pump cannot tell you how much milk you are making.

If you have concerns about milk supply, please call or see a lactation specialist.

Problems with pumps should be reported to the manufacturer and the U.S. Food and Drug Administration (FDA). The FDA's Manufacturer and User Facility

Device Experience Database (MAUDE) contains prior complaints filed about pumps. Visit www.fda.gov/cdrh/maude.html for more information.

See also **Automatic electric breast pumps; Battery operated breast pump; Hand expression of breastmilk; Manual pump**

▶ Breast, rash and skin lesions

DEFINITION Red bumps or infected patches of skin on the breast or nipple can reflect infectious or allergic conditions. Because of the serious nature of some infectious conditions, including *Herpes*, women reporting rashes or lesions on the breast should be seen immediately by medical personnel.

Ask about

Onset.

Age of baby.

Known history of herpes lesions or other skin conditions.

EMERGENT CARE NEEDED?

Are any of the following present?

History of herpes lesions on the nipple or breast.

Rash or lesions plus fever, aching, chills, malaise in mother or baby.

Rash or lesion on the breast with a history of herpes elsewhere on mother or partner's body.

IF YES, *Seek emergency care now.*

PROMPT CARE NEEDED?

Are any of the following present?

Pain during breastfeeding.

Trauma to nipple or breast from feeding.

IF YES, *Call lactation care provider now.*

SELF CARE INFORMATION

Practice good attachment:

Watch for feeding cues and offer the breast as soon as they are seen.

Wait for baby to open mouth wide (greater than a 100° angle).

Pull baby in so that chin touches the breast first, and nipple enters the mouth along the top of the tongue; this should result in a wide open mouth full of breast tissue.

Lips should be flanged outward.

Baby's lips should look off center when compared with the areola; the bottom lip should be farther away from the nipple than the top lip.

IMPORTANT CONDITIONS TO REPORT

History of other skin conditions.

Known skin reactions.

Rash or lesions may appear on the nipple and breast for several reasons, including eczema, psoriasis, topical allergy or sensitivity, poison ivy, chicken pox, poor latch, trauma, damage from nipple shields, **abscess**, or **blebs**.

Emergency differential diagnosis is crucial in women with history of herpes lesions on the nipple. As herpes can be fatal to the newborn, breastfeeding should be discontinued on the affected nipple until differential diagnosis is obtained. *Active herpes or chicken pox lesions on the nipple and breast are potentially life threatening for the baby.* Herpes lesions elsewhere on the body do not contraindicate breastfeeding. However, parents should practice very careful handwashing techniques to avoid touching lesions and then touching the baby.

See also Bleb; Blisters on nipple or breast; Contraindicated conditions; Nipple pain

► Breast reduction

DEFINITION A procedure that decreases the size of the breast by removing fat and glandular tissue from the breast. Reduction surgery is likely to alter a woman's ability to make milk.

Ask about

Onset.
Type of procedure.

ASSESSMENT

PROMPT MEDICAL CARE NEEDED?

Are any of the following present?

Inadequate stooling pattern (less than three stools daily) in newborn period after fourth day.

Inadequate weight gain (less than 0.5 oz daily) in the early months.

Inadequate feeding (less than ten times daily in the newborn period).

IF YES, *Call pediatric care provider now.*

SELF CARE INFORMATION

Monitor baby's feeding, stooling, and urination daily.

Practice skin-to-skin contact frequently.

Feed baby at first sign of hunger cues (signs that say "feed me" include hand-to-face or hand-to-mouth movements, lip smacking, seeking with lips, rooting, and head bobbing).

Feed baby at least 10–12 times per 24 hours.

Listen for signs of baby swallowing.

Allow baby to end feedings.

Expect at least 3–4 infant stools per 24 hours after the first 4 days of life.

Good positioning and attachment are crucial to reduce nipple pain.

If baby is fed away from the breast, hand express or pump milk to maintain supply.

IMPORTANT CONDITIONS TO REPORT

Inadequate feeding (less than 10 feedings daily in the newborn).

Inadequate stooling pattern (less than three stools daily after fourth day).

Ongoing concerns.

Notes

It is not possible to predict the degree of lactation success prenatally. Women who are interested in breastfeeding should be considered to do so with ongoing, proactive monitoring of milk transfer and baby's growth.

Surgical techniques that include complete removal of the nipple are more likely to impact innervation of the nipple (and thus the production of appropriate hormones through neuroendocrine pathways). Post-surgical nipple sensation may indicate the extent to which innervation has been altered.

Pedicle techniques which preserve nipple attachment may have a lesser impact on potential for milk production.

See also **Breast surgery; Insufficient milk supply**

▶ Breast refusal

DEFINITION Sudden rejection of the breast by the baby.

Ask about

Onset.
Age of baby.

ASSESSMENT

EMERGENT CARE NEEDED?
Are any of the following present?
   Extreme **lethargy or irritability** in baby.
   Sudden change in baby's muscle tone (extremely floppy or stiff).
   Sudden disinterest in feeding.
   Unable to wake baby.
   Doesn't calm, even with cuddles.

IF YES,   *Seek emergency care now.*

PROMPT CARE NEEDED?
Are any of the following present?
   Refusal to feed.
   Repeated refusal of one breast.

IF YES,   *Call lactation care provider today.*

SELF CARE INFORMATION
   Express milk from the refused breast(s) as many times daily as baby would
      generally nurse.
   Practice skin-to-skin contact with baby, particularly at sleepy times.
   Do not force baby to the breast.
   Make sure baby is adequately fed (give expressed milk via cup, spoon, or dropper).

Persistent or recurrent refusal.

Presence of ear infection or teething.

Notes

Rarely, babies experience life threatening infections or events that cause extreme lethargy and disinterest in feeding. They may be suddenly floppy or stiff. These symptoms indicate a medical emergency.

Occasionally, babies suddenly refuse to nurse from one or both breasts. This is often considered a **nursing strike**, rather than weaning. Typically it is an indication that something is troubling the baby. Troubles can range from stuffy nose, teething, and ear infection to a negative reaction to mother–baby separation or family stress. Strategies for overcoming nursing strike include not forcing nursing, offering lots of cuddling and holding, having mom lie down beside a sleepy baby and offering the breast, having mom and baby take a bath together, and applying "peer pressure" by bringing an older baby in contact with other nursing babies. When nursing strike persists, the baby should be examined to rule out ear infection or other contributing factors.

Mother may need assistance with expressing milk to continue her milk supply during this phase. She may be helped by exploring her reaction to the baby's refusal to nurse.

A mother whose baby refuses the same breast consistently and without explanation should be referred for breast evaluation, and should be routinely monitored for breast cancer. Cancer has been diagnosed as late as five years after persistent breast refusal. This phenomenon is referred to as **Goldsmith's sign**.[56]

See also Goldsmith's sign; Nursing strike; Refusal of infant to breastfeed

Footnotes

[56]Saber, A., Dardik, H., Ibrahim, I.M., & Wolodiger, F. (1996). The milk rejection sign: a natural tumor marker. *The American Surgeon, 62,* 998–999.

▶ Breast shells

DEFINITION Hard plastic devices designed to be worn between the breast and the bra in order to surround the nipples with air and to hold clothing away from the breast.

Mothers who request breast shells may be experiencing nipple or breast pain and should be referred to the lactation care provider for evaluation.

Breast shells have been recommended for women with inverted nipples. However, research does not support claims that these devices alter nipple inversion.

Repeated use of breast shells has been associated with increased risk of mastitits, perhaps due to the pressure placed on the breast.

See also Breast pain; Inverted nipples; Nipple pain

▶ Breast stimulation

DEFINITION Massage and stroking of the breast to trigger the flow of milk by increasing the hormones of lactation.

Nursing babies are the best breast stimulators.

When mothers are separated from their babies, gentle manual stimulation of the breast and nipple may assist with milk collection.[57]

See also Alternate breast massage; Hand expression of breastmilk; Milk production

Footnotes

[57]Jones, E., Dimmock, P.W., & Spencer, S.A. (2001). A randomised controlled trial to compare methods of milk expression after preterm delivery. *Archives of Disease in Childhood, Fetal & Neonatal Edition, 85*(2), F91–F95.

▶ Breast storage capacity

DEFINITION Referring to the potential milk holding space within the breast.

> **Notes**
>
> Research has identified a wide range of internal storage capacity among women.[58] Storage capacity may be the controlling factor in frequency of feeding, as mothers with larger capacity may be able to go longer between feedings.
>
> Women with small breasts may be told that they will have trouble making enough milk. Research does not support this belief. Fat deposits are the major contributor to breast size.
>
> Mothers should be encouraged to follow baby's **feeding cues** to determine feeding frequency, rather than any external schedule. Signs that say "feed me" include hand-to-face or hand-to-mouth movements, lip smacking, seeking with lips, rooting, and head bobbing. Crying is a late indicator of hunger and should not be used to determine feeding needs.

See also Feeding cues; Milk production

Footnotes

[58]Cregan, M.D., & Hartmann, P.E. (1999). Computerized breast measurement from conception to weaning: clinical implications. *Journal of Human Lactation, 15*(2), 89–96.

▶ Breast structure

DEFINITION Refers to the tissues within the breast that contribute to the production of milk.

> **Notes**
>
> Internal breast structure involved in making milk includes millions of clusters of **alveoli** or milk-making cells connected via ductules and **ducts** that carry milk to pores in the nipples. The average breast is thought to have 9 ducts connecting to separate **lobes** of milk making tissue, articulated with 9 pores in the surface of the nipple.[59]

External breast structure includes the breast, nipple, areola (circle of dark pigment surrounding the nipple), and **Montgomery's glands** (sebaceous and alveolar tissue providing lubrication and protection to the nipple–areolar complex).

The breast is supported by **Cooper's ligaments.**

Milk is manufactured with nutrients carried to the breast through the arteries, arterioles, and capillaries of the intercostal (rib cage area) and thoracic arteries. Extensive lymphatic drainage of the breast helps maintain the health of mammary tissue. Sensation of the nipples and breasts is provided through extensive branching of the fourth, fifth, and sixth intercostal nerves.

Breast tissue tends to extend into the axillary (armpit) area.

Normal variations in breast structure include size and number of the breasts, nipples, areola, and Montgomery's glands. Women may have extra "accessory" breast or nipple tissue anywhere on the ventral surface of their trunk, as well as in the axillary, groin, and upper thigh area.

Women with small breasts may be told that they will have trouble making enough milk. Research does not support this at all. Fat deposits are the major contributor to breast size.

See also Milk production

Footnotes

[59]Ramsay, D.T., Kent, J.C., Hartmann, R.A., & Hartmann, P.E. (2005). Anatomy of the lactating human breast redefined with ultrasound imaging. *Journal of Anatomy, 206*(6), 525–534.

▶ Breast surgery

DEFINITION Surgical procedures of many types, including breast **biopsy**, **abscess** drainage, **augmentation** or **reduction**, may impact breastfeeding.

Notes

Medical and lactation evaluation are indicated for breastfeeding women who have had breast surgery.

See also Augmentation surgery; Biopsy, breast; Breast augmentation; Breast reduction

▶ Breathing, sucking, swallowing

DEFINITION These three reflexes must be coordinated in order for feeding to be successful.

Ask about

Gestational age of baby at birth.

ASSESSMENT

EMERGENT CARE NEEDED?
Are any of the following present?
Sputtering, choking, or gagging at the breast in the newborn.

IF YES, *Seek medical care within 2 to 4 hours.*

Notes

Newborn babies who are unable to coordinate breathing, sucking, and swallowing should be referred for immediate medical evaluation. If untreated, babies may be at risk for aspiration.

Coordination of the suck, swallow, and breathe reflexes is thought to occur around 32 weeks gestation, although it has been observed as early as 28 weeks in some babies.

In the older baby, problems with these reflexes may reflect nasal congestion, gastroesophageal reflux, overabundant milk supply, or overactive milk ejection. Routine medical and lactation evaluation is indicated.

See also Weak suck; Uncoordinated suckling

▶ Bromocriptine (Parlodel®)

DEFINITION A medication once used to dry up the milk of women who did not wish to breastfeed. Several deaths were attributed to bromocriptine use. This drug is no longer approved for this use.

> **Notes**
>
> The American Academy of Pediatrics lists bromocriptine in the Table 5 (drugs associated with significant side effects and should be given with caution).[60] Hale lists bromocriptine as a category L5 (contraindicated) drug.[61]

See also Weaning

Footnotes

[60]American Academy of Pediatrics Committee on Drugs. (2001). Transfer of drugs and other chemicals into human milk. *Pediatrics, 108,* 776–789.

[61]Hale, T.W. (2004). *Medications and mothers milk* (pp. 98–99). Amarillo, TX: Pharmasoft Publishing.

▶ Bronchus-associated lymphoid tissue (BALT)

DEFINITION Immunologically active tissue found within the lungs.

> **Notes**
>
> The breast is thought to act as an extension of bronchus-associated lymphoid tissue (BALT). When a pathogen is breathed into the lung, BALT tissue responds by triggering the production of an immunoglobulin to attach the pathogen. The breast may also respond to the BALT trigger by manufacturing and releasing appropriate immunoglobulins to fight the organism through the milk.

See also **Bioactive components of breastmilk**

▶ Burping

DEFINITION Referring to the practice of placing baby upright after feeding (or between sides when breastfeeding) and patting baby's back gently to encourage the release of air from the stomach.

> **Notes**
>
> Babies who take in a lot of air with their milk may need help with burping after feeding. Babies who feed calmly at the breast, without periods of crying or gasping, may not need to be burped. Mothers who work diligently at burping with no success may feel frustrated. In this event, they should be relieved of burping duty.
>
> Babies who spit up routinely should be gently burped or held in an upright position after feeding to assist them in removing gas from their stomachs with minimal milk loss.

▶ Cabbage

DEFINITION A vegetable of the Cruciferae (mustard) plant family, cabbage is known for causing intestinal gas due to the abundance of indigestible carbohydrates (fiber) it contains.[62]

> **Notes**
>
> There is little evidence that any vegetables that mothers consume negatively affect their babies. Gas and flatulence are normal occurrence in the newborn, as in all humans.
>
> Adults associate eating cabbage and other cruciferous vegetables with gas, due to difficulty digesting complex sugars in these foods. These sugars do not pass into the nursing baby's gastrointestinal tract in the same form (at least until the baby eats solid foods), so there is unlikely to be any effect for baby.
>
> Many mothers will put themselves on increasingly restrictive diets, without seeking help for their baby's symptoms.
>
> Clinicians should carefully evaluate a mother's concerns and her baby's symptoms to distinguish normal gas from colic or other digestive difficulty.

See also Maternal diet

▶ Cabbage leaves for engorgement

DEFINITION The use of cabbage leaves in the bra has been suggested as a treatment for breast engorgement. Research has not identified any difference between cabbage leaves and cool gel packs in reducing engorgement.[62]

> **Notes**
>
> Cabbage has been acknowledged as a carrier of *Listeria monocytogenes,* which can cause a serious infection, *Listeriosis.* Therefore, in the event that cool applications are needed, cool gel packs are recommended rather than cabbage.

See also Engorgement

Footnotes

[62]Snowden, H.M., Renfrew, M.J., & Woolridge, M.W. (2005). Treatments for breast engorgement during lactation. *Cochrane Database of Systematic Reviews, 2.*

▶ Caffeine

DEFINITION A chemical alkaloid with central nervous system stimulant properties. Caffeine is found in coffee beans, tea leaves, and cacao, among other plants. Breastfeeding mothers should moderate their caffeine usage. Caffeine use can result in physical dependence.

> **Notes**
>
> Caffeine is considered "usually compatible with breastfeeding" by the American Academy of Pediatrics, who note further that no effect has been seen in babies of mothers who have moderate intake of caffeine (defined as two to three cups daily, presumably of coffee).[63] Hale lists caffeine as a L2 (safer) drug.[64]

> Mothers of premature babies and babies with cardiac problems should limit caffeine intake and should report what they do consume to baby's pediatric care provider. This is due to the routine practice of giving caffeine to premature babies in order to treat apnea.
>
> Asthmatic women who take theophylline may need to be monitored for cumulative effects of this drug in combination with any dietary caffeine.
>
> Rarely, mother's caffeine consumption may cause irritability or sleeplessness in her baby.
>
> Caffeine content of coffee, tea, soda, and chocolate varies widely with brand and brewing method.

See also Medications

Footnotes

[63]American Academy of Pediatrics Committee on Drugs. (2001). Transfer of drugs and other chemicals into human milk. *Pediatrics, 108,* 776–789.

[64]Hale, T.W. (2004). *Medications and mothers milk* (pp. 112–113). Amarillo, TX: Pharmasoft Publishing.

▶ Calcium

DEFINITION An important mineral for bone health, proper functioning of heart, muscles, and nerves, and blood clotting. The recommended dietary allowance for calcium in lactating women older than 19 years of age is 1000 mg per day. Women younger than 18 years require 1300 mg.

Notes

It is not possible to increase the calcium content of a mother's milk by increasing her calcium intake.

Extra calcium during lactation will not prevent bone loss, which is recovered during weaning.[65] However, calcium is an important mineral for women to consume throughout their life in order to preserve bone density and health.

Women who entered pregnancy with **osteoporosis** or other bone density problems, and women who do not consume dairy foods should receive medical evaluation or dietary counseling during this time.

The following table provides the calcium content averages of various foods:

Selected Calcium Rich Foods	Calcium (mg)
Lowfat yogurt, 8 oz	400
Sardines with bones, 3 oz	345
Lowfat milk, 8 oz	300
Cheddar cheese, 1 oz	200
Collards, 1/2 c	180
Tofu (with calcium sulfate), 4 oz	145
Kale, 1/2 c	100
American cheese, 1 oz	100

See also Bone loss; Bone mineral density (BMD); Osteoporosis

Footnotes

[65]Kalkwarf, H.J. (2004). Lactation and maternal bone health. *Advances in Experimental Medicine and Biology*, *554*, 101–114.

▶ Caloric density of breastmilk

DEFINITION The number of calories per unit of measure. Human milk is considered to average around 20 calories per ounce, although there is a range of published values, reflecting the difficulty of finding representative samples of milk. Fat content in milk varies throughout the day and within each feeding, depending on diurnal variation as well as how full the breast is and how well the baby or pump is eliciting the milk rejection reflex, which flushes fat down through the breast.

Notes

Women may question the nutrient, fat, or caloric content of their milk. It is very rare for the nutrient composition of human milk to be inadequate. Routine testing of the fat or other content of milk is not recommended, due to diurnal variation and the difficulty of collecting a representative sample.

Evaluation of baby's growth, stooling pattern, feeding frequency, milk transfer, and mechanics should occur when doubts arise about milk adequacy.

See also Weight gain, baby–high; Weight gain, baby–low

▶ Caloric intake of baby

DEFINITION The amount of energy, as measured by kilocalories, consumed by the infant daily. The Dietary Reference Intakes (DRI) for infants between 0 and 6 months are 570 kcals for males and 520 kcals for females. The DRI for infants between 6 and 12 months are 743 kcals for males and 676 kcals for females.

Notes

When babies are allowed to feed in response to hunger cues, breastmilk typically provides adequate calories for the baby. When feedings are shortened by mother, are infrequent (less than 10 times per 24 hours), or delayed by pacifier use, babies may not have an opportunity to remove an adequate amount of milk from the breast. Ongoing inadequate milk removal will decrease overall milk production.

It is very rare for the caloric composition of human milk to be inadequate. Routine testing of the fat or other content of milk is not recommended, due to diurnal variation and the difficulty of collecting a representative sample.

Evaluation of baby's growth, stooling pattern, feeding frequency, milk transfer and mechanics should occur when doubts arise about milk adequacy.

See also Caloric density of breastmilk; Weight gain, baby–high; Weight gain, baby–low

▶ Caloric intake of mother

DEFINITION The amount of energy, as measured by kilocalories, consumed by the mother daily. The recommended dietary intake for breastfeeding women is 500 additional calories daily during lactation than they consumed to maintain their weight before pregnancy.

Nutrient rich foods such as fresh fruits, vegetables, whole grains, lean protein, and other nutrient-dense foods are the backbone of a healthful diet.

Postpartum weight loss is a goal of most women. Encourage nursing mothers to lose weight gradually while consuming a healthful diet, in order to maintain their energy levels. Moderate dieting has no effect on nutrient composition of milk. Extreme dieting may deplete women's energy stores, but rarely affects milk production. Similarly, research indicates that increasing calories has no effect on milk production.

Research studies have demonstrated no negative effect for infant growth when breastfeeding mothers lost weight gradually (less than 1–2 lb per week on average).

See also **Weight loss, mother**

▶ Cancer of the breast

DEFINITION Malignant growth within the tissues of the breast. Unexplained and unusual lumps in the lactating breast must be examined by medical personnel.

Notes

While masses in the lactating breast are often associated with plugged milk ducts, other types of growths, including cancerous ones, are possible. When lumps in the breast do not resolve within 24–48 hours, a complete breast evaluation should be performed. Women who have previously been diagnosed and treated for breast cancer can breast-feed. Those who have had past breast surgery may experience decreased milk production in the segments of the breast that were surgically involved.

When cancer is identified in the lactating breast, weaning is generally indicated because of the nature of the drugs and other therapies used to treat cancer.

Breastfeeding reduces the risk of developing breast cancer in the mother, and possibly the child.

See also **Abrupt weaning; Biopsy, breast; Breast, lumps; Breast refusal; Breast surgery; Goldsmith's sign**

▶ Candidiasis

DEFINITION Overgrowth of *Candida albicans,* a common fungus. Symptoms of yeast infection of the breast include red, shiny looking skin on the nipple and/or areola, flaky skin, and sharp, itching pain that persists between feedings. Infant symptoms of yeast overgrowth or "thrush" include white patches on the inner buccal surface (cheek) or tongue, and occasionally pain on latch. Infants may also have diaper area yeast overgrowth.

Ask about

Onset.
Medications taken in last month.

ASSESSMENT

PROMPT CARE NEEDED?
Are any of the following present?
Sharp, stabbing, persistent nipple pain (not just during feedings).
Presence of white patches in infant's mouth.

IF YES, *Seek medical care today.*

ROUTINE CARE NEEDED?
Are any of the following present?
Nipple pain only during feeding.

IF YES, *Call lactation care provider today.*

SELF CARE INFORMATION
Finish all medication.
If administering nystatin suspension to the infant, pour a dose into a clean cup or spoon. Half of the dose should be used for each side of the mouth. Suspension may be applied with a cotton swab. A clean swab should be used for each application. Take care not to introduce used swabs into the bottle of suspension.
If baby uses artificial nipples, pacifiers, etc., these should be boiled at least daily and replaced after completion of yeast treatment.

IMPORTANT CONDITIONS TO REPORT

Persistent symptoms.

Recurrent symptoms.

Notes

Candida overgrowth may follow or increase after antibiotic treatment.

Recommended treatment for Candidiasis is topical antifungal (nystatin).

If symptoms are not relieved by topical treatment, feeding evaluation should occur to rule out positioning or attachment problems that may be contributing to pain.

Medical evaluation should rule out other conditions resulting in redness and pain, including **eczema**, reaction to surface allergens, trauma, **Raynaud's phenomenon**, and concomitant bacterial infection.

Subsequent treatment with oral antifungals such as ketaconazole and fluconazole may resolve symptoms.

Lactation evaluation should rule out contributing problems with latch and distortion of nipple in baby's mouth.

See also Nipple pain

► Cardiac problems

DEFINITION   Referring to diseases and disorders of the heart and circulatory system.

Ask about

Onset.

History of heart problems.

ASSESSMENT

EMERGENT CARE NEEDED?

Are any of the following present?

A bluish tinge to the baby's mouth and lips during feeding.

IF YES,   *Seek emergency care now.*

IMPORTANT CONDITIONS TO REPORT

Worsening, persistence, or recurrence of symptoms.

Notes

Women with cardiac problems may breastfeed their babies. Any medications taken should be evaluated for their transfer into milk.

Babies with cardiac problems benefit from receiving their mother's milk. They may have problems sustaining attachment to the breast, and suckling may be weak and ineffective.

However, breastfeeding is less physiologically stressful than bottle feeding. Heart, oxygen saturation, and respiratory rates are more optimal during breastfeeding than while bottle feeding.

Mothers may benefit from pumping or expressing milk after feeding to maintain an adequate milk supply.

Lactation consultation is recommended to evaluate effective positions and techniques.

▶ Caries, nursing bottle

DEFINITION Decay of the teeth caused by the presence of sugary fluids in the mouth during bed and nap time.

Notes

This phenomenon rarely happens with children falling asleep at the breast due to the different fluid dynamics of breastfeeding.

Breastfed children with strong family history of excess caries may be at greater risk for developing caries while nursing.

See also Nursing bottle caries

▶ Casein

DEFINITION The tough, curd-like protein fraction of all mammalian milk. (Whey is the name for the more liquid proteins in milk.)

> **Notes**
>
> The casein–whey ratio of human milk is typically 40–60 as compared with cow's milk at 80–20. This difference is thought to account for some of the difficulty in digesting cow's milk and cow's milk-based formulae as well as for the colic related with cow's milk feeding. (Many cow's milk-based formulae have been chemically altered to reduce the casein/whey ratio.)

See also Colic

▶ CCK
See also Cholecystokinin

▶ Celiac disease and breastfeeding

DEFINITION   Celiac disease is a permanent intolerance of gluten, a protein found in wheat, rye, barley, and possibly oats. This autoimmune disease causes damage to the intestinal wall and interferes with nutrient absorption.
Mothers and babies with this disorder can breastfeed.

> **Notes**
>
> Because celiac disease is a genetic disorder, children of mothers with this disorder are at greater risk. People with celiac disease are at increased risk for developing diabetes and other autoimmune diseases.
> Research has shown that the risk of developing celiac disease is reduced when babies are still breastfeeding at the time of introduction of gluten in the baby's diet.[66] In children who have inherited celiac disease, extended breastfeeding may delay the development of celiac disease and reduce its severity.

See also Autoimmune diseases

Footnotes
[66]Ivarsson, A., Hernell, O., Stenlund, H., & Persson, L.A. (2002). Breast-feeding protects against celiac disease. *American Journal of Clinical Nutrition, 75*, 914–921.

▶ Central nervous system (CNS)

DEFINITION Referring to the brain and spinal cord.

▶ Cereals for baby

DEFINITION Referring to pulverized grain foods prepared for babies. Often these cereals are iron enriched.

> ### Notes
>
> Rice cereal is typically the first cereal to be introduced to infants at or after 6 months of age. Iron-fortified cereals are a good source of additional iron needed by babies at about 6 months.
>
> Recent research suggests that early introduction of cereals (before 4 months of age) may trigger eczema, celiac disease, and type 1 diabetes in genetically susceptible children.
>
> Parents should be encouraged to delay introducing their baby to cereal and other solid foods until 6 months of age.

See also Baby food; Complementary feeding; Mixed feeding; Starting solid foods

▶ Certified lactation counselor/consultant (CLC)

DEFINITION Breastfeeding care provider who has completed a course of study resulting in certification as a lactation counselor or consultant.

See also ALPP; IBCLC; IBLCE; ILCA

▶ Cesarean birth

DEFINITION   Delivery of baby via surgical incision made through the abdomen and uterus.

Ask about

Date of cesarean.
Age of baby.
Feeding status.

ASSESSMENT

EMERGENT CARE NEEDED?

Are any of the following present?

Baby refuses to feed for more than six hours.
Exclusively breastfed baby stools less than once daily in the newborn period.
Extreme **lethargy or irritability** in baby.
Sudden change in baby's muscle tone (extremely floppy or stiff) or repetitive jerking movements (e.g., seizure activity).
Baby shows sudden disinterest in feeding.
Unable to wake baby.
Doesn't calm, even with cuddles.

IF YES,   *Call pediatrician now.*

PROMPT CARE NEEDED?

Are any of the following present?

Difficulty finding comfortable feeding positions after surgery.
Concerns about adequacy of milk supply.
Concerns about adequacy of infant growth.

IF YES,   *Call lactation care provider today.*

SELF CARE INFORMATION

Practice skin-to-skin contact frequently.

Feed baby at first sign of hunger cues (signs that say "feed me" include hand-to-face or hand-to-mouth movements, lip smacking, seeking with lips, rooting, and head bobbing).

Feed baby at least 10–12 times per 24 hours.

Listen for signs of baby swallowing.

Allow baby to end feedings.

Expect at least 3–4 infant stools per 24 hours after the first 4 days of life.

Good positioning and attachment are crucial to reduce nipple pain.

If feedings are missed, hand express or pump milk to maintain supply.

IMPORTANT CONDITIONS TO REPORT

Ongoing difficulty with breastfeeding.

Ongoing concerns about infant growth.

Notes

Mothers and babies who experience Cesarean birth have greater risk of being separated in the hospital, as well as experiencing delayed skin-to-skin contact, delayed breastfeeding initiation, delayed development of mature milk, and early supplementation. Mothers should be monitored to ensure they are healing well after surgery and receiving appropriate pain relief.

A wide range of drugs are used to relieve pain. An up-to-date drug reference should be consulted to determine the safety and possible side effects of individual drugs.

Newborn and premature babies are at greater risk of side effects due to limited ability to clear drugs from their systems.

Face-to-face lactation counseling can assist mothers in finding comfortable breastfeeding positions and learning their babies' feeding cues.

See also Anesthesia; Analgesia; Childbirth

▶ Chemical contaminants in breastmilk

DEFINITION   All foods, including breastmilk, may contain traces of chemical contaminants present in the environment. Breastmilk is one of the easiest and least painful body tissues to sample. For this reason, it is used to monitor population exposure to chemicals. According to the American Academy of Pediatrics, low level exposure to contaminants should not contraindicate breastfeeding.[67]

Ask about

Known contaminant exposure.
Age of baby.

<table>
<tr><td colspan="2" align="center">**ASSESSMENT**</td></tr>
<tr><td colspan="2">**EMERGENT CARE NEEDED?**
Sudden exposure of mother to toxic chemical.</td></tr>
<tr><td>IF YES,</td><td>*Seek emergency care now.*</td></tr>
<tr><td colspan="2">**PROMPT CARE NEEDED?**
History of high level exposure to toxic chemicals in a breastfeeding woman.</td></tr>
<tr><td>IF YES,</td><td>*Seek medical care today.*</td></tr>
<tr><td colspan="2">**ROUTINE CARE NEEDED?**
General questions about environmental exposure.</td></tr>
<tr><td>IF YES,</td><td>*Call lactation care provider today.*</td></tr>
</table>

IMPORTANT CONDITIONS TO REPORT

Known history of environmental or workplace exposure to toxic chemicals.
Any negative effects of past exposure.

Notes

Women who know they have been exposed to specific chemicals or pollutants should consult with their physician regarding need for analysis of the contaminant content of their milk. Several contaminants are addressed in the American Academy of Pediatrics's drug reference.[68]

Many researchers have looked for negative effects of toxin exposure via breastmilk and have found only benefits for breastfed babies, as compared with formula fed babies.

See also DDT in breastmilk; Pesticides and pollutants in breastmilk

Footnotes

[67] AAP Section on Breastfeeding. (2005). Breastfeeding and the use of human milk. *Pediatrics, 115*, 497.

[68] AAP Committee on Drugs. (2001). Transfer of drugs and other chemicals into human milk. *Pediatrics, 108*, 776–789.

▶ ## Chemotherapy

DEFINITION   Drugs and chemical agents used to destroy cancer cells. These drugs are typically contraindicated in breastfeeding as they may be toxic to the infant.

> **Notes**
>
> An up-to-date drug reference should be consulted to determine the safety and possible side effects of individual drugs.
>
> Mothers who must undergo **abrupt weaning** to begin cancer treatment or receive surgery or radiation may benefit from practical and emotional support from lactation and medical specialists.

See also Abrupt weaning; Breast cancer

Drug References

AAP Committee on Drugs. (2001). The transfer of drugs and other chemicals into human milk. *Pediatrics, 108*, 776–789.

Briggs, G.G., Freeman, R.K., & Yaffee, S.J. (Eds.). (2002). *Drugs in pregnancy and lactation* (6th ed.). Philadelphia: Lippincott, Williams and Wilkins.

Hale, T.W. (2004). *Medications and mothers milk*. Amarillo, TX: Pharmasoft Publishing.

Lawrence, R.A., & Lawrence, R.M. (2005). *Breastfeeding: A guide for the medical profession* (6th ed.). St. Louis: Mosby.

▶ Chicken pox, mother-to-child transmission

DEFINITION   Referring to the characteristic lesions resulting from infection with *Varicella zoster*, a virus of the herpes family. This highly infectious virus is passed via droplet and direct contact with lesions. Exposure can be dangerous for the newborn. If mother is judged safe to be with her infant and she has no lesions on the breast area, breastfeeding is considered safe.

Ask about

Onset.
Age of baby.
Infection of any household members.

ASSESSMENT

EMERGENT CARE NEEDED?
Are any of the following present?
Eruption of chicken pox in a newborn infant.
Presence of chicken pox lesions on the breast and nipple area.

IF YES,   *Call pediatrician now.*

Notes

Mothers and other family members who are infected in the early perinatal period may infect their infants by passing droplets and allowing infant contact with lesions. Infection risk may be decreased by administering varicella-zoster immunoglobulin (VZIG) to the infant.

If a breastfeeding mother is separated from her baby, she should be encouraged to express or pump her milk eight or more times daily to maintain her milk supply. If she has no lesions on the breast or nipple area, her milk may be given to the baby. Careful handwashing should be practiced to avoid involving the breast or collected milk.

If only siblings are infected, baby and mother should be isolated and continue breastfeeding.

See Lawrence & Lawrence for an excellent protocol for *Varicella zoster* in the peripartum.[69]

See also Acute infection

Footnotes

[69]Lawrence, R.A., & Lawrence, R.M. (2005). *Breastfeeding: A guide for the medical profession* (6th ed., pp. 653–655). St. Louis: Mosby.

▶ Child

DEFINITION   A young person up to the age of puberty.

▶ Childbirth

DEFINITION   The process of giving birth to a baby.

> **Notes**
>
> Several maternity care practices increase the chances of breastfeeding success:
> Prenatal childbirth and breastfeeding education.
> Nurturing, supportive care during the birth process.
> Use of non-pharmacologic pain relief methods (massage, hydrotherapy, acupressure, hypnotherapy, etc.) during labor.
> Immediate and ongoing skin-to-skin contact with infant after delivery.
> Continuous rooming-in.
> Ongoing education and support while mother and baby learn how to breastfeed, including feeding cues, comfortable positioning and latch, how to express milk, and how to find breastfeeding support after discharge.
> Avoidance of unnecessary supplementation, use of bottles, pacifiers, etc.

See also Analgesia; Anesthesia; Cesarean birth; Doula; Epidural anesthesia

▶ Child spacing

DEFINITION   Intentional or natural delay in period of time between sequential births.

Women who are exclusively breastfeeding a young baby are likely to experience a lack of menses (**amenorrhea**). Women may be amenorrheic for more than one year while breastfeeding.

Birth intervals of two to three years or more are recommended to allow time for mother's body to recover and replenish nutrient stores.

Women who wish to become pregnant again may wish to breastfeed less intensively to trigger resumption of their menses. Nutritionally appropriate foods should be offered to the baby when mother begins to **wean**.

See also Amenorrhea; Birth intervals; (LAM) Lactational Amenorrhea Method; Weaning

▶ Chlamydia

DEFINITION   A sexually transmitted infection caused by *Chlamydia trachomatis*. Symptoms in women may include redness of the vagina, discomfort, and vaginal discharge. Pelvic inflammatory disease may result from infection. Mothers with this condition may breastfeed.

Newborns may contract *Chlamydia trachomatis* through the birth process, resulting in chlamydial conjunctivitis or pneumonia. *Chlamydia trachomatis* has not been known to pass through the milk of an infected mother. Weaning and mother–baby separation are not indicated.

An up-to-date drug reference should be consulted to determine the safety and possible side effects of drugs.

See also Sexually transmitted infections

Drug References

AAP Committee on Drugs. (2001). The transfer of drugs and other chemicals into human milk. *Pediatrics, 108,* 776–789.

Briggs, G.G., Freeman, R.K., & Yaffee, S.J. (Eds.). (2002). *Drugs in pregnancy and lactation* (6th ed.). Philadelphia: Lippincott, Williams and Wilkins.

Hale, T.W. (2004). *Medications and mothers milk.* Amarillo, TX: Pharmasoft Publishing.

Lawrence, R.A., & Lawrence, R.M. (2005). *Breastfeeding: A guide for the medical profession* (6th ed.). St. Louis: Mosby.

Choanal atresia

DEFINITION   A congenital condition marked by blockage or narrowing of the nasal airway. Babies born with this condition may have difficulty breathing and coordinating breastfeeding with breathing.

ASSESSMENT

EMERGENT CARE NEEDED?

Are any of the following present?

Newborn baby unable to breathe while feeding.

Newborn breastfeeding baby breaking suction every few seconds to breathe.

Blue tinged lips and mouth during feeding.

IF YES,   *Seek emergency care now.*

PROMPT CARE NEEDED?

Are any of the following present?

Breastfeeding mother of baby with known or diagnosed choanal atresia.

IF YES,   *Call lactation care provider today.*

IMPORTANT CONDITIONS TO REPORT

Ongoing feeding difficulties.

> **Notes**
>
> Surgery is often performed to open up the nasal airway. Until surgery is performed, babies may have difficulty feeding at the breast. Babies with this condition are at risk for aspiration.
>
> When feeding at the breast is not possible, mothers can be helped to express their milk to be fed to baby. After corrective surgery, babies may be fed at the breast.

See also Breast pump; Hand expression of milk

▶ Chocolate

DEFINITION   Foods made from the cacao seed. Moderate chocolate intake is compatible with breastfeeding. Chocolate contains small amounts of theobromine, a mild stimulant similar to caffeine.

> **Notes**
>
> The American Academy of Pediatrics lists chocolate on Table 7 (Food and Environmental Agents: Effects on Breastfeeding), and warns of increased irritability and bowel movements with consumption of more than one pound of chocolate daily by mother.[70]

See also Maternal diet

Footnotes
[70]AAP Committee on Drugs. (2001). The transfer of drugs and other chemicals into human milk. *Pediatrics, 108,* 782.

Drug References
Briggs, G.G., Freeman, R.K., & Yaffee, S.J. (Eds.). (2002). *Drugs in pregnancy and lactation* (6th ed.). Philadelphia: Lippincott, Williams and Wilkins.

Hale, T.W. (2004). *Medications and mothers milk.* Amarillo, TX: Pharmasoft Publishing.

Lawrence, R.A., & Lawrence, R.M. (2005). *Breastfeeding: A guide for the medical profession* (6th ed.). St. Louis: Mosby.

▶ C-hold

DEFINITION   Referring to a breastfeeding technique where the breast is supported by the mother's hand with the thumb resting above the nipple, and the remainder of the hand is below the nipple, thus making the shape of the letter "C."

Notes

In supporting the breast, it is crucial that the mother's fingers are held beyond the areas of the breast where the baby's lips should seal. The C-hold may be a good way to hold the breast, although breast holding is not required after the early days of breastfeeding.

The mother's hand should not change the natural way the breast falls, but merely support the breast in its natural "angle of the dangle" so that its weight is off the baby's chin and milk can flow directly from the alveoli to the baby.

See also **Cigarette hold, Scissor hold**

▶ Cholecystokinin (CCK)

DEFINITION   A hormone produced in the gut wall in response to the presence of fat and protein rich food passing from the stomach to the small intestine. The presence of CCK causes the gallbladder to contract, sending bile to the duodenum to emulsify and aid in the digestion of fats and fat soluble vitamins. CCK also triggers production of pancreatic enzymes that digest protein.

Notes

The presence of CCK in the gut is thought to give an overall sense of satiety or fullness, along with temporary sedation.

▶ Cholera

DEFINITION   An acute infectious disease caused by *Vibrio cholerae*. Symptoms of cholera are excessive watery diarrhea, vomiting, cramping of the muscles, and mineral imbalance. Breastfeeding greatly reduces the risk of cholera infection. When a mother is infected with cholera, breastfeeding may continue.

▶ Chronic illness

DEFINITION   Diseases or disorders that reoccur or last for a long time. Breastfeeding is known to reduce the severity or risk of developing several chronic illnesses, including eczema, asthma, diabetes, multiple sclerosis, and celiac disease.

> ### Notes
>
> While breastfeeding is universally recommended, parents with a family history of chronic illness should be strongly encouraged to consider breastfeeding to decrease their child's risk.
>
> Exclusive breastfeeding (offering no food or drink other than breastmilk to the young baby) offers the highest level of protection against chronic diseases.

▶ Cigarette hold

DEFINITION   Referring to a breastfeeding technique where the breast and nipple are held between the mother's index and middle fingers, as a smoker might hold a cigarette. This position can be difficult for breastfeeding, as mother's fingers may be in the way of the baby's mouth.

> ### Notes
>
> The mother's fingers may compress the breast tissue, possibly restricting the flow of milk or causing local tissue injury. The **C-hold** may be a better way to hold the breast, although breast holding is generally not required after the early days of breastfeeding.
>
> The mother's hand should not change the natural way the breast falls, but merely support the breast in its natural "angle of the dangle" so that its weight is off the baby's chin and milk can flow directly from the alveoli to the baby.

See also C-hold; Scissor hold

▶ CIMS

See also Coalition for Improving Maternity Services (CIMS)

▶ Circumcision

DEFINITION   The cultural or religious practice of removing the foreskin of the penis.

> **Notes**
>
> After circumcision, breastfeeding babies should be offered skin-to-skin contact and the breast for comfort as well as nourishment. Breastfeeding has been demonstrated to reduce pain.
>   Feeding problems seen following circumcision should be referred for medical evaluation.

▶ Circumoral cyanosis

DEFINITION   A state where the skin and mucous membranes around the mouth turn purplish-blue, reflecting lack of oxygenation in the blood.

Ask about

Onset.
Medical conditions of baby.

EMERGENT CARE NEEDED?

Are any of the following present?

Circumoral cyanosis during feeding or at other times.

Cyanosis of the hands and feet beyond the first few days of life.

Acrocyanosis is common and normal in newborns.

IF YES, *Seek medical care now.*

IMPORTANT CONDITIONS TO REPORT

Medications used.

See also Acrocyanosis; Cyanosis

▶ CLC

See also Certified lactation counselor/consultant

▶ Cleft lip and palate (CL/CP)

DEFINITION Congenital disruption of the formation of structures of the mouth and face, resulting in crevices in oral structures.

Clefts may occur on one (unilateral) or both (bilateral) sides of the mouth.

Cleft lip (CL) can occur with or without clefts of the palate.

Cleft palate (CP) can involve the hard and/or soft palate (the roof of the mouth) and the alveolar (gum) ridge.

Palate clefts can also occur under the skin, with a coverage of intact skin. This is called a submucosal cleft.

The severity of the cleft will control the difficulty of feeding.

Ask about

Type and location of cleft.

EMERGENT CARE NEEDED?

Are any of the following present?

Choking spells or dusky color of skin during feeding sessions.

IF YES, *Seek medical care now.*

PROMPT CARE NEEDED?

Are any of the following present?

Learning to breastfeed a baby with CL/CP.

Problems breastfeeding a baby with CL/CP.

IF YES, *Call lactation care provider today.*

SELF CARE INFORMATION

With unilateral cleft lip, hold baby in an upright or semi-upright position for feeding.

Compress the breast gently into the baby's mouth to assist in milk removal.

Pump or hand express after feedings and store the collected milk to be fed to the baby.

Notes

A dental device called an obturator may make breastfeeding easier for babies with hard palate clefts.

Severe clefts may make it impossible to feed at the breast until repair surgery is completed. However, mothers should be encouraged to express their milk and feed it to their babies with a cleft palate feeder.

Breastmilk offers protection against ear infection, which babies with clefts are more prone to develop.

See also Obturator; Palate

▶ Clenching or clamping onto the nipple/areola

DEFINITION   Painful pressure applied by the baby's mouth on the nipple or areola. Clenching or clamping may indicate pain, excessive rate of flow, or inappropriate latch technique. Clenching and clamping can cause pain and trauma to the nipple.

Ask about

Onset.
Age of baby.
Presence of nipple trauma.

ASSESSMENT

PROMPT CARE NEEDED?

Are any of the following present?

Persistent clenching or clamping.
Nipple pain on feeding.
Excessive stooling (more than six times per day).
Fussy, gassy baby.

IF YES,   *Call lactation care provider today.*

SELF CARE INFORMATION

Practice good attachment:

Watch for feeding cues and offer the breast as soon as it is seen.
Wait for baby to open mouth wide (greater than a 100° angle).
Pull baby in so that chin touches the breast first, and nipple enters the mouth along the top of the tongue; this should result in a wide open mouth on breast.
Lips should be flanged outward.
Baby's lips should look off center when compared with the areola; the bottom lip should be farther away from the nipple than the top lip.

IMPORTANT CONDITIONS TO REPORT

Ongoing pain.

See also Nipple pain

▶ Clicking sounds during breastfeeding

DEFINITION   Noises such as suction breaks or tongue clicks that occur during feeding. Clicking indicates that there is open space inside the baby's mouth. This is most often due to poor positioning and attachment.

Ask about

Onset.
Age of baby.

ASSESSMENT

EMERGENT CARE NEEDED?

Are any of the following present?

Extreme **lethargy or irritability** in baby.

Sudden change in baby's muscle tone (extremely floppy or stiff) or repetitive jerking movements (e.g., seizure activity).

Baby shows sudden disinterest in feeding.

Unable to wake baby.

Doesn't calm, even with cuddles.

IF YES,   *Seek emergency care now.*

PROMPT MEDICAL CARE NEEDED?

Are any of the following present?

Low urinary and/or bowel output.

Nasal regurgitation.

Tight lingual frenulum with feeding difficulty.

Cyanosis and/or choking during feeding.

IF YES, *Seek medical care within 2 to 4 hours.*

PROMPT LACTATION CARE NEEDED?

Are any of the following present?

Tight lingual frenulum in breastfeeding baby (tongue-tied baby).

Nipple or breast pain.

History of recurrent breast infection.

Milk supply problems.

Poor growth of breastfed infant.

Clicking sounds that do not resolve with changes in positioning.

IF YES, *Call lactation care provider today.*

ROUTINE CARE NEEDED?

Are any of the following present?

Ongoing problems with clicking.

IF YES, *Call lactation care provider today.*

SELF CARE INFORMATION

Practice good attachment:

Watch for hunger cues and offer the breast as soon as it is seen.

Place baby so that nose is opposite nipple.

Wait for baby to open mouth wide (greater than a 100° angle).

Pull baby in so that chin touches the breast first, and nipple enters the mouth along the top of the tongue; this should result in a wide open mouth on breast.

Lips should be flanged outward.

Baby's lips should look off center when compared with the areola; the bottom lip should be farther away from the nipple than the top lip.

See also Ankyloglossia; Cleft lip and palate

▶ Closet nursing

DEFINITION   Breastfeeding a baby or child secretly, usually due to fear of disapproval of continued breastfeeding.

SELF CARE INFORMATION

Long term breastfeeding is a great gift to baby's health.

Seek mother-to-mother support via La Leche League or other peer support network.

See also Nursing during pregnancy; Tandem nursing; Weaning

Footnotes

[72]AAP Section on Breastfeeding. (2005). Breastfeeding and the use of human milk. *Pediatrics, 115*, 499.

▶ Clothing, breastfeeding

DEFINITION   Clothing specially designed for the nursing mother, including bras, shirts, and dresses designed to provide easy, comfortable access to the breast while protecting modesty.

Notes

Breastfeeding clothing is available from a number of retail establishments. A quick Internet search on "breastfeeding clothing" will identify multiple options.

See also Bras

▶ Cluster feeding

DEFINITION   The tendency of young babies to have a cycle of short, closely spaced feedings interspersed with periods of rest or sleep. This means babies may nurse four or five times in three hours, rest for three hours, and then nurse again four to five times in three to four hours. This is a typical pattern that is associated with good milk production and growth.

Notes

Although 10–12 feedings are expected in 24 hours, they are rarely evenly spaced throughout 24 hours. Mothers should be encouraged to respond to feeding cues, supporting a clustered feeding pattern. This allows babies to maximize the amount of milk produced.

▶ Clutch hold

DEFINITION   Another name for the "football hold." A breastfeeding position in which the baby is tucked under the mother's arm, with its feet behind her back, and attaches to the breast next to her arm. Mother supports the baby's torso with her forearm, holding the baby's neck in the palm of her hand.

> **Notes**
>
> This is a good position for mothers recovering from Cesarean delivery, those with large breasts, and premature babies.

See also Cradle hold; Football hold

▶ ## CMV

DEFINITION   Cytomegalovirus. A virus of the herpes family that is widespread in the population and can be dormant in the body for years. CMV infection has no obvious symptoms, with rare exception of an illness similar to mononucleosis.

SELF CARE INFORMATION
Practice routine, careful handwashing with soap and water, especially when handling children and diapers.

> **Notes**
>
> There is some risk of negative effects to babies born to women who had their first infection with CMV during pregnancy. According to the Centers for Disease Control and Prevention, "during a pregnancy when a woman *who has never had CMV infection* becomes infected with CMV, there is a potential risk that after birth the infant may have CMV-related complications, the most common of which are associated with hearing loss, visual impairment, or diminished mental and motor capabilities. On the other hand, infants and children *who acquire CMV after birth* have few, if any, symptoms or complications."[73]
>
> It is appropriate for mothers with CMV infection to breastfeed their full term healthy babies.
>
> In the event that a mother with CMV infection has a preterm baby, careful consideration of the benefits of breastfeeding versus the risk of CMV transmission must be made. See the American Academy of Pediatrics's 2005 statement for more guidance.[74]

Footnotes

[73]National Center for Infectious Diseases. (2005). *Cytomegalovirus (CMV) infection.* Retrieved March 14, 2005, from http://www.cdc.gov/ncidod/diseases/cmv.htm.

[74]AAP Section on Breastfeeding. (2005). Breastfeeding and the use of human milk. *Pediatrics, 115,* 497.

▶ CNS

See also Central nervous system (CNS)

▶ Coalition for Improving Maternity Services (CIMS)

DEFINITION   "Established in 1996, the Coalition for Improving Maternity Services (CIMS) is a collaborative effort of numerous individuals and more than 50 organizations representing over 90,000 members. Our mission is to promote a wellness model of maternity care that will improve birth outcomes and substantially reduce costs."[71]

Notes

The Coalition for Improving Maternity Services
P.O. Box 2346
Ponte Vedra Beach, FL 32004
Phone: 888-282-2467
E-mail: info@motherfriendly.org
Web site: www.motherfriendly.org
CIMS administers the Mother-Friendly Childbirth Initiative (MFCI).

Footnotes

[71]The Coalition for Improving Maternity Services. (2005). Welcome to CIMS. Retrieved June 30, 2005 from http://www.motherfriendly.org.

▶ Co-bedding

DEFINITION The practice of a parent or parents sleeping in the same bed with their baby.

SELF CARE INFORMATION

Babies should not share a bed with a smoker, someone under the influence of alcohol or medications that could make them difficult to rouse, or someone who is extremely fatigued.

Babies should never sleep alone or with another person on a waterbed, sofa, reclining chair, saggy mattress, or bean bag.

Parents who share an adult bed with their baby should ensure that there are no gaps between the mattress and the frame or between the mattress and the wall in which the baby could become stuck. There should be no pillows, fluffy comforters (duvets), stuffed animals, or other suffocation/choking hazards on the baby's sleeping surface (whether in own bed or an adult bed).

No other child should share a bed with the co-bedding infant.

> **Notes**
>
> According to the American Academy of Pediatrics, "Mother and infant should sleep in proximity to each other to facilitate breastfeeding."[75]

See also Co-sleeping; SIDS (suddent infant death syndrome)

Footnotes

[75]AAP Section on Breastfeeding. (2005). Breastfeeding and the use of human milk. *Pediatrics, 115*, 500.

▶ Cocaine

DEFINITION A drug produced from coca leaves that creates a feeling of euphoria. Cocaine is an addictive illicit drug.

Footnotes

[76]AAP Committee on Drugs. (2001). The transfer of drugs and other chemicals into human milk. *Pediatrics, 108,* 778.

[77]Hale, T.W. (2004). *Medications and mothers milk.* Amarillo, TX: Pharmasoft Publishing, 198–199.

▶ Coffee

DEFINITION   A beverage made from coffee beans that contains several aromatic and active chemicals, including caffeine, a CNS stimulant. Breastfeeding mothers should moderate their caffeine usage. Caffeine use is addictive.

Notes

Caffeine is considered "usually compatible with breastfeeding" by the American Academy of Pediatrics.[78] The authors note further that no effect has been seen in babies of mothers who have moderate intake of caffeine (defined as two to three cups daily, presumably of coffee). Hale lists caffeine as a L2 (safer) drug.[79]

Mothers of premature babies and babies with cardiac problems should limit caffeine intake and report what they do consume to baby's pediatric care provider. This is due to the routine practice of giving caffeine to premature babies to treat apnea.

Asthmatic women who take theophylline may need to be monitored for cumulative effects of this drug in combination with any dietary caffeine.

Rarely, mother's caffeine consumption may cause irritability or sleeplessness in her baby.

Caffeine content of coffee varies with brand and brewing method.

See also Caffeine

Footnotes

[78]AAP Committee on Drugs. (2001). The transfer of drugs and other chemicals into human milk. *Pediatrics, 108*, 780.

[79]Hale, T.W. (2004). *Medications and mothers milk.* Amarillo, TX: Pharmasoft Publishing, 112–113.

Drug References

Briggs, G.G., Freeman, R.K., & Yaffee, S.J. (Eds.). (2002). *Drugs in pregnancy and lactation* (6th ed.). Philadelphia: Lippincott, Williams and Wilkins.

Lawrence, R.A., & Lawrence, R.M. (2005). *Breastfeeding: A guide for the medical profession* (6th ed.). St. Louis: Mosby.

▶ Colds

DEFINITION   An acute viral infection characterized by inflammation of the upper respiratory tract, runny nose, and cough. Mothers and babies with colds should continue breastfeeding.

Notes

Over-the-counter medications used to treat colds should be reviewed in a drug reference. In general, long acting or extra strength preparations should be avoided due to their long half-life in the body.

Some antihistamine and decongestant drugs are noted to result in a dramatic decrease in milk supply during the time they are in circulation. Care should be taken to avoid these medications during lactation, particularly pseudoephedrine.

If breastfeeding mother and baby are receiving cold medication, care should be taken to avoid overdosing the baby.

See also Acute infection, Over-the-counter drugs

▶ Colic, infantile

DEFINITION   A condition of infancy described by the classic "rule of three": bouts of high pitched crying lasting more than three hours per day, for more than three days per week, and for more than three weeks in a well-nourished, otherwise healthy baby.[80] Colic typically starts after 2 weeks of age and resolves by 4 months.

Ask about

Age of baby.
Diet of baby.
Weight gain of baby.

ASSESSMENT

EMERGENT CARE NEEDED?

Are any of the following present?

Difficulty breathing.

IF YES, *Seek emergency care now.*

Are any of the following present?

Hives.

Vomiting.

Diarrhea.

Blood in the stools.

Irritability and excessive crying.

IF YES, *Seek medical care now.*

ROUTINE CARE NEEDED?

Are any of the following present?

Education needed about mixed feeding.

IF YES, *Call lactation care provider today.*

IMPORTANT CONDITIONS TO REPORT

Signs of dehydration (scanty, dark urine).
Difficulty breathing.
Eczema.
Hives.
Vomiting.

Diarrhea.

Blood in the stools.

Irritability and excessive crying.

SELF CARE INFORMATION

Solid foods do not help babies sleep through the night.

Try comfort techniques such as rocking, singing, skin-to-skin contact, bathing, seeking a quiet, calm environment, and going out for a walk.

> **Notes**
>
> Medical evaluation should rule out organic problems such as rectal fissure, otitis media, and fractures.
>
> This problem occurs evenly among exclusively breastfed, mixed fed, and formula fed infants, and is thus thought to have largely developmental causes.
>
> In breastfed babies, a trial of removing dairy foods from mother's diet may be conducted for 10–14 days to determine if symptoms improve. If not, mothers should resume their normal diet.

See also Allergy in the breastfed infant

Footnotes

[80]Wessel, M.A., Cobb, J.C., Jackson, E.B., Harris, G.S. Jr., & Detwiler, A.C. (1954). Paroxysmal fussing in infancy, sometimes called colic. *Pediatrics, 14,* 421–435.

▶ Collection and storage of breastmilk

DEFINITION   Procedure by which milk is safely expressed and stored.

> **Notes**
>
> Milk collection may be done by hand or pump expression.
>
> Begin all milk collection by washing hands, pump, and collection device carefully.
>
> Massage breasts and stimulate nipples prior to expressing.
>
> Label containers with date of expression and name of infant (if it will be used in a multi-child setting).

Glass and hard plastic containers with tight lids are recommended. All containers should be food-grade. Plastic bags designed for milk storage may be used, but it may be difficult to prevent spillage and puncture of these bags.

For the full-term, healthy baby, milk can be safely stored:[81]
    Up to four hours at room temperature (less than 75° F), but should be refrigerated immediately if possible (with frozen gel pack in an insulated lunch bag or cooler if refrigerator is not available).
    72 hours in the refrigerator.
    Up to three months in the freezer section of a refrigerator/freezer.
    Up to six months in a deep freezer.
    Milk that will not be used fresh within 72 hours should be frozen as soon as possible.

Thaw milk in its container.
Milk can be safely thawed by:
    Placing frozen containers in the refrigerator overnight.
    Holding frozen containers under lukewarm running tap water.
    Placing frozen containers in lukewarm water.

Hot water is not recommended due to potential nutrient loss.
Milk should never be boiled or microwaved.
Milk does not need to be overly warm before fed to infant.
For the preterm or ill infant, request individual milk storage and handling guidelines from the hospital newborn intensive care unit.

See also Containers for milk storage; Storing expressed milk; Thawing expressed milk

Footnotes

[81]Arnold, L.D.W. (2004). *Safe storage of expressed breastmilk for the healthy infant and child.* East Sandwich, MA: Health Education Associates.

▶ Colostrum

DEFINITION   Milk produced in the breast under the influence of the hormones of pregnancy. Colostrum is a yellowish, thick milk rich in immunoglobulins and other nutrients. The transition to mature milk begins with the delivery of the placenta.

The composition of milk changes gradually from colostrum to transitional milk to mature milk over the next two to four days.

When mothers report that their milk has not "come in" or changed by day five following delivery, lactation consultation is indicated.

Prolonged production of colostrum may indicate retained placental fragments.

> **Notes**
>
> It is normal to note some dried colostrum on the nipple or clothing during pregnancy.

See also Breastmilk secretion; Retained placental fragments

► Comfort nursing

DEFINITION   Offering the breast to calm an upset baby or child.

See also Nonnutritive sucking

► Complementary feeding

DEFINITION   A term used to indicate appropriate addition of solid foods to the baby's diet at and after 6 months of age.

The American Academy of Pediatrics (AAP), the United States Breastfeeding Committee (USBC), the United Nations Children's Fund (UNICEF), and the World Health Organization (WHO) recommend exclusive (full) breastfeeding for about the first six months of life.

Researchers have shown that flavors from the foods the mother eats in pregnancy and during lactation pass into the milk. When foods taste familiar, baby is more likely to accept them.

In addition to age, signs of readiness may include increased interest in table foods, ability to sit, ability to pick up objects and put them in the mouth, and decreased tongue thrusting (automatically pushing foods out of the mouth with the tongue).

Ask about

Age of baby.

Reason for wanting to start solid foods.

ASSESSMENT

PROMPT CARE NEEDED?

Are any of the following present?

Breastfed baby under 5 months of age.

Mother concerned about baby's weight gain.

Decreased stooling or urination.

IF YES, *Seek medical care today and call lactation care provider today.*

ROUTINE CARE NEEDED?

Are any of the following present?

Breastfed baby around 6 months of age.

Mother has questions about starting solids.

IF YES, *Call lactation care provider today.*

SELF CARE INFORMATION

Babies are not equally interested in starting solid foods; if the baby is not interested, wait a few days and try again.

When babies start solid foods around 6 months, they do not usually have a prolonged time on the semi-liquid foods that were popular when the recommendation for starting solids was for younger babies.

Move the baby onto family foods as appropriate.

IMPORTANT CONDITIONS TO REPORT

Difficulty breathing.

Difficulty swallowing.

Rapid progression of symptoms.

See also Allergy in the breastfed infant; Solid foods for breastfed infants

▶ Components of breastmilk

DEFINITION   Referring to the nutrients and other substances that constitute human milk. Breastmilk is a rich and changing mix of macronutrients and micronutrients, as well as immunoglobulins, white blood cells, minerals, growth factors, and enzymes.

Notes

The nutrient and energy content of human milk is largely controlled by metabolic processes.
   It is very rare for the nutrient composition of human milk to be inadequate.
Routine testing of the fat or other content of milk is not recommended, due to diurnal variation and the difficulty of collecting a representative sample.
   Evaluation of baby's growth, stooling pattern, and feeding frequency and mechanics should occur when doubts arise about milk adequacy.

See also Antibodies in breastmilk; Anti-infective agents in breastmilk; Anti-inflammatory agents in breastmilk

▶ Concerns about milk supply

DEFINITION   Concern about insufficient amount of milk produced by the breast.
   Women typically have concerns about milk supply, many of which are not based in actual insufficiency. However, mothers with this concern should be carefully evaluated.
   Maternal, infant, and environmental factors all contribute to milk supply problems.
   Milk supply can be increased. This is accomplished by increasing stimulation and removal of milk from the breast.

Ask about

Onset.
Age of baby.

EMERGENT CARE NEEDED?

Are any of the following present?

Meconium bowel movements after 5 days of life.

Fewer than 3 bowel movements daily in breastfed newborn after the first two days of life.

No urine in six hours.

Brick dust urine (uric acid crystals) after 2 days of life.

Dark colored urine.

Fewer than 4 urinations daily in the breastfed newborn after day 5.

Noticeably sunken fontanelles (soft spot on top of head).

Decreased activity.

Baby below birthweight at 10–14 days.

Cessation of weight gain.

IF YES, *Seek pediatric care now.*

PROMPT CARE NEEDED?

Are any of the following present?

Scanty or infrequent urination, less than 6 urinations per day after day 5 of life.

IF YES, *Seek pediatric care today.*

Are any of the following present?

Identified milk supply problem.

Concern about possible milk supply problems.

IF YES, *Call lactation care provider today.*

SELF CARE INFORMATION

Ensure baby is feeding 10–12 times per 24 hours.

Express milk after feeding.

IMPORTANT CONDITIONS TO REPORT

Persistent problems.

Recurrent problems.

See also Increasing milk supply

▶ Constipation

DEFINITION Delayed or infrequent passage of hard, dry stool. In the breastfed infant, more than three stools are expected daily. Fewer stools indicate need for medical evaluation of baby.

Ask about

Onset.
Age of baby.
Foods fed to baby.

ASSESSMENT

EMERGENT CARE NEEDED?

Are any of the following present?

Less than one stool per day in breastfed newborn.
Lethargic baby.

IF YES, *Seek emergency care now.*

PROMPT CARE NEEDED?

Are any of the following present?

Fewer than three stools per day in breastfed newborn.
Straining or grunting with stool.

IF YES, *Seek pediatric care now.*

ROUTINE CARE NEEDED?

Are any of the following present?

Concern about infrequent stooling in older baby with adequate weight gain.

IF YES, *Call pediatrician today.*

IMPORTANT CONDITIONS TO REPORT
No improvement of symptoms.
Ongoing problems with stooling.

Notes

Constipation is not normal in the breastfeeding infant.

See also Botulism, infantile

▶ Containers for milk storage

DEFINITION Safe vessels for preserving expressed milk.

Notes

Glass and hard plastic containers with tight lids are recommended. All containers should be food-grade. Plastic bags designed for milk storage may be used, but it may be difficult to prevent spillage and puncture of these bags.[82]

See also Collection and storage of breastmilk; Milk storage bags

Footnotes
[82]Arnold, L.D.W. (2004). *Safe storage of expressed breastmilk for the healthy infant and child.* East Sandwich, MA: Health Education Associates.

► Contraception

DEFINITION   Devices and drugs used to reduce fertility.

Many contraceptive methods are compatible with breastfeeding, including all barrier methods (condoms, foam, diaphragms, and cervical caps), intrauterine devices (IUDs), and progestin-only hormonal methods.* Combined estrogen/progestin methods are generally not recommended as they may reduce milk supply and affect infant growth.

The **Lactational Amenorrhea Method (LAM)** is a form of natural family planning which is 98% effective in the first six months following the birth of a baby, so long as the mother's menses have not returned, her baby is exclusively breastfed, and there are no long periods of time between feedings, day and night. Once the baby is older than 6 months, or any of the above criteria is no longer true, LAM is no longer effective and mothers should utilize other forms of birth control.

Notes

*Progestin-only injectibles are intended for use in breastfeeding women only at six weeks post-delivery, or when full milk supply is developed. Use prior to that time may decrease milk supply due to high circulating progestin levels, simulating a state of pregnancy.

See also **Amenorrhea; Birth interval; Lactational Amenorrhea Method (LAM); Progestin-only contraceptives; Natural family planning**

► Contraindicated conditions

DEFINITION   Diseases, conditions, or medications in the mother or infant that make it inadvisable to breastfeed.

According to the Centers for Disease Control, Breastfeeding is NOT advisable if one or more of the following conditions is true:

1. An infant diagnosed with galactosemia, a rare genetic metabolic disorder

2. The infant whose mother:
   - Has been infected with the human immunodeficiency virus (HIV)
   - Is taking antiretroviral medications
   - Has untreated, active tuberculosis
   - Is infected with human T-cell lymphotropic virus type I or type II
   - Is using or is dependent upon an illicit drug
   - Is taking prescribed cancer chemotherapy agents, such as antimetabolites that interfere with DNA replication and cell division
   - Is undergoing radiation therapies; however, such nuclear medicine therapies require only a temporary interruption in breastfeeding.[83]

Footnotes

[83]Centers for Disease Control and Prevention. (2005). Breastfeeding: Infectious diseases and specific conditions affecting human milk: When should a mother avoid breastfeeding? Retrieved November 7, 2005 from http://www.cdc.gov/breastfeeding/disease/contraindicators.htm.

▶ Contraindicated medications

DEFINITION   Drugs taken by the mother that make it inadvisable to breastfeed.

According to the American Academy of Pediatrics[84], breastfeeding is rarely contraindicated by medication use, except for "mothers who are receiving diagnostic or therapeutic radioactive isotopes or have had exposure to radioactive materials (for as long as there is radioactivity in the milk); mothers who are receiving antimetabolites or chemotherapeutic agents or a small number of other medications until they clear the milk; [and] mothers who are using drugs of abuse ('street drugs')."

Notes
An up-to-date drug reference should be consulted to determine the safety and possible side effects of individual drugs.
Newborn and premature babies are at greater risk of drug side effects due to limited ability to clear drugs from their systems.

Footnotes

[84]AAP Section on Breastfeeding. (2005). Breastfeeding and the use of human milk. *Pediatrics, 115,* 497.

Drug References

AAP Committee on Drugs. (2001). The transfer of drugs and other chemicals into human milk. *Pediatrics, 108,* 776–789.

Briggs, G.G., Freeman, R.K., & Yaffee, S.J. (Eds.). (2002). *Drugs in pregnancy and lactation* (6th ed.). Philadelphia: Lippincott, Williams and Wilkins.

Hale, T.W. (2004). *Medications and mothers milk.* Amarillo, TX: Pharmasoft Publishing.

Lawrence, R.A., & Lawrence, R.M. (2005). *Breastfeeding: A guide for the medical profession* (6th ed.). St. Louis: Mosby.

▶ ## Cooper's ligaments

DEFINITION   Connective tissue within the breast that suspends the tissue.

▶ ## Corticosteroids

DEFINITION   Hormones produced by the adrenal glands. These hormones are also synthesized and used as medications to reduce inflammation and treat many autoimmune disorders.

Notes

A wide range of corticosteroid preparations are in use. Potency varies widely. An up-to-date drug reference should be consulted to determine the safety and possible side effects of individual drugs.

Newborn and premature babies are at greater risk of drug side effects due to limited ability to clear drugs from their systems.

Drug References

American Academy of Pediatrics Committee on Drugs. (2001). Transfer of drugs and other chemicals into human milk. *Pediatrics, 108,* 776–789.

Briggs, G.G., Freeman, R.K., & Yaffee, S.J. (Eds.). (2002). *Drugs in pregnancy and lactation* (6th ed.). Philadelphia: Lippincott, Williams, and Wilkins.

Hale, T.W. (2004). *Medications and mothers milk.* Amarillo, TX: Pharmasoft Publishing.
Lawrence, R.A., & Lawrence, R.M. (2005). *Breastfeeding: A guide for the medical profession* (6th ed.). St. Louis: Mosby.

▶ Co-sleeping

DEFINITION   The practice of a parent or parents sleeping in close proximity to their baby. Co-sleeping does not necessarily denote bedsharing. Co-sleeping is supportive of breastfeeding.

SELF CARE INFORMATION

Babies should not share a bed with a smoker, someone under the influence of alcohol or medications that could make them difficult to rouse, or someone who is extremely fatigued.

Babies should never sleep alone or with another person on a waterbed, sofa, reclining chair, saggy mattress, or bean bag.

Parents who share an adult bed with their baby should ensure that there are no gaps between the mattress and the frame or between the mattress and the wall in which the baby could become stuck. There should be no pillows, fluffy comforters (duvets), stuffed animals, or other suffocation/choking hazards on the baby's sleeping surface (whether in own bed or an adult bed).

No other child should share a bed with the co-sleeping infant.

Notes

According to the American Academy of Pediatrics, "Mother and infant should sleep in proximity to each other to facilitate breastfeeding."[85]

See also Co-bedding; SIDS (sudden infant death syndrome)

Footnotes

[85]AAP Section on Breastfeeding. (2005). Breastfeeding and the use of human milk. *Pediatrics, 115,* 500.

▶ Cow's milk

DEFINITION   The fluid produced by the mammary glands of the lactating cow. Cow's milk is not recommended for children younger than 1 year of age.

Notes

Breastmilk and infant formula are the only appropriate milks for babies younger than 1. While cow's milk-based formula is an appropriate substitute for breastmilk, unaltered cow's milk is not, as it may lead to mineral and nutrient imbalance and bleeding in the gut.

Between 1 and 2 years of age, whole cow's milk may be offered to children. Low-fat and skim milk should not be offered until children are older than 2.

Concern about infant allergy is much more predominant than actual allergy. The American Academy of Pediatrics reports that the prevalence of infant cow's milk allergy is two to three percent. The overall prevalence of childhood food allergy is four to six percent.[86]

Counseling and education should include comfort techniques for the irritable baby and coping methods for parents.[87]

Breastfeeding babies may react to cow's milk protein in their mother's diet.

See also Allergy in the breastfed infant; Colic, infantile

Footnotes

[86]AAP Committee on Nutrition. (2000). Hypoallergenic infant formulas. *Pediatrics, 106*, 346.

[87]Ziegler, R.S. (2003). Food allergen avoidance in prevention of food allergy in infants and children. *Pediatrics, 111*, 1662–1671.

▶ Cradle hold

DEFINITION   A breastfeeding position in which baby is placed across the mother's lap and turned toward the mother. In this position, the weight of the baby is often carried on the arm of the mother on the same side as the breast that is being nursed.

This position is also called the "Madonna" position.

▶ Creams and ointments

DEFINITION   Topical preparations that have been made for several purposes, such as to protect the skin, to decrease itching, to clean the skin (antiseptics), and to moisturize the skin.

Women with questions about creams may be experiencing nipple or breast pain.

Ask about

Nipple discomfort.

ASSESSMENT

ROUTINE CARE NEEDED?
Are any of the following present?
　　Sore nipples.
　　Painful breastfeeding.
　　Skin rash, breakouts, or itching on the breast, areola, and nipple.

IF YES,   *Call lactation care provider today and call obstetric care provider today.*

IMPORTANT CONDITIONS TO REPORT
Symptoms worsen or persist.
Signs of infection.
Feeding or stooling expectations are not met.

SELF CARE INFORMATION
Most ointments and creams are not intended for ingestion. When a mother puts an ointment or cream on her areola or nipple, her baby will be exposed to the ingredients during nursing.
Only use ointments and creams on the breast that are recommended for this purpose. Never use a product that has been prescribed for another problem.
Mothers can have reactions to ointments and creams. Report any changes immediately.

See also Breast pain; Herpes simplex virus; Nipple pain; Sore nipples

▶ Crib death

DEFINITION The unexpected death of a healthy appearing baby under the age of 1.

Crib death is also called SIDS (sudden infant death syndrome) and cot death.

SIDS is rare in the first month of life and most cases occur before 6 months of age.

In the United States there are more SIDS cases in the fall and winter seasons as compared to the spring and summer months.

The National "Back to Sleep" Campaign encourages parents to put their babies asleep on their back. Since initiation of this campaign, the number of babies to die from SIDS per year has been reduced by 50%.

About 2200 babies die per year from SIDS in the United States.

SIDS is sudden and silent. The baby shows no signs of suffering.

The risk of SIDS increases if babies are not put to sleep on their backs, if they are overheated, if they are exposed to secondhand smoke, and if they have unsafe bedding.

SELF CARE INFORMATION

Learn about safe sleeping practices for babies.

Protect the baby from second hand smoke.

See also Co-bedding; Co-sleeping

▶ Cross cradle position

DEFINITION   A variation on the cradle or Madonna hold, where the mother's arms are switched so that the weight of the baby is supported by the opposite arm to the breast the baby is suckling. The mother supports the baby's back with her forearm, with her hand cradling baby's neck. The other hand supports her breast if needed. Once baby is successfully latched on, the mother can switch her arms to hold the baby in cradle.

> **Notes**
>
> This position is helpful in the early postpartum period when baby's head needs more support. It also helps mothers to remember to start feedings with the baby right in front of the nipple, rather than tucked in the crook of her arm (which is where women instinctively place the baby in the cradle or Madonna hold).

See also Cradle hold; Clutch hold; Football hold

▶ Cross nursing

DEFINITION   One woman breastfeeding another woman's baby. Cross nursing is not recommended due to fears of infection, which can pass from nurse to nursling or the reverse.

See also Wet nursing

▶ Crying

DEFINITION   A behavioral state involving tears and other signs of distress. Crying is the most agitated state for babies.

Infants have a predictable sequence of states of awareness including deep sleep, light sleep (with rapid eye movements), quiet alert, awake, active alert, and crying.

Light sleep, quiet alert, and awake states are the best times to initiate feeding. Crying is a late feeding cue.

Onset.

Age of baby.

ASSESSMENT

EMERGENT CARE NEEDED?

Are any of the following present?

Respiratory distress.

Lethargy or loss of muscle tone.

Fear that a parent will harm crying baby.

IF YES, *Seek emergency care now.*

PROMPT CARE NEEDED?

Are any of the following present?

Projectile vomiting.

Fever.

Crying for longer than three hours.

IF YES, *Seek medical care now.*

Are any of the following present?

Crying before or during feedings.

Intermittent crying.

Concern about foods mother is eating.

IF YES, *Call lactation care provider today.*

SELF CARE INFORMATION

Comfort techniques for irritable baby (rocking, singing, skin-to-skin contact, bathing, seeking quiet, calm environment, etc.).

Notes

Crying is a calorically expensive event for babies. Parents should be encouraged to comfort crying babies.

See also Allergy in the breastfed infant; Feeding cues

▶ Cup-feeding

DEFINITION   An alternative feeding method for delivering liquid to infants. Cup-feeding is the internationally recommended method of supplementing breastfed infants, due to ease of cleaning the cup and the avoidance of introducing baby to an artificial nipple shape.

▶ Custody and breastfeeding

DEFINITION   Referring to legal custody shared between parents and the complications of meeting the needs of the breastfeeding baby in this situation.

Ask about

Age of baby.
Length of mother–baby separation.

ASSESSMENT

PROMPT CARE NEEDED?
   Are any of the following present?
      Mother wishes to maintain milk supply during separation from baby.

IF YES,   *Call lactation care provider today.*

SELF CARE INFORMATION
   Express milk on the same schedule the baby would normally feed during separation
      to maintain milk supply.
   Monitor fullness of breasts closely.

▶ Cyanosis

DEFINITION A state where the skin and mucous membrane turn purplish-blue, reflecting lack of oxygenation in the blood.

Ask about

Onset.
Medical conditions of baby.

ASSESSMENT

EMERGENT CARE NEEDED?
Are any of the following present?
Circumoral cyanosis during feeding (cyanosis around the mouth) or at other times.
Cyanosis of the hands and feet beyond the first few days of life.
(Acrocyanosis is common and normal in newborns.)

IF YES, *Seek medical care now.*

IMPORTANT CONDITIONS TO REPORT
Medications used.

See also Acrocyanosis; Circumoral cyanosis

▶ Cystic breasts

DEFINITION A common breast condition in women including variable lumpiness, tenderness, and palpable cysts (pockets of fluid). Symptoms may change during the menstrual period. This benign condition is compatible with breastfeeding.

New lumps in the breast should be medically examined to rule out **plugged ducts** and other problems.

See also Breast lumps; Fibrocystic breasts; Plugged breasts

▶ Cystic fibrosis and breastfeeding

DEFINITION   A chronic genetic disease that affects all the respiratory and digestive tracts, creating thick mucus that can cause obstruction leading to difficult respiration and digestion.

Infants and children with cystic fibrosis may have stunted growth and frequent infections. Breastfeeding is recommended for children with this condition, as it may boost their immune systems and decrease negative outcomes.

▶ Cytokine

DEFINITION   Immunoactive proteins, including interleukin, interferon, and others that are secreted by the cells of the immune system to regulate immune response.

▶ Cytomegalovirus (CMV)

DEFINITION   A virus of the herpes family that is widespread in the population and can be dormant in the body for years. CMV infection has no obvious symptoms, with rare exception of an illness similar to mononucleosis.

SELF CARE INFORMATION

Practice routine, careful handwashing with soap and water, especially when handling children and diapers.

> **Notes**
>
> There is some risk of negative effects to babies born to women who had their first infection with CMV during pregnancy. According to the Centers for Disease Control and Prevention, "during a pregnancy when a woman *who has never had CMV infection* becomes infected with CMV, there is a potential risk that after birth the infant may have CMV-related complications, the most common of which are associated with hearing loss, visual impairment, or diminished mental and motor capabilities. On the other hand, infants and children *who acquire CMV after birth* have few, if any, symptoms or complications."[88]
>
> In the event that a mother with CMV infection has a preterm baby, careful consideration of the benefits of breastfeeding vs the risk of CMV transmission must be made. See the American Academy of Pediatrics's 2005 statement for more guidance.[89]

Footnotes

[88]National Center for Infectious Diseases. (2005). *Cytomegalovirus (CMV) infection.* Retrieved March 14, 2005, from http://www.cdc.gov/ncidod/diseases/cmv.htm.

[89]AAP Section on Breastfeeding. (2005). Breastfeeding and the use of human milk. *Pediatrics, 115*, 497.

▶ Daily Reference Intakes (DRI)

DEFINITION   Values of the amount of nutrients needed by healthy people. This new terminology replaces the concept of RDA (recommended dietary allowances), which offered population estimates of the amount of nutrients needed to avoid deficiency. The DRIs look at nutrient needs from the point of view of promoting health rather than avoiding deficiency.

Dairy products for baby

DEFINITION Foods made from cow's milk. Cow's milk is not recommended for children younger than 1.

> **Notes**
>
> Breastmilk and infant formula are the only appropriate milks for babies younger than 1. While cow's milk-based formula is an appropriate substitute for human milk, unaltered cow's milk is not, as it may lead to mineral and nutrient imbalance and bleeding in the gut.
>
> Unless there is a family history of cow's milk allergy, babies may be introduced to small amounts of yogurt, cheese, and other dairy foods after 8 months of age.
>
> Between 1 and 2 years of age, whole cow's milk may be offered to children. Low-fat and skim milk should not be offered until children are older than 2.
>
> Concern about infant allergy is much more predominant than actual allergy. The American Academy of Pediatrics reports that the prevalence of infant cow's milk allergy is two to three percent.[90] The overall prevalence of childhood food allergy is four to six percent.[91]
>
> Breastfeeding babies may react to cow's milk protein in their mother's diet.

See also Allergy in the breastfed infant; Colic, infantile; Cow's milk

Footnotes

[90]AAP Committee on Nutrition. (2000). Hypoallergenic infant formulas. *Pediatrics, 106*, 346.

[91]Ziegler, R.S. (2003). Food allergen avoidance in prevention of food allergy in infants and children. *Pediatrics, 111*, 1662–1671.

Dancer hand position

DEFINITION A technique used to assist the baby with low muscle tone or depressed reflexes in maintaining positioning at the breast. This technique keeps the weight of the breast off the baby's jaw and gives some support to the baby's facial muscles.

In this position, the mother's hand slides up under the breast to hold the weight of the breast cupped in her hand. She supports baby's chin and jaw with the web of tissue between her thumb and forefinger, and uses her thumb and index finger to cup the baby's cheeks, giving support.

See also Down syndrome; Neurological dysfunction; Uncoordinated sucking

▶ Day care

DEFINITION   A substitute care provider or group of providers who care for a child while the parents go to work or school. Breastfeeding mothers should be supported in expressing and collecting their milk to be given to babies in day care.

Ask about

Onset of separation.
Age of baby.

ASSESSMENT

ROUTINE CARE NEEDED?
   Are any of the following present?
      Mother–baby separation anticipated.
      Mother wishes to express milk for baby.

IF YES,   *Call lactation care provider today.*

SELF CARE INFORMATION
   Frequent milk expression is ideal.

IMPORTANT CONDITIONS TO REPORT
   Decreasing milk supply.
   Questions about collection and storage.

See also Decreasing milk supply; Working women

▶ DDT in breastmilk

DEFINITION   All foods, including breastmilk, may contain traces of chemical contaminants present in the environment, such as the insecticide DDT. According to the American Academy of Pediatrics, no effects of DDT have been noted in the breast-fed infant (Table 7).[92]

Notes

Breastmilk is one of the easiest and least painful body tissues to sample. For this reason, it is used to monitor population exposure to chemicals.

Women who know they had high level exposure to specific chemicals or pollutants should consult with their physician regarding analysis of the contaminant content of their milk.

Many researchers have looked for negative effects of toxin exposure via breastmilk and have found only benefits for breastfed babies, as compared with formula fed babies.

See also Contaminants in breastmilk

Footnotes

[92]AAP Committee on Drugs. (2001). The transfer of drugs and other chemicals into human milk. *Pediatrics, 108*, 782.

Drug References

Briggs, G.G., Freeman, R.K., & Yaffee, S.J. (Eds.). (2002). *Drugs in pregnancy and lactation* (6th ed.). Philadelphia: Lippincott, Williams and Wilkins.

Hale, T.W. (2004). *Medications and mothers milk.* Amarillo, TX: Pharmasoft Publishing.

Lawrence, R.A., & Lawrence, R.M. (2005). *Breastfeeding: A guide for the medical profession* (6th ed.). St. Louis: Mosby.

▶ Decrease in milk supply

DEFINITION   Insufficient amount of milk produced by the breast. Maternal, infant, and environmental factors all contribute to milk supply problems.

Milk supply can be increased. This is accomplished by increasing stimulation and removal of milk from the breast.

Mothers of hospitalized infants and employed mothers may experience a decrease in milk supply when pumping.

Concerns about milk supply always warrant evaluation.

Ask about

Onset.
Age of baby.

ASSESSMENT

EMERGENT CARE NEEDED?

Are any of the following present?

Meconium bowel movements after 5 days of life.

Fewer than 3 bowel movements daily in breastfed newborn after the first two days of life.

No urine in six hours.

Brick dust urine (uric acid crystals) after 2 days of life.

Dark colored urine.

Fewer than 4 urinations daily in the breastfed newborn after day 5.

Noticeably sunken fontanelles (soft spot on top of head).

Decreased activity.

Baby below birthweight at 10–14 days.

Cessation of weight gain.

IF YES,   *Seek medical care within 2 to 4 hours.*

PROMPT CARE NEEDED?

Are any of the following present?

Scanty urination.

IF YES,   *Call pediatric care provider today.*

SELF CARE INFORMATION
Ensure baby is feeding 10–12 times per 24 hours.
Express milk after feeding.

IMPORTANT CONDITIONS TO REPORT
Persistent problems.
Recurrent problems.

See also Increasing milk supply

▶ Decreasing supplemental formula

DEFINITION   Reducing the amount of formula used as breastmilk supply increases. Decreases in supplemental formula should be made gradually and with careful monitoring to ensure adequate growth and nutrition of baby.

Ask about

Reason for supplementation.
Age of baby.

ASSESSMENT

PROMPT CARE NEEDED?
Are any of the following present?
Desire to begin decreasing formula supplementation.
Continued decrease in supplementation.

IF YES, *Call lactation care provider today.*

SELF CARE INFORMATION

Ensure adequate breast stimulation by expressing milk every time baby is supplemented.

Bring baby to a pediatric care provider for frequent weight checks.

IMPORTANT CONDITIONS TO REPORT

Decrease in stooling pattern of baby.

Concerns about milk production.

> **Notes**
>
> Decrease in supplementation should not be made without review and approval of the medical care provider who ordered supplementation.

See also Milk transfer-estimating; Test weighing

▶ Deep breast pain

DEFINITION   Uncomfortable sensations in the breast. Pain is not an expected part of breastfeeding and indicates need for feeding evaluation.

There can be many reasons for pain in the breast, including breast infection or inflammation, clogs, or cysts. Poor latch-on or positioning can also cause pain.

Pinched nerves and lymphatic congestion may contribute to deep pain.

Candida infection has been suggested as a cause of deep pain. However, research has not confirmed this suggestion.

Ask about

Onset.

Location of pain.

Whether unilateral or bilateral.

PROMPT CARE NEEDED?

Are any of the following present?

Persistent deep pain with feeding.

Persistent deep pain between feedings.

Constant deep pain.

Pain combined with color change of nipple(s).

Pain with visible fissure or bleeding of the nipple(s).

IF YES, *Call lactation care provider today.*

Notes

Breastfeeding should not be painful. Advise mothers to seek medical or lactation care for breast pain.

See also Breast pain; Latch-on; Mastitis; Sore nipples

► Dehydration and breastfeeding

DEFINITION Depletion of the water stores in the body, due to a number of causes including lack of adequate fluid intake, diarrhea, and vomiting. Infants and young children can become dehydrated quickly. Severely dehydrated women may make less milk, but mild dehydration has little effect on milk production and content.

Ask about

Onset.

Age of baby.

EMERGENT CARE NEEDED?

Are any of the following present?

Meconium bowel movements after 5 days of life.

Fewer than 3 bowel movements daily in breastfed newborn after the first two days of life.

No urine in six hours.

Brick dust urine (uric acid crystals) after 2 days of life.

Dark colored urine.

Fewer than 4 urinations daily in the breastfed newborn after day 5.

Noticeably sunken fontanelles (soft spot on top of head).

Decreased activity.

Baby below birthweight at 10–14 days.

Cessation of weight gain.

Diarrhea or vomiting lasting more than a few hours.

IF YES, *Seek medical care within 2 to 4 hours.*

PROMPT CARE NEEDED?

Are any of the following present?

Scanty urination.

IF YES, *Call pediatric care provider today.*

SELF CARE INFORMATION

Ensure baby is feeding 10–12 times per 24 hours.

Practice skin-to-skin care as much as possible.

IMPORTANT CONDITIONS TO REPORT

Persistent problems.

Recurrent problems.

▶ Demerol® (Meperidine)

DEFINITION A narcotic analgesic drug often administered during childbirth. This drug is known to decrease the infant's early feeding behaviors.

SELF CARE INFORMATION

If this drug was given to mother during the birth process, extended skin-to-skin contact should be practiced until the infant shows feeding cues.

IMPORTANT CONDITIONS TO REPORT

Feeding difficulties.

See also Childbirth

▶ Depo-Provera® contraceptive (Medroxyprogesterone)

DEFINITION   A low dose progestin injection used to provide birth control.

> **Notes**
>
> Progestin-only injectibles are intended for use in breastfeeding women only at six weeks post-delivery, or when full milk supply is developed. Use prior to that time may decrease milk supply due to high circulating progestin levels, simulating a state of pregnancy.

See also Birth control; Progestin-only contraceptives

▶ Depression

DEFINITION   Symptoms of depression are not unusual for women during the early days postpartum. Depending upon the population studied, between 30% to 84% of women experience some form of mood disorder during this period.[93]

> **Ask about**

Onset.
Age of baby.
Past history of depression.

ASSESSMENT

EMERGENT CARE NEEDED?

Are any of the following present?

Suicidal thoughts.

Thoughts of harming baby.

IF YES, *Seek emergency care now.*

PROMPT CARE NEEDED?

Are any of the following present?

Persistent sadness.

Inability to function.

IF YES, *Seek medical care within 2 to 4 hours.*

ROUTINE CARE NEEDED?

Are any of the following present?

Ongoing breastfeeding in a woman with depression.

IF YES, *Call lactation care provider today.*

SELF CARE INFORMATION

Mood swings are normal in the postpartum period, but may become more severe. Seek support.

Practice skin-to-skin contact frequently.

Feed baby at first sign of hunger cues (signs that say "feed me" include hand-to-face or hand-to-mouth movements, lip smacking, seeking with lips, rooting, and head bobbing).

Feed baby at least 10–12 times per 24 hours.

Listen for signs of baby swallowing.

Allow baby to end feedings.

Expect at least 3–4 infant stools per 24 hours after the first 4 days of life.

Good positioning and attachment are crucial to reduce nipple pain.

If feedings are missed, hand express or pump milk to maintain supply.

IMPORTANT CONDITIONS TO REPORT

Exacerbation of symptoms.

Nonresolution of symptoms.

Past history of depression, mood disorders, premenstrual syndrome, or thyroid disorders.

Notes

Symptoms of depression can progress to other postpartum mood disorders. It is important to encourage mothers to report any worsening of symptoms.

Women who experienced depression during pregnancy and those with a prior history of depression, mood disorders, or premenstrual syndrome are at greater risk for postpartum depression.

Hypothyroidism, anemia, and other physical disorders share many symptoms with postpartum depression.

Many antidepressant medications are considered compatible with breastfeeding. Consult an up-to-date drug reference for more info.

See also Anemia; Baby blues; Postpartum depression; Hypothyroidism

Footnotes

[93]Kendall-Tackett, K.A., & Kantor, G.K. (1993). *Postpartum depression: A comprehensive approach for nurses.* Newbury Park, CA: Sage.

Drug References

American Academy of Pediatrics Committee on Drugs. (2001). Transfer of drugs and other chemicals into human milk. *Pediatrics, 108,* 776–789.

Briggs, G.G., Freeman, R.K., & Yaffee, S.J. (Eds.). (2002). *Drugs in pregnancy and lactation* (6th ed.). Philadelphia: Lippincott, Williams, and Wilkins.

Hale, T.W. (2004). *Medications and mothers milk.* Amarillo, TX: Pharmasoft Publishing.

Lawrence, R.A., & Lawrence, R.M. (2005). *Breastfeeding: A guide for the medical profession* (6th ed.). St. Louis: Mosby.

▶ **DHA**

DEFINITION   Docosahexanoic acid in breastmilk. A long-chain polyunsaturated fatty acid (LCPUFA) found naturally in human milk. These fatty acids assist in the development of nerve and brain tissue, and may account for some of the differences between formula and breastfed children in terms of IQ, test scores, and visual acuity.

Notes

While LCPUFAs have been added to formula in recent years, there is little evidence of beneficial outcomes in children who have consumed them. Supplements are also being marketed for mothers to consume during pregnancy and lactation, also with little evidence of efficacy.

See also Arachidonic acid; Fat in breastmilk; LCPUFAs

▶ Diabetes and breastfeeding

DEFINITION A chronic disease causing high levels of sugar in the blood. It is caused by too little insulin, or resistance to insulin. There are three major types of diabetes:

Type 1, which is usually diagnosed in childhood. The pancreas makes little or no insulin, requiring daily injections of this hormone that regulates sugar metabolism.

Type 2, usually occurring in adulthood. The pancreas does not make enough insulin and/or the body's cells become resistant to the insulin in circulation. This type of diabetes may be managed by careful diet, and often with use of oral medications. Type 2 diabetes is becoming increasingly common.

Gestational diabetes is the condition of high blood sugar levels occurring during pregnancy in a woman without prior diabetes.

Women with all of these conditions can breastfeed their babies.

Ask about

Onset.
Type of diabetes.

EMERGENT CARE NEEDED?

Are any of the following present?

Insulin shock in the breastfeeding woman.

IF YES, *Seek emergency care now.*

PROMPT CARE NEEDED?

Are any of the following present?

Difficulty maintaining blood glucose levels during breastfeeding.

IF YES, *Seek medical care today.*

ROUTINE CARE NEEDED?

Are any of the following present?

Ongoing breastfeeding in the diabetic woman.

IF YES, *Call lactation care provider today.*

SELF CARE INFORMATION

Women with diabetes are more prone to infection. Monitor breasts and nipples daily for any red, infected, or painful areas.

If insulin dependent, be aware that less insulin may be required during breastfeeding—watch for signs of low blood sugar.

IMPORTANT CONDITIONS TO REPORT

Any symptoms of infection.

Difficulty regulating blood sugar.

Notes

Women with diabetes should be encouraged to breastfeed. Breastfeeding is known to reduce the risk of developing diabetes in susceptible individuals (e.g., children of diabetic mothers).

Research suggests that women who have experienced gestational diabetes are less likely to progress to diabetes if they breastfeed their babies.

See also Autoimmune diseases

▶ **Diarrhea and breastfeeding**

DEFINITION   Frequent loose, watery stools. Diarrhea is typically caused by a virus. Diarrhea can be serious in infants and young children, as they can become dehydrated quickly.

Ask about

Onset.
Age of baby.

ASSESSMENT

EMERGENT CARE NEEDED?

Are any of the following present?

Diarrhea episodes in a baby younger than 3 months of age.

Meconium bowel movements after 5 days of life.

Fewer than 3 bowel movements daily in breastfed newborn after the first two days of life.

No urine in six hours.

Brick dust urine (uric acid crystals) after 2 days of life.

Dark colored urine.

Fewer than 4 urinations daily in the breastfed newborn after day 5.

Noticeably sunken fontanelles (soft spot on top of head).

Decreased activity.

Baby below birthweight at 10–14 days.

Cessation of weight gain.

IF YES,   *Seek medical care within 2 to 4 hours.*

PROMPT CARE NEEDED?

Are any of the following present?

Scanty urination.

Sporadic diarrhea.

IF YES,   *Call pediatric care provider today.*

SELF CARE INFORMATION

Ensure baby is feeding 10–12 times per 24 hours.

Practice careful handwashing before and after handling baby, changing diapers, and going to the bathroom.

IMPORTANT CONDITIONS TO REPORT

Persistent problems.

Recurrent problems.

> **Notes**
>
> Diarrhea in the nursing mother is of concern for proper functioning of her body, but not for the manufacture of milk.

See also Acute infection; Blood in stool; Dehydration; Stooling patterns

▶ Diet of the mother

DEFINITION   Referring to foods eaten by the mother on a daily basis.

> **Notes**
>
> Mothers can produce enough milk, and milk of good quality, even when the mother's supply of nutrients is limited.[94] Rules about eating or not eating certain foods during lactation are not warranted, may be hard to follow, and may decrease the mother's enjoyment of breastfeeding. However, there may be individual cases where certain foods affect the baby. Most commonly, the mother's drinking of liquid cow's milk has been associated with colic symptoms in some babies. If this is the case, improvement may be seen after the mother eliminates cow's milk from her diet for at least a week. Mothers should seek further information about diet and breastfeeding on an individual basis.

See also Allergy in the breastfed infant; Macrobiotic diet; Maternal diet—vegetarian

Footnotes

[94]National Academy of Sciences Subcommittee on Nutrition. (1991). *Nutrition during lactation*. Washington, DC: National Academy Press.

▶ # Dimpled nipple

DEFINITION A condition in which the center of the nipple is retracted toward the chest wall. This condition may affect one or both nipples, and may be cause for pain in the breastfeeding woman.

Ask about

Onset of nipple condition.

ASSESSMENT

EMERGENT CARE NEEDED?

Are any of the following present?

Sudden occurrence of dimpled nipples.

IF YES, *Seek medical care today.*

PROMPT CARE NEEDED?

Are any of the following present?

Preexisting dimpled nipple with pain.

Ongoing problems with dimpled nipple.

IF YES, *Call lactation care provider today.*

SELF CARE INFORMATION

Keep area around dimpled nipple dry, changing pads frequently.

IMPORTANT CONDITIONS TO REPORT

Worsening of condition.

Symptoms of infection.

See also Inverted nipple

▶ Disabilities, mothers with

DEFINITION Referring to mothers living with a physical or mental challenge.

Ask about

Type of disability.
Age of baby.

ASSESSMENT

PROMPT CARE NEEDED?

Are any of the following present?

Mother with disabilities learning to breastfeed.

Ongoing breastfeeding support needed.

IF YES, *Call lactation care provider today.*

SELF CARE INFORMATION

Set up a feeding station in the home where nonperishable snacks, drinks of water, baby changing equipment, handwipes, and telephone can be at the ready.

IMPORTANT CONDITIONS TO REPORT

Concern about feeding adequacy or comfort.

Notes

Breastfeeding is often an ideal feeding choice for mothers with disabilities, as it requires little preparation for feeding.

▶ Discharge from nipple

DEFINITION   Visible evidence of blood or other secretion from the nipple.

Ask about

Onset.
Age of baby.
History of trauma or surgery to the breast.

ASSESSMENT

EMERGENT CARE NEEDED?

Are any of the following present?

Persistent bleeding from nipple between feedings.

Symptoms of infection (redness or pus at the site of bleeding, fever, chills, achiness, or malaise).

Appearance of nipple discharge in nonpregnant, nonlactating women.

IF YES,   *Seek medical care within 2 to 4 hours.*

PROMPT CARE NEEDED?

Are any of the following present?

Bleeding during feedings.

Pain on latch.

IF YES,   *Call lactation care provider today.*

SELF CARE INFORMATION

Practice good attachment:

Watch for feeding cues and offer the breast as soon as it is seen.

Wait for baby to open mouth wide (great than a 100° angle).

Pull baby in so that chin touches the breast first, and nipple enters the mouth along the top of the tongue; this should result in a wide open mouth on breast.

Lips should be flanged outward.

Baby's lips should look off center when compared with the areola; the bottom lip should be farther away from the nipple than the top lip.

IMPORTANT CONDITIONS TO REPORT
Any substance or item being used to decrease pain.
Worsening symptoms.
Persistent symptoms.

See also Bleeding, breast; Nipple pain; Intraductal papilloma

▶ Distractibility

DEFINITION A characteristic of babies older than 4 months whose attention is easily diverted away from feeding at the breast.

SELF CARE INFORMATION
Try feeding baby in a dark, quiet room.

▶ Diurnal variation

DEFINITION Changes that happen on a daily cycle. For example, prolactin levels appear to be naturally higher during the night and lower during the day.

▶ Docosahexanoic acid in breastmilk (DHA)

DEFINITION A long-chain polyunsaturated fatty acid (LCPUFA) found naturally in human milk. These fatty acids assist in the development of nerve and brain tissue, and may account for some of the differences between formula and breastfed children in terms of IQ, test scores, and visual acuity.

> **Notes**
>
> While LCPUFAs have been added to formula in recent years, there is little evidence of beneficial outcomes in children who have consumed them. Currently these products are also marketed for mothers during pregnancy/lactation, also with little, if any, evidence.

► Domperidone

DEFINITION   A dopamine agonist drug similar to metoclopramide used to control gastrointestinal symptoms. This drug is used "off label" in other countries to increase milk supply, but is not currently available in the United States. The Food and Drug Administration (FDA) has warned that this drug has not been approved for increasing milk supply in any country and is not approved for any use in the U.S.[95]

See also Metoclopramide (Reglan®)

Footnotes

[95]U.S. Food and Drug Administration. (2004). *FDA talk paper: FDA warns against women using unapproved drug, Domperidone, to increase milk production.* Retrieved March 17, 2005, from http://www.fda.gov/bbs/topics/ANSWERS/2004/ANS01292.html.

► Donor milk

DEFINITION   Excess milk obtained from breastfeeding mothers. In the United States, donor milk should be obtained only from a member milk bank of the Human Milk Banking Association of North America.

Notes

Informal donation of milk from one mother to another cannot be condoned, as it is possible to pass infectious agents through the milk.

Donor milk from a recognized human milk bank will have gone through several different screening processes (history and serology of the donor, bacteriology of the milk before and after heat treatment, etc.) and will be heat treated to remove most pathogens.

The uses of donor milk are many, including providing nourishment to preterm or chronically ill infants, such as those with feeding intolerance, malabsorption, cardiac problems, metabolic problems, and diarrhea.

Use of donor milk in preterm infants is thought to reduce the risk of necrotizing enterocolitis.

A prescription is necessary in order for donor milk to be dispensed from the milk bank.

There is a processing cost associated with obtaining donor milk; this fee may be waived or reduced if cost prohibitive.
Human Milk Banking Association of North America (HMBANA)
1500 Sunday Drive, Suite 102
Raleigh, NC 27607
Phone: 919-861-4530 ext. 226
Web site: www.hmbana.org

See also Cross nursing; Milk banks

▶ Double pumping

DEFINITION A system that allows both breasts to be pumped simultaneously. Double pumping generally takes less time and may stimulate more milk production. This technique is particularly helpful for mothers of preterm or ill babies, and others who are separated from their babies routinely.

Notes

Double pump kits can be purchased. All rental grade electric pumps are available with double pump kits. Some personal use pumps are available with double pump kits.

▶ Doula

DEFINITION A person who accompanies the family during the peripartum period, offering support and nurturing care as the mother gives birth and develops a relationship with her new baby. Doula care has been shown to reduce the risk of prolonged labor, need for analgesia, and Cesarean birth. Doula care has also been shown to increase exclusive breastfeeding.

Doulas can be found by contacting:
ALACE (The Association of Labor Assistants & Childbirth Educators)
P.O. Box 390436
Cambridge, MA 02139
Phone: 617-441-2500
E-mail: info@alace.org
Web site: www.alace.org

DONA (Doulas of North America)
P.O. Box 626
Jasper, IN 46547
Phone: 888-788-DONA
E-mail: doula@dona.org
Web site: www.dona.org

▶ Down syndrome (DS)

DEFINITION   A congenital genetic disorder that usually results in mild to moderate mental retardation and other conditions, including decreased muscle tone, and often heart defects and gastrointestinal problems. Babies with Down syndrome benefit from breastfeeding, as do mothers with this syndrome.

Ask about

Age of baby.

ASSESSMENT

EMERGENT CARE NEEDED?
Are any of the following present?
Circumoral cyanosis (blue tinge around lips).
Vomiting in the newborn with DS.

IF YES,   *Seek emergency care now.*

PROMPT CARE NEEDED?

Are any of the following present?

Beginning breastfeeding with DS baby.

Difficulty with breastfeeding DS baby.

| IF YES, | *Call lactation care provider today.* |

ROUTINE CARE NEEDED?

Are any of the following present?

Ongoing feeding concerns with DS baby.

| IF YES, | *Report to lactation care provider.* |

SELF CARE INFORMATION

Because of baby's low muscle tone, milk expression may be required after feeding to maximize milk removal (which will increase milk manufacture).

Feeding cues may be more subtle; ensure that baby is feeding 10–12 times per 24 hours.

Avoid pacifier and bottle nipple use.

Practice skin-to-skin contact as much as possible.

IMPORTANT CONDITIONS TO REPORT

Vomiting.

Feeding difficulties.

Notes

Growth and development of babies with DS should be closely monitored. Vomiting in babies with DS in the newborn period is of special concern because of the increased risk of intestinal obstruction.

See also Breast pump; Dancer hand position; Haberman feeder; Hand expression of breastmilk; Muscle tone

▶ DRI

DEFINITION   Daily Reference Intakes. Values of the amount of nutrients needed by healthy people. This new terminology replaces the concept of RDA (recommended dietary allowances), which offered population estimates of the amount of nutrients needed to avoid deficiency. The DRIs look at nutrient needs from the point of view of promoting health rather than avoiding deficiency.

▶ Drugs and breastfeeding

DEFINITION   Many factors influence whether a drug the mother takes will be found in her milk, the amount of the drug that is found in the milk, and the effect of the drug on the baby. Some drugs can also affect the milk supply.

Ask about

Age of baby.
Weight of baby.
History of taking drug (i.e., was the drug taken during pregnancy?).
How long the drug will be taken.

ASSESSMENT

ROUTINE CARE NEEDED?
   Are any of the following present?
      Drug compatibility with lactation.

IF YES,   *Consult up-to-date drug references and call lactation provider today.*

SELF CARE INFORMATION

Do not self-medicate while breastfeeding without discussing the drug with your health care provider. This includes prescription, over-the-counter, and street drugs, as well as herbs, tinctures, vitamins, minerals, and other nutritional supplements.

Tell every health care provider that you are breastfeeding.

If you are prescribed a drug that is not compatible with breastfeeding, ask if there is an alternative drug that is.

IMPORTANT CONDITIONS TO REPORT

Any changes in the baby's behavior or appearance.

Any changes in your milk supply.

Notes

An up-to-date drug reference should be consulted to determine the safety and possible side effects of individual drugs.

Newborn and premature babies are at greater risk of drug side effects due to limited ability to clear drugs from their systems.

See also Medications

Drug References

AAP Committee on Drugs. (2001). The transfer of drugs and other chemicals into human milk. *Pediatrics, 108,* 776–789.

Briggs, G.G., Freeman, R.K., & Yaffee, S.J. (Eds.). (2002). *Drugs in pregnancy and lactation* (6th ed.). Philadelphia: Lippincott, Williams and Wilkins.

Hale, T.W. (2004). *Medications and mothers milk.* Amarillo, TX: Pharmasoft Publishing.

Lawrence, R.A., & Lawrence, R.M. (2005). *Breastfeeding: A guide for the medical profession* (6th ed.). St. Louis: Mosby.

▶ Drugs, contraindicated

DEFINITION   Drugs taken by the mother that make it inadvisable to breastfeed.

According to the American Academy of Pediatrics, breastfeeding is rarely contraindicated by medication use, except for "mothers who are receiving diagnostic or therapeutic radioactive isotopes or have had exposure to radioactive materials (for as long as there is radioactivity in the milk); mothers who are receiving antimetabolites or chemotherapeutic agents or a small number of other medications until they clear the milk; [and] mothers who are using drugs of abuse ('street drugs')."

Notes

An up-to-date drug reference should be consulted to determine the safety and possible side effects of individual drugs.

> Newborn and premature babies are at greater risk of drug side effects due to limited ability to clear drugs from their systems.

Footnotes

[96]AAP Section on Breastfeeding. (2005). Breastfeeding and the use of human milk. Pediatrics, *115*, 497.

Drug References

AAP Committee on Drugs. (2001). The transfer of drugs and other chemicals into human milk. *Pediatrics, 108*, 776–789.

Briggs, G.G., Freeman, R.K., & Yaffee, S.J. (Eds.). (2002). *Drugs in pregnancy and lactation* (6th ed.). Philadelphia: Lippincott, Williams and Wilkins.

Hale, T.W. (2004). *Medications and mothers milk.* Amarillo, TX: Pharmasoft Publishing.

Lawrence, R.A., & Lawrence, R.M. (2005). *Breastfeeding: A guide for the medical profession* (6th ed.). St. Louis: Mosby.

▶ Dry-up medication

DEFINITION Medications such as bromocriptine (Parlodel®) were once used to dry up the milk of women who did not wish to breastfeed. Several deaths were attributed to bromocriptine use. This drug is no longer approved for use as dry-up medication.

Notes

The American Academy of Pediatrics lists bromocriptine in the Table 5 (drugs associated with significant side effects and should be given with caution).[97] Hale lists bromocriptine as a category L5 (contraindicated) drug.[98]

See also Weaning

Footnotes

[97]AAP Committee on Drugs. (2001). The transfer of drugs and other chemicals into human milk. *Pediatrics, 108*, 779.

[98]Hale, T.W. (2004). *Medications and mothers milk.* Amarillo, TX: Pharmasoft Publishing, 98.

▶ Ducts and ductules

DEFINITION   The tubes and tubules within the breast that carry milk from the alveoli through the breast tissue and out through the nipple pores.

See also Plugged ducts

▶ Ear infection

DEFINITION   An infection or inflammation of the middle ear, also called "otitis media." The inflammation may begin with an infection that causes a sore throat, cold, or other respiratory or breathing problem. Babies who are breastfed have a lower incidence of otitis media compared to babies who are not.

Ask about

Age of baby.
History of sore throat, cold, respiratory, or breathing problem.
Change in breastfeeding behavior.

ASSESSMENT

PROMPT CARE NEEDED?

   Are any of the following present?

   Unusual irritability.

   Difficulty sleeping.

   Tugging or pulling at one or both ears.

   Fever.

   Fluid draining from one or both ears.

IF YES,   *Seek medical care today.*

PROMPT LACTATION CARE NEEDED?

   Are any of the following present?

   Difficulty breastfeeding.

   Crying at the breast or pulling away and crying after a few sucks.

   Baby has been treated for ear infection but continues to fret or cry at the breast.

IF YES,   *Call lactation care provider today.*

SELF CARE INFORMATION

Even after the otitis media has resolved, the baby may be uncomfortable nursing or may remember the pain of nursing. Changing positions may help. If the problem persists, have the ears checked again by the health care provider.

Keep the breasts soft and express excess milk during the time the baby is not nursing well.

IMPORTANT CONDITIONS TO REPORT

Less urination or stooling.

Continued symptoms of otitis media after treatment.

Continued problems with breastfeeding after treatment is initiated.

See also Acute infection

▶ Eczema

DEFINITION   An allergic inflammation of the skin characterized by itching, redness, and scaling.

Ask about

Onset.

Age of baby.

Medications used.

ASSESSMENT

PROMPT CARE NEEDED?

Are any of the following present?

Eczema on the breast.

Eczema on the baby.

Questions about medications.

IF YES,   *Seek medical care today.*

IMPORTANT CONDITIONS TO REPORT

Allergy and eczema in parents and siblings.

Infant symptoms of blood in stool, wheezing, hives, facial swelling, runny nose, vomiting, and irritability.

Notes

Research has identified that exclusive breastfeeding reduces the risk of atopic eczema in susceptible children.

In adults, atopic eczema is typically treated with topical steroid creams. The specific cream indicated should be examined in an up-to-date drug reference to ensure it is safe for use by the breastfeeding mother.

Steroid cream use is of greater concern when the affected area is on the breast where the baby's mouth will be placed, as the baby will then absorb the steroid both through direct contact and through the milk.

In the breastfed baby, atopic eczema may be a symptom of food allergy, related to an allergen in food that the mother or baby is consuming. Mother and baby should avoid consuming offending allergens such as cow's milk, fish, eggs, peanuts, and tree nuts.

Infantile symptoms of an allergic reaction include hives, facial swelling, runny nose, wheezing, eczema, vomiting, irritability (colic), blood in the stool, and **anaphylaxis**. Treatment centers on identification and avoidance of the proteins that are triggering the allergic reaction.

Babies born into allergic families are more likely to develop allergy, particularly those with two allergic parents or one allergic parent and an allergic sibling. Exclusive breastfeeding is the optimal feeding choice for these babies in particular.

Hypoallergenic formula is recommended when supplementing babies with documented allergy and has been suggested as a preferable supplemental formula in babies with a strong family history (biparental, parental, and/or sibling) of allergy.[99]

See also Allergy in the breastfed baby

Footnotes

[99]AAP Committee on Nutrition. Hypoallergenic infant formulas. (2000). *Pediatrics, 106,* 348.

Drug References

AAP Committee on Drugs. (2001). The transfer of drugs and other chemicals into human milk. *Pediatrics, 108,* 776–789.

Briggs, G.G., Freeman, R.K., & Yaffee, S.J. (Eds.). (2002). *Drugs in pregnancy and lactation* (6th ed.). Philadelphia: Lippincott, Williams and Wilkins.

Hale, T.W. (2004). *Medications and mothers milk.* Amarillo, TX: Pharmasoft Publishing.

Lawrence, R.A., & Lawrence, R.M. (2005). *Breastfeeding: A guide for the medical profession* (6th ed.). St. Louis: Mosby.

▶ Electronic scales

DEFINITION   Sensitive weighing devices which can be used to monitor growth of infants, and when highly sensitive, used to estimate the amount of milk transferred from the breast to the baby during a feeding.

Ask about

Age of baby.
Reason for needing scale.

ASSESSMENT

EMERGENT CARE NEEDED?

Are any of the following present?

Newborn with greater than ten percent weight loss.

Infant who does not wake for feedings.

Baby below birthweight at 10 days.

Cessation of weight gain.

Fewer than three bowel movements daily in breastfed newborn after first 2 days of life.

Inadequate urination or dark urine.

IF YES,   *Seek medical care within 2 to 4 hours.*

PROMPT CARE NEEDED?

Are any of the following present?

Concerns about milk supply.

History of inadequate milk transfer.

Baby with a known diagnosis that could negatively impact milk supply (e.g., Down syndrome, clefts, prematurity).

Mother with a history of breast surgery.

Mother with two inverted nipples.

IF YES, *Call lactation care provider today.*

ROUTINE CARE NEEDED?
Are any of the following present?

Scale rental with none of above indicators.

IF YES, *Manufacturer, distributor, equipment sales.*

SELF CARE INFORMATION

Frequent feedings are the key to adequate milk production. Expect 10–12 feedings per 24 hours.

If using an electronic scale to estimate weight gain, be sure to weigh baby before and after feedings wearing the same clothing, without changing the diaper.

Track intake over several feedings and average the results. The amount of milk consumed normally varies widely from feed to feed.

IMPORTANT CONDITIONS TO REPORT

Inadequate weight gain.

Ongoing concerns.

Notes

Scales with breastmilk intake function can be rented from breast pump distributors.

See also Milk transfer—estimating; Test weighing; Weight gain—baby

▶ Employment and breastfeeding

DEFINITION   Mothers who work for pay may do so away from home or in the home. Employed mothers may be separated from their baby or have the baby nearby.

In the United States, more than half of the mothers with babies under the age of 1 year are employed.

Ask about

Amount of separation—hours per day, days per week.
Start date of work.
Age of baby.
Mother's plans to continue breastfeeding.
Mother's plans to express milk.
Accommodations at work for expressing and saving milk.
How the baby will be fed away from the mother.

ASSESSMENT

ROUTINE CARE NEEDED?
Are any of the following present?
Information about managing work and breastfeeding.

IF YES, *Call lactation care provider.*

SELF CARE INFORMATION

Stress does not seem to affect milk supply but frequent milk removal is needed to maintain or improve the milk supply.
Milk can be collected and frozen in the early weeks to supplement milk collected after mother's return to work.
Milk supply is best maintained by using a pump that is intended for that purpose.
Select child care facilities carefully.
Expressed milk is a raw food and should be refrigerated immediately if possible.
The timing of return to work and the number of hours spent away from the baby affect the duration of breastfeeding more than the type of work a woman does.

IMPORTANT CONDITIONS TO REPORT

Problems with expressing milk (check that the equipment is working properly).
Breast problems.
Problems with the infant accepting expressed milk.

See also Collection and storage of milk; Day care; Decreasing milk supply

▶ Ending a feeding

DEFINITION Babies make a seal at the breast with their lips and tongue. In addition, the chin is drawn into the breast and held there firmly during suckling.

In order to "take the baby off of the breast" the mother needs to break the seal. She can do this by inserting her clean finger into the corner of the baby's mouth or by pressing down onto her breast to break the seal.

SELF CARE INFORMATION

Satisfied babies end feedings by themselves. Feedings should not be timed or routinely ended by mother.

IMPORTANT CONDITIONS TO REPORT

Nipple pain.
Baby does not end feeding.
Deep breast pain.

▶ Engorgement

DEFINITION Swelling in the breast associated with increase in the flow of blood and lymph to the breast, as well as the manufacture of milk. More common in the first days postpartum, engorgement may also occur whenever feedings are infrequent.

Ask about

Onset.
Age of baby.
Feeding pattern.

EMERGENT CARE NEEDED?

Are any of the following present?

Symptoms of infection (fever, aching, chills, and malaise).

Red streaks on the breast.

IF YES, *Seek medical care within 2 to 4 hours.*

PROMPT CARE NEEDED?

Are any of the following present?

Baby unable to latch onto breast.

Engorgement not resolving after latch-on.

IF YES, *Call lactation care provider today.*

SELF CARE INFORMATION

Consider soaking breasts in warm water before feedings or applying cool gel packs between feedings.

Gently hand express to soften breasts before feedings.

Nonprescription anti-inflammatory agents may also be helpful.

IMPORTANT CONDITIONS TO REPORT

Lack of resolution in 24–48 hours.

Symptoms of infection (fever, chills, aching, redness, and malaise).

Notes

Engorgement is best resolved by softening the breast so that baby can latch onto the breast. Nursing the baby offers more relief than does pumping.

See also Breast infection; Hand expression of breastmilk

▶ Environmental contaminants

DEFINITION   All foods, including breastmilk, may contain traces of chemical contaminants present in the environment. Breastmilk is one of the easiest and least painful body tissues to sample. For this reason, it is used to monitor population exposure to chemicals. According to the American Academy of Pediatrics, low-level exposure to contaminants should not contraindicate breastfeeding.[100]

Ask about

Known contaminant exposure.
Age of baby.

ASSESSMENT

EMERGENT CARE NEEDED?
Are any of the following present?
Sudden exposure of mother to toxic chemical.

IF YES, *Seek emergency care now.*

PROMPT CARE NEEDED?
Are any of the following present?
History of high level exposure to toxic chemicals in a breastfeeding woman.

IF YES, *Call maternal medical care provider today.*

ROUTINE CARE NEEDED?
Are any of the following present?
General questions about environmental exposure.

IF YES, *Call lactation care provider.*

IMPORTANT CONDITIONS TO REPORT
Known history of environmental or workplace exposure to toxic chemicals.
Any negative effects of past exposure.

Notes

Women who know they have been exposed to specific chemicals or pollutants should consult with their physician regarding analysis of the contaminant content of their milk. Several contaminants are addressed in the American Academy of Pediatrics's drug reference.

> Many researchers have looked for negative effects of toxin exposure via breastmilk and have found only benefits for breastfed babies, as compared with formula fed babies.

See also DDT in breastmilk; Pesticides and pollutants in breastmilk

Footnotes
[100]AAP Section on Breastfeeding. (2001). Breastfeeding and the use of human milk. *Pediatrics, 115,* 497.

▶ Enzymes in breastmilk

DEFINITION   Proteins such as lipoprotein lipase and amylase that assist in metabolism, digestion, and growth are found in human milk.

▶ Epidermal growth factor

DEFINITION   A component in human milk that triggers the growth of the skin cells lining the gastrointestinal and respiratory tracts.

▶ Epidural anesthesia and breastfeeding

DEFINITION   Administration of drugs to the spinal cord to cause partial loss of sensation during childbirth and painful procedures.

SELF CARE INFORMATION
When mothers receive pain medications during the birth process, extended skin-to-skin contact should be practiced until the infant shows feeding cues.

IMPORTANT CONDITIONS TO REPORT
Feeding difficulties.

See also Analgesia; Anesthesia; Childbirth; Demerol; Medications

Drug References

AAP Committee on Drugs. (2001). The transfer of drugs and other chemicals into human milk. *Pediatrics, 108,* 776–789.

Briggs, G.G., Freeman, R.K., & Yaffee, S.J. (Eds.). (2002). *Drugs in pregnancy and lactation* (6th ed.). Philadelphia: Lippincott, Williams and Wilkins.

Hale, T.W. (2004). *Medications and mothers milk.* Amarillo, TX: Pharmasoft Publishing.

Lawrence, R.A., & Lawrence, R.M. (2005). *Breastfeeding: A guide for the medical profession* (6th ed.). St. Louis: Mosby.

▶ Epilepsy and breastfeeding

DEFINITION   A disorder of the electrical rhythm in the central nervous system, characterized by seizures. Mothers and babies with epilepsy can breastfeed.

IMPORTANT CONDITIONS TO REPORT

Any unusual symptoms in the baby of the epileptic mother.

> **Notes**
>
> A number of drugs are used to treat epilepsy. An up-to-date drug reference should be consulted to determine the safety and possible side effects of individual drugs.
>
> Newborn and premature babies are at greater risk of side effects due to limited ability to clear drugs from their systems.
>
> Breastfeeding is thought to provide gradual withdrawal for the baby exposed to mother's epilepsy medications in utero.

Drug References

AAP Committee on Drugs. (2001). The transfer of drugs and other chemicals into human milk. *Pediatrics, 108,* 776–789.

Briggs, G.G., Freeman, R.K., & Yaffee, S.J. (Eds.). (2002). *Drugs in pregnancy and lactation* (6th ed.). Philadelphia: Lippincott, Williams and Wilkins.

Hale, T.W. (2004). *Medications and mothers milk.* Amarillo, TX: Pharmasoft Publishing.

Lawrence, R.A., & Lawrence, R.M. (2005). *Breastfeeding: A guide for the medical profession* (6th ed.). St. Louis: Mosby.

▶ Exclusive breastfeeding

DEFINITION Giving no other food or drink to a breastfed infant.

▶ Exercise and breastfeeding

DEFINITION Physical exertion is a normal part of the life of lactating women around the globe. There is no reason for lactating women to refrain from exercise. For comfort, mothers may want to select a well-fitting supportive bra that does not compress their breasts.

▶ Expression of mothers' milk

DEFINITION Removal of milk from the breast via compression and vacuum. Expression may be accomplished by hand or pump.

Ask about

Reason mother plans to express milk.

ASSESSMENT

PROMPT CARE NEEDED?

Are any of the following present?

Imminent separation of mother and baby.

IF YES, *Call lactation care provider today.*

SELF CARE INFORMATION

Wash hands before beginning.

Practice hand expression when baby is latched onto one breast.

Gently massage and then compress the breast.

Your skill will improve with practice.

Store expressed milk in the refrigerator, a cooler with ice packs, or the freezer if it will not be used within 48 hours.

Follow safe milk storage guidelines.

IMPORTANT CONDITIONS TO REPORT

Questions or problems with this technique.

See also Breast pump; Collection and storage of breastmilk

▶ Failure to thrive (FTT)

DEFINITION A condition in which a child's size and growth rate is significantly below that of average children. There are multiple causes for FTT ranging from organic problems such as metabolic disorders, cerebral palsy, and organ defects, as well as psychological and social causes. FTT occurs in both formula fed and breastfed infants.

Ask about

Onset.

Age of baby.

Feeding method.

EMERGENT CARE NEEDED?

Are any of the following present?

Meconium bowel movements after 5 days of life.

Fewer than 3 bowel movements daily in breastfed newborn after the first two days of life.

No urine in six hours.

Brick dust urine (uric acid crystals) after 2 days of life.

Dark colored urine.

Fewer than 4 urinations daily in the breastfed newborn after day 5.

Noticeably sunken fontanelles (soft spot on top of head).

Decreased activity.

Baby below birthweight at 10–14 days.

Cessation of weight gain.

IF YES, | *Seek medical care within 2 to 4 hours.*

PROMPT CARE NEEDED?

Are any of the following present?

Concern about inadequate infant growth.

IF YES, | *Call pediatric care provider today.*

Are any of the following present?

Diagnosed FTT in a breastfed child.

IF YES, | *Referral to growth and nutrition department.*

Are any of the following present?

Continued breastfeeding in a child diagnosed with FTT.

IF YES, | *Call lactation care provider today.*

SELF CARE INFORMATION

Practice skin-to-skin contact frequently.

Watch for hunger cues (signs that say "feed me" include hand-to-face or hand-to-mouth movements, lip smacking, seeking with lips, rooting, and head bobbing).

Feed baby at first sign of hunger cues.

Expect 10–12 unscheduled feedings in 24 hours.

Allow baby to end feedings.

IMPORTANT CONDITIONS TO REPORT

Infant disinterest in feeding.

Ongoing problems with milk supply.

> **Notes**
>
> Growth expectations are different in breastfed infants after the first 6 months of age. Because growth charts are based on mixed fed children, breastfeeding babies may appear to fall a few percentiles on the charts sometime between 4 and 12 months of age. This should be individually evaluated, but such an occurrence may be an artifact of the charts.

See also Milk supply, inadequate

▶ Fasting and breastfeeding

DEFINITION   Going without food for periods of six hours or more. Fasting may be performed in preparation for certain medical tests (e.g., blood glucose), as a religious observance (e.g., during Ramadan for Muslims), or as a misguided weight loss plan. Short term fasting is not thought to have a negative effect on milk production. Breastfeeding women should continue to drink to satisfy thirst during a period of fasting (unless not allowed in the case of fasting before blood work or surgery).

SELF CARE INFORMATION

If fasting is considered for religious purposes, check with your religious leader. For example, in many areas, breastfeeding women are exempted from the requirement to fast during Ramadan.

If fasting is recommended for a surgical procedure for baby, ask the surgeon or anesthesiologist how long baby should fast before surgery. Fasting is typically recommended for four hours prior to surgery for breastfed infants.

See also Maternal diet

▶ Fathers and breastfeeding

DEFINITION   The father of the baby plays an important role in the mother's opinion of and success with breastfeeding.

▶ Fatigue, maternal

DEFINITION   Exhaustion, weariness, or lack of energy. May be the result of lack of sleep. May also be associated with anemia, depression, infection, underactive or overactive thyroid, pain, and the use of some drugs (including prescription drugs).

Ask about

Onset of symptom of fatigue.
Age of baby.
Weight gain of baby.

ASSESSMENT

EMERGENT CARE NEEDED?
Are any of the following present?

Fever.

Confusion.

Dizziness.

Blurred vision.

Swelling, weight gain, and little or no urine.

IF YES,   *Seek emergency care now.*

PROMPT CARE NEEDED?

Are any of the following present?

Ongoing fatigue.

Constipation.

Intolerance to cold.

Dry skin.

Headache.

Sadness or depression.

Insomnia.

IF YES, *Seek medical care today.*

ROUTINE CARE NEEDED?

Are any of the following present?

Questions about frequency of nighttime and daytime nursings.

Concern about weight gain pattern of baby.

Questions about fatigue and breastfeeding.

IF YES, *Call lactation care provider today.*

SELF CARE INFORMATION

Although tiredness is common postpartum, fatigue should be investigated since it can be a nonspecific symptom of other problems.

IMPORTANT CONDITIONS TO REPORT

Fatigue that is not relieved by sleep.

See also Anemia; Hypothyroidism; Postpartum depression

▶ Fat in breastmilk

DEFINITION   A calorie rich nutrient in human milk. Fat is composed of fatty acids of different lengths. The long-chain fats in human milk are particularly noted for their beneficial effects on the growth of brain and nerve cells.

Age of baby.
Questions about milk supply.
Adequacy of growth.

ASSESSMENT

PROMPT CARE NEEDED?

Are any of the following present?
Concern about inadequate infant growth.

IF YES, *Call pediatric care provider today.*

Are any of the following present?
Slow weight gain in a breastfed child.

IF YES, *Call lactation care provider.*

SELF CARE INFORMATION

Practice skin-to-skin contact frequently.
Watch for hunger cues (signs that say "feed me" include hand-to-face or hand-to-mouth movements, lip smacking, seeking with lips, rooting, and head bobbing).
Feed baby at first sign of hunger cues.
Expect 10–12 unscheduled feedings in 24 hours.
Allow baby to end feedings.

IMPORTANT CONDITIONS TO REPORT

Infant disinterest in feeding.
Ongoing problems with milk supply.

Notes

Fat content in milk varies throughout the day and within each feeding, depending on how full the breast is, as well as how well the baby or pump is eliciting the milk ejection reflex, which flushes fat down through the breast.

It is very rare for the caloric composition of human milk to be inadequate. Routine testing of the fat or other content of milk is not recommended, due to diurnal variation and the difficulty of collecting a representative sample.

See also Arachidonic acid; Docosahexaenoic acid in breastmilk; Caloric density of milk

▶ Fat-soluble vitamins in breastmilk

DEFINITION   Organic chemicals required by the body in small amounts. Vitamins are divided into two groups: fat-soluble and water-soluble. Vitamins A, D, E, and K are the fat-soluble vitamins found in human milk.

> **Notes**
>
> According to the American Academy of Pediatrics, "All breastfed infants should receive 200 IU of oral vitamin D drops daily beginning during the first 2 months of life and continuing until the daily consumption of vitamin D-fortified formula or milk is 500 mL."[101]

Footnotes
   [101] AAP Section on Breastfeeding. (2005). Breastfeeding and the use of human milk. *Pediatrics, 115,* 500.

▶ FDA
See also Food and Drug Administration (FDA)

▶ Feeding cues

DEFINITION   Infant behaviors that indicate hunger and satiety (fullness).
   Adults can learn to read feeding cues to aid in breastfeeding and the overall development of the parent–child relationship.

SELF CARE INFORMATION
   Practice frequent skin-to-skin contact with baby to learn feeding cues.
   Signs that say "feed me" include hand-to-face or hand-to-mouth movements, lip smacking, seeking with lips, rooting, and head bobbing.
   Signs of fullness include removing mouth from nipple with relaxed body tone, falling asleep during feeding, and general bodily relaxation.

▶ Feeding methods, alternate

DEFINITION   Ways of supplementing a breastfed baby that avoid introduction of a bottle.

Ask about

Reason for supplementation or alternate feeding.

ASSESSMENT

PROMPT CARE NEEDED?
>   *Are any of the following present?*
>   Baby unable to withdraw milk from the breast.

IF YES,   *Seek medical care within 2 to 4 hours.*

>   *Are any of the following present?*
>   Need or desire to supplement baby.

IF YES,   *Call lactation care provider today.*

SELF CARE INFORMATION
   Clean devices carefully according to product literature.

IMPORTANT CONDITIONS TO REPORT
   Difficulty with feeding method.

   See also At-breast supplementation; Bottle feeding; Cup-feeding; Feeding tube devices; Finger-feeding; Gavage feeding; Tube feeding

▶ Feeding pattern of breastfed infants

DEFINITION   The observed method or schedule of seeking nutrition. Observation of breastfed newborns indicates that while most babies nurse 10–12 times or more over 24 hours, they tend to do so in a clustered feeding pattern. That is, young babies tend to have a cycle of short, closely spaced feedings interspersed with periods of rest or sleep. This pattern is associated with good milk production and growth.

Age of baby.

Current feeding pattern.

ASSESSMENT

EMERGENT CARE NEEDED?

Are any of the following present?

Sudden disinterest in feeding.

Extreme **lethargy** in baby.

Sudden change in baby's muscle tone (extremely floppy or stiff).

IF YES, *Seek emergency care now.*

PROMPT MEDICAL CARE NEEDED?

Are any of the following present?

Meconium bowel movements after 5 days of life.

Fewer than 3 bowel movements daily in breastfed newborn after the first two days of life.

No urine in six hours.

Brick dust urine (uric acid crystals) after 2 days of life.

Dark colored urine.

Fewer than 4 urinations daily in the breastfed newborn after day 5.

Noticeably sunken fontanelles (soft spot on top of head).

Decreased activity.

Baby below birthweight at 10–14 days.

Cessation of weight gain.

IF YES, *Seek pediatric care within 2 to 4 hours.*

PROMPT LACTATION CARE NEEDED?

Are any of the following present?

Fewer than eight feedings per day in a newborn.

Concerns about adequacy of milk supply.

Young baby waking frequently at night to feed.

IF YES, *Call lactation care provider today.*

SELF CARE INFORMATION

Practice skin-to-skin contact frequently.

Watch for hunger cues (signs that say "feed me" include hand-to-face or hand-to-mouth movements, lip smacking, seeking with lips, rooting, and head bobbing).

Feed baby at first sign of hunger cues.

Practice good attachment.

Expect 10–12 feedings per 24 hours (feedings may occur in clusters—3 or 4 feedings in 2 hours, followed by a few hours of rest, then more clusters, rest, etc.).

Listen for signs of baby swallowing.

Allow baby to end feedings.

Expect at least 3–4 infant stools per 24 hours after the first 4 days of life.

Good positioning and attachment are crucial to reduce nipple pain.

If feedings are missed, hand express or pump milk to maintain supply.

IMPORTANT CONDITIONS TO REPORT

Inadequate feeding (less than 10 feedings daily in the newborn).

Inadequate stooling pattern (less than three stools daily).

See also Cluster feeding

▶ Feeding tube devices

DEFINITION   Administration of extra fluids (expressed breastmilk or formula) to the baby through a tube. Tube devices may be attached to the breast (at-breast feeding), a finger (finger-feeding), or inserted into the baby's stomach through the nose (gavage feeding).

Ask about

Reason for device.

PROMPT CARE NEEDED?

Are any of the following present?

Baby unable to withdraw milk from the breast.

IF YES, *Seek pediatric care within 2 to 4 hours.*

Are any of the following present?

Need or desire to use a feeding tube device with a breastfed baby.

Problems with a feeding tube device.

IF YES, *Call lactation care provider today.*

SELF CARE INFORMATION

Clean devices carefully according to product literature.

IMPORTANT CONDITIONS TO REPORT

Difficulty with feeding method.

Notes

At-breast supplementation is useful when a baby is not receiving an adequate amount of milk from the breast. This may be due to a temporary or permanent problem with milk supply on the part of the mother. It may also result from weak or inefficient suckling on the part of the baby, due to temporary or permanent conditions (e.g., prematurity, undernourishment, Down syndrome, cardiac problems).

Gavage feeding is typically practiced in hospital settings and can be a supportive step toward full breastfeeding with the ill or premature baby.

See also At-breast supplementation; Bottle feeding; Cup-feeding; Feeding methods, alternate; Finger-feeding; Gavage feeding

▶ Fenugreek

DEFINITION   An herb frequently used in teas and syrups. Fenugreek has been sold as a galactagogue (substance that increases milk), but there is currently little scientific evidence of this effect. Fenugreek may interfere with the absorption of many medications.

▶ Fertility

DEFINITION   Referring to a woman's ability to conceive and carry a child. Breastfeeding is associated with decreased fertility in the first six months following birth. This is due to amenorrhea, a period of cessation of menses (monthly flow of blood from the uterus).

Ask about

Age of infant.
Feeding pattern.

ASSESSMENT

PROMPT CARE NEEDED?

Are any of the following present?

Desire to extend lactational amenorrhea.

IF YES,   *Call lactation provider today.*

ROUTINE CARE NEEDED?

Are any of the following present?

Concern about prolonged lack of menses.
Concern about contraceptive usage.
Desire to conceive again.

IF YES,   *Schedule routine medical visit.*

SELF CARE INFORMATION

Characteristics of breastfeeding thought to increase the chances of amenorrhea include baby younger than 6 months, **exclusive breastfeeding,** unrestricted feeding (at least 10–12 feedings per day), avoidance of pacifiers, and **co-sleeping**. Once any of these criteria is no longer true, secure another family planning method (unless pregnancy is desired at this time).

IMPORTANT CONDITIONS TO REPORT

Past fertility problems.
Resumption of menstrual period.

Notes

Women who continue to breastfeed exclusively during the first 6 months of their baby's life are likely to experience amenorrhea (that is, no menstrual period). Many breastfeeding women experience amenorrhea of a year or more, as long as they continue to breastfeed frequently.

Lactational Amenorrhea Method (LAM) is a form of natural family planning which is 98% effective in the first six months following the birth of a baby, so long as the mother's menses have not returned, her baby is exclusively breastfed, and there are no long periods of time between feedings, day and night. Once the baby is older than 6 months, or any of the above criteria is no longer true, LAM is no longer effective and mothers should utilize other forms of birth control.

See also Bellagio Consensus; Contraception; Lactational Amenorrhea Method (LAM); Menstrual cycle; Natural family planning

▶ Fever and breastfeeding

DEFINITION Elevated body temperature is a sign of inflammation or infection. There is no reason to stop breastfeeding during a fever, except in the case of contraindicated infections.*

Fever can also follow epidural anesthesia.

Fever in a breastfeeding woman may be a symptom of inflammatory process in the breast.

Ask about

Onset.
Age of baby.

EMERGENT CARE NEEDED?

Are any of the following present?

About baby:

Extreme **lethargy**.

Sudden change in muscle tone (extremely floppy or stiff).

Sudden disinterest in feeding.

Unable to wake baby.

IF YES, *Seek emergency care now.*

PROMPT CARE NEEDED?

Are any of the following present?

About mother:

Fever higher than 100°F (37.7°C).

Extreme breast discomfort.

Flulike aching throughout body.

Extreme exhaustion.

Visible or palpable breast **abscess**.

About baby:

Extreme discomfort.

Fever higher than 100°F (37.7°C) in a baby younger than three months of age.

Vomiting and diarrhea that last for more than a few hours in a child of any age.

Rash accompanied by a fever.

A cold that gets worse and includes a fever.

Ear pain or drainage from an ear.

Sore throat or problems swallowing.

Sharp or persistent pains in the abdomen or stomach.

Fever and vomiting at the same time.

Not eating for more than a day in the older baby who is eating solid foods.

IF YES, *Seek medical care now.*

ROUTINE CARE NEEDED?

Are any of the following present?

Fever higher than 100°F (37.7°C) in an older baby or child.

Any cough or cold that does not get better in several days.

IF YES, *Call pediatric care provider today.*

SELF CARE INFORMATION

Feed baby at least 10–24 times per 24 hours.

Soften breasts between feedings with gentle hand expression.

Finish full course of antibiotics prescribed (unless told to stop by a physician).

Continue nonprescription pain relief as recommended.

Continue to monitor for symptoms of recurring breast infection (redness, heat, fever, chills, pain).

IMPORTANT CONDITIONS TO REPORT

Symptoms worsen or persist.

Signs of infection.

Notes

Rarely, babies experience life threatening infections or events that cause extreme lethargy and disinterest in feeding. They may be suddenly floppy or stiff. These symptoms indicate a medical emergency, as they may reflect botulism or other life threatening infection.

Many mothers experiencing **mastitis** may mistake symptoms of mastitis for flu. When a mother calls to ask for recommendations of safe flu medications, remember to ask her if she has any red, painful, hot spots on her breasts. See **Mastitis** for more information.

Few infections are incompatible with breastfeeding.

*Infections in the breastfeeding mother that are not compatible with breastfeeding include **HIV, HTLV-1,** and active **herpes** lesion on the nipple and/or other area that will be in contact with baby's mouth.[102]

Mothers with certain infections may breastfeed once a period of treatment is initiated. These infections include tuberculosis, hepatitis, and Lyme disease. The Centers for Disease Control and Prevention and state health departments can provide further information.

See also Breast infection; Mastitis

Footnotes
[102]AAP Section on Breastfeeding. (2005). Breastfeeding and the use of human milk. *Pediatrics, 115*, 496–506.

▶ Fibroadenoma and breastfeeding

DEFINITION   A benign tumor found in the breast. Fibroadenomas are compatible with breastfeeding.

SELF CARE INFORMATION
Routine breast self exam should be performed monthly.
Continue breast screening as recommended by medical care provider.

IMPORTANT CONDITIONS TO REPORT
New lumps.
Changes to existing lumps.

See also Breast lumps

▶ Fibrocystic breasts

DEFINITION   A common breast condition in women including variable lumpiness, tenderness, and palpable cysts (pockets of fluid). Symptoms may change during the menstrual period. This benign condition is compatible with breastfeeding.

> **Notes**
>
> New lumps in the breast should be medically examined to rule out **plugged ducts** and other problems.
>   Women who have experienced fibrocystic breasts may misdiagnose plugged ducts and other breastfeeding problems as fibrocystic changes.

See also Breast lumps; Plugged ducts

▶ Finger-feeding

DEFINITION A feeding technique that includes taping or otherwise attaching a feeding tube to a parent or health care provider's finger, and inserting the finger into
the baby's mouth. Expressed breastmilk or formula contained in the feeding syringe
is then allowed to flow into the baby's mouth in response to suckling motions.

Efficacy and safety of finger-feeding have not been established.

Finger-feeding offers no known advantage to at-breast feeding or cup-feeding.
Whenever possible, infants requiring supplementation should be fed with an at-
breast device to maximize stimulation of milk and maternal control of feeding.

▶ Flat nipples

DEFINITION A nipple that does not change in protruberance when the areola is
compressed.

Ask about

Appearance of nipple.
Action of nipple when the areola is compressed.
Nipple changes during pregnancy and lactation.
Diagnosis of "flat" nipple.

ASSESSMENT

PROMPT MEDICAL CARE NEEDED?
Are any of the following present?
Meconium bowel movements after 5 days of life.
Fewer than 3 bowel movements daily in breastfed newborn after the first
two days of life.
No urine in six hours.
Brick dust urine (uric acid crystals) after 2 days of life.

Dark colored urine.

Fewer than 4 urinations daily in the breastfed newborn after day 5.

Noticeably sunken fontanelles (soft spot on top of head).

Decreased activity.

Baby below birthweight at 10–14 days.

Cessation of weight gain.

IF YES, *Seek pediatric care within 2 to 4 hours.*

PROMPT LACTATION CARE NEEDED?

Are any of the following present?

Poor feeding.

Poor milk transfer.

Inadequate weight gain.

Problems with latch-on.

Concern about milk supply.

IF YES, *Call lactation care provider today.*

SELF CARE INFORMATION

Training flat nipples to stand out during pregnancy has not been demonstrated to be effective.

Mothers with "flat" nipples should be encouraged to express milk early and frequently until baby is able to facilitate nipple stretching well into the mouth.

IMPORTANT CONDITIONS TO REPORT

Poor feeding.

Poor milk transfer.

Inadequate weight gain.

Problems with latch-on.

See also **Milk transfer; Weight gain**

▶ **Flu, maternal**

DEFINITION Flu, or influenza, is a viral infection. This condition is compatible with breastfeeding.

SELF CARE INFORMATION

Examine your breasts and nipples for any sign of inflammation.
Continue to breastfeed.

IMPORTANT CONDITIONS TO REPORT

Any redness, pain, or tenderness of the breast.

> **Notes**
>
> Symptoms of flu (fever, body aches, and chills) may also indicate breast inflammation or infection.

See also **Fever and breastfeeding; Mastitis**

▶ Fluid needs of breastfeeding mother

DEFINITION   Amount of water and watery liquids required daily for lactation. Mothers should drink to satisfy thirst during lactation for their own health. Only in severe dehydration would fluid status affect milk production.

> **Notes**
>
> Research indicates that increasing maternal fluids has no effect on volume or composition of milk produced.

▶ Fluoride and breastfeeding

DEFINITION   A compound of the trace mineral fluorine. Fluoride helps harden the teeth during formation and protects erupted teeth from decay.

Footnotes

[103]AAP Section on Breastfeeding. (2005). Breastfeeding and the use of human milk. *Pediatrics, 115*, 500.

▶ Flutter sucking

DEFINITION   A light, fast sucking associated with little or no milk transfer. This phenomenon is also called nonnutritive suckling.

See also Nonnutritive suckling; Uncoordinated suck

▶ Food allergies and breastfeeding

DEFINITION   An abnormal immune reaction to substances that are eaten.

Ask about

Onset.
Age of baby.
Known allergies.

EMERGENT CARE NEEDED?

Are any of the following present?

Difficulty breathing.

Difficulty swallowing.

Swelling of tongue.

IF YES, *Seek emergency care now.*

PROMPT CARE NEEDED?

Are any of the following present in the baby?

Swelling of the face, hands, or feet.

Persistent rash, headache, or fever.

Persistent diarrhea, nausea, or vomiting.

Bloody stool.

IF YES, *Seek pediatric care within 2 to 4 hours.*

ROUTINE CARE NEEDED?

Are any of the following present in the baby?

Suspected reaction to food.

Occasional nausea, vomiting, or diarrhea.

Persistent runny nose.

Wheezing.

Mild rash or itching.

IF YES, *Call pediatric care provider today.*

SELF CARE INFORMATION

Monitor symptoms.

Possibility of developing allergy to other proteins.

Comfort techniques for irritable baby (rocking, singing, skin-to-skin contact, bathing, seeking quiet, calm environment, etc.).

IMPORTANT CONDITIONS TO REPORT

Family history of allergy.

Symptoms worsen, persist, or reoccur.

If breathing or other extreme symptoms are reported, refer to emergency care immediately.

Babies born into allergic families are more likely to develop allergy, particularly those with two allergic parents or one allergic parent and an allergic sibling. Exclusive breastfeeding is the optimal feeding choice for these babies in particular. Should the baby develop allergy symptoms, mother may be counseled to avoid consuming offending allergens such as cow's milk, fish, eggs, peanuts, and tree nuts.

Mothers who have not chosen breastfeeding may **relactate** for their allergic infant. Other allergic infants are fed hypoallergenic formula.

In the event that the allergic response is to a solid food, that food should not be fed to baby and should be avoided by the breastfeeding mother until a medical care provider directs her to reintroduce the allergen.

Rarely, babies develop allergies to foreign protein fragments consumed by their breastfeeding mother. The most potent allergens in the United States diet include cow's milk, fish, eggs, peanuts, and tree nuts. Infantile symptoms of an allergic reaction include hives, facial swelling, runny nose, wheezing, eczema, vomiting, irritability (colic), blood in the stool, and **anaphylaxis**. Treatment centers on identification and avoidance of the proteins that are triggering the allergic reaction.

If supplementation is required, babies with documented allergy should be fed hypoallergenic formula identified by a medical care provider.

Concern about infant allergy is much more predominant than actual allergy. The American Academy of Pediatrics reports that the prevalence of infant cow's milk allergy is two to three percent.[104] The overall prevalence of childhood food allergy is four to six percent.[105]

Counseling and education should include comfort techniques for the irritable baby and coping methods for parents.

See also Atopic eczema

Footnotes

[104]AAP Committee on Nutrition. (2000). Hypoallergenic infant formulas. *Pediatrics, 106,* 346–349.

[105]Ziegler, R.S. (2003). Food allergen avoidance in prevention of food allergy in infants and children. *Pediatrics, 111,* 1662–1671.

▶ Food and Drug Administration (FDA)

DEFINITION   A U.S. federal agency that regulates foods, drugs, medical devices, biologic agents, animal feed and drugs, cosmetics, and radiation-emitting products.

Problems with drugs, formula, pumps, and other devices should be reported to the manufacturer and the FDA's Center for Devices and Radiological Health.

The FDA's Manufacturer and User Facility Device Experience Database (MAUDE) database contains prior complaints filed about devices. Visit www.fda.gov/cdrh/maude.html for more information.

The FDA's Center for Food Safety and Applied Nutrition (CFSAN) regulates infant formula. Visit www.cfsan.fda.gov for more safety updates and other information.

Notes

U.S. Food and Drug Administration
5600 Fishers Lane
Rockville, MD 20857-0001
Phone: 888-INFO-FDA
Web site: www.fda.gov

▶ Food restrictions postpartum

DEFINITION   The thought that certain substances should not be eaten by nursing mothers for fear that they will alter the quality or acceptability of her milk.

There are no foods that should be forbidden during lactation. Mother's milk is indeed flavored by the foods she consumes, as is amniotic fluid.

IMPORTANT CONDITIONS TO REPORT
Concerns about infant's behavior related to mother's diet should be evaluated by infant's medical care provider.

See also Food allergies and breastfeeding; Maternal diet

▶ Football hold

DEFINITION   Another name for the "clutch hold." A breastfeeding position in which the baby is tucked under the mother's arm, with its feet behind her back, and attaches to the breast next to her arm. Mother supports the baby's torso with her forearm, holding the baby's neck in the palm of her hand.

Notes

This is a good position for mothers recovering from Cesarean delivery, those with large breasts, and premature babies.

See also Clutch hold; Cradle hold

▶ Foremilk

DEFINITION   Refers to the milk that flows from the breast at the beginning of a feeding.

Notes

There is an outdated belief that foremilk is always low in fat. Fat content in milk varies throughout the day and within each feeding, depending on how full the breast is, as well as how well the baby or pump is eliciting the milk ejection reflex, which flushes fat down through the breast.

There is no scientific evidence to support the common advice that mothers should keep the baby at the breast longer to get more hindmilk. The baby can regulate its calorie intake when allowed to feed and stop feeding according to its own feeding cues.

It is very rare for the caloric composition of human milk to be inadequate. Routine testing of the fat or other content of milk is not recommended, due to diurnal variation and the difficulty of collecting a representative sample.

See also Caloric density of breastmilk; Fat in breastmilk; Hindmilk

▶ Formula, infant

DEFINITION   A food patterned on breastmilk, which is the only suitable replacement for human milk in the first year of baby's life.

Formula may also be called artificial baby milks, manufactured baby milk, infant formula, artificial milks, formulated baby milks, or breastmilk substitutes.

Formula may be used to supplement breastfeeding when desired by the mother or when medically indicated.

Ask about

Age of baby.
Age of baby when supplements started.
Type of supplements.
How supplements are fed.
Amount of supplement per 24 hours.
Reactions from supplement.

ASSESSMENT

EMERGENT CARE NEEDED?

Are any of the following present?

Signs of dehydration (scanty, dark urine).
Difficulty breathing.

IF YES,   *Seek emergency care now.*

PROMPT CARE NEEDED?

Are any of the following present?

Eczema.
Hives.
Vomiting.
Diarrhea.
Blood in the stools.
Irritability and excessive crying.
Meconium bowel movements after 5 days of life.

Fewer than 3 bowel movements daily in breastfed newborn after the first two days of life.

No urine in six hours.

Brick dust urine (uric acid crystals) after 2 days of life.

Dark colored urine.

Fewer than 4 urinations daily in the breastfed newborn after day 5.

Noticeably sunken fontanelles (soft spot on top of head).

Decreased activity.

Baby below birthweight at 10–14 days.

Cessation of weight gain.

IF YES, *Seek pediatric care within 2 to 4 hours.*

ROUTINE CARE NEEDED?

Are any of the following present?

Education needed about formula feeding.

Education wanted about decreasing amount of supplement.

Education wanted about increasing milk volume.

IF YES, *Call lactation care provider today.*

SELF CARE INFORMATION

Complementary feedings are those that are added to breastfeeding.

IMPORTANT CONDITIONS TO REPORT

Ongoing symptoms.

Notes

Formula is regulated by the FDA Center for Food Safety and Applied Nutrition (CFSAN). Visit www.cfsan.fda.gov for more information.

For medical indications for formula use, consult a reference such as the Academy of Breastfeeding Medicine's "Protocol #3: Hospital guidelines for the use of supplementary feedings in the healthy term breastfed neonate," which can be accessed on the Internet at www.bfmed.org/protocol/supplementation.pdf.

See also Decreasing supplemental formula; Increasing milk supply

▶ Fortification of human milk for premature infants

DEFINITION   The practice of adding minerals and fats to expressed breastmilk to increase its nutrient content. Calcium, phosphorus, zinc, and iron are among the nutrients added.

In the United States, commercially available "human milk" fortifiers are made with cow's milk products.

> **Notes**
>
> Fortifiers are typically used only for very low birthweight infants in neonatal care unit settings.

See also Lactoengineering; Premature infants; Preterm milk properties

▶ Freezing and storing human milk

DEFINITION   Safe methods for preserving expressed milk.

> **Notes**
>
> Glass and hard plastic containers with tight lids are recommended. All containers should be food-grade. Plastic bags designed for milk storage may be used, but it may be difficult to prevent spillage and puncture of these bags.
>
> Milk can be safely stored:
>
> Up to four hours at room temperature (lower than 75° F), but should be refrigerated immediately if possible (with frozen gel pack in an insulated lunch bag or cooler if refrigerator is not available).
>
> 72 hours in the refrigerator.
>
> Up to three months in the built-in freezer section of a refrigerator.
>
> Up to six months in a deep freezer.
>
> Milk that will not be used fresh within 72 hours should be frozen as soon as possible.[106]

See also Collection and storage of breastmilk; Milk storage bags

Footnotes

[106]Arnold, L.D.W. (2004). *Safe storage of expressed breastmilk for the healthy infant and child.* East Sandwich, MA: Health Education Associates.

▶ # Frenotomy

DEFINITION A procedure that releases the restriction of the frenulum, the tissue that holds the tongue to the bottom of the mouth.

▶ # Frenulum, lingual

DEFINITION The membrane attaching the tongue to the bottom of the mouth.

When the frenulum is tight, it can restrict the movement of the tongue, resulting in breastfeeding problems for some mothers and babies.

Ask about

Age of baby.
Appearance of tongue.

ASSESSMENT

PROMPT MEDICAL CARE NEEDED?

Are any of the following present?

Meconium bowel movements after 5 days of life.

Fewer than 3 bowel movements daily in breastfed newborn after the first two days of life.

No urine in six hours.

Brick dust urine (uric acid crystals) after 2 days of life.

Dark colored urine.

Fewer than 4 urinations daily in the breastfed newborn after day 5.

Noticeably sunken fontanelles (soft spot on top of head).

Decreased activity.

Baby below birthweight at 10–14 days.

Cessation of weight gain.

IF YES, *Seek pediatric care within 2 to 4 hours.*

PROMPT LACTATION CARE NEEDED?

Are any of the following present?

Tight lingual frenulum in baby.

Nipple or breast pain or damage.

History of recurrent breast infection.

Milk supply problems.

Poor growth of breastfed infant.

IF YES, *Call lactation care provider today.*

SELF CARE INFORMATION

Practice skin-to-skin contact frequently.

Watch for hunger cues (signs that say "feed me" include hand-to-face or hand-to-mouth movements, lip smacking, seeking with lips, rooting, and head bobbing).

Feed baby at first sign of hunger cues.

Practice good attachment:

Offer the breast as soon as it is seen.

Wait for baby to open mouth wide (greater than a 100° angle).

Pull baby in so that chin touches the breast first, and nipple enters the mouth along the top of the tongue; this should result in a wide open mouth full of breast.

Lips should be flanged outward.

Baby's lips should look off center when compared with the areola; the bottom lip should be farther away from the nipple than the top lip.

IMPORTANT CONDITIONS TO REPORT

Unresolved symptoms.

Ongoing concerns.

Insufficient intake or output of the baby.

See also Nipple pain

▶ Frequency of feedings

DEFINITION   The number of feedings in a period of time.

Expectation for breastfeeding is 10–12 feedings per 24 hours.

Observation of breastfed newborns indicates that while most babies nurse 10–12 times per day, they tend to do so in a clustered feeding pattern. That is, young babies tend to have a cycle of short, closely spaced feedings interspersed with periods of rest or sleep. This pattern is associated with good milk production and growth.

Ask about

Age of baby.
Current feeding pattern.

ASSESSMENT

EMERGENT CARE NEEDED?

Are any of the following present?

Sudden disinterest in feeding.

Extreme **lethargy** in baby.

Sudden change in baby's muscle tone (extremely floppy or stiff).

IF YES,   *Seek emergency care now.*

PROMPT MEDICAL CARE NEEDED?

Are any of the following present?

Meconium bowel movements after 5 days of life.

Fewer than 3 bowel movements daily in breastfed newborn after the first two days of life.

No urine in six hours.

Brick dust urine (uric acid crystals) after 2 days of life.

Dark colored urine.

Fewer than 4 urinations daily in the breastfed newborn after day 5.

Noticeably sunken fontanelles (soft spot on top of head).

Decreased activity.

Baby below birthweight at 10–14 days.

Cessation of weight gain.

IF YES, *Seek pediatric care within 2 to 4 hours.*

PROMPT LACTATION CARE NEEDED?

Are any of the following present?

Fewer than eight feedings per day in a breastfed newborn.

Concerns about adequacy of milk supply.

IF YES, *Call lactation care provider today.*

ROUTINE CARE NEEDED?

Are any of the following present?

Baby waking frequently at night to feed.

IF YES, *Call lactation care provider.*

SELF CARE INFORMATION

Practice skin-to-skin contact frequently.

Watch for hunger cues (signs that say "feed me" include hand-to-face or hand-to-mouth movements, lip smacking, seeking with lips, rooting, and head bobbing).

Feed baby at first sign of hunger cues.

Practice good attachment.

Expect 10–12 feedings per 24 hours (feedings may occur in clusters—3 or 4 feedings in 2 hours, followed by a few hours of rest, then more clusters, rest, etc.).

Listen for signs of baby swallowing.

Allow baby to end feedings.

Expect at least 3–4 infant stools per 24 hours after the first 4 days of life.

Good positioning and attachment are crucial to reduce nipple pain.

If feedings are missed, hand express or pump milk to maintain supply.

IMPORTANT CONDITIONS TO REPORT

Inadequate feeding (less than 10 feedings daily in the newborn).

Inadequate stooling pattern (less than three stools daily).

See also Ankyloglossia; Cluster feeding; Feeding pattern of breastfed infants

▶ **FTT**

DEFINITION Failure to thrive. A condition in which a child's size and growth rate is significantly below that of average children. There are multiple causes for FTT ranging from organic problems such as metabolic disorders, cerebral palsy, and organ defects, as well as psychological and social causes. FTT occurs in both formula fed and breastfed infants.

Ask about

Onset.
Age of baby.
Feeding method.

ASSESSMENT

EMERGENT CARE NEEDED?
Are any of the following present?

Meconium bowel movements after 5 days of life.
Fewer than 3 bowel movements daily in breastfed newborn after the first two days of life.
No urine in six hours.
Brick dust urine (uric acid crystals) after 2 days of life.
Dark colored urine.
Fewer than 4 urinations daily in the breastfed newborn after day 5.
Noticeably sunken fontanelles (soft spot on top of head).
Decreased activity.
Baby below birthweight at 10–14 days.
Cessation of weight gain.

IF YES,　*Seek pediatric care within 2 to 4 hours.*

PROMPT CARE NEEDED?

Are any of the following present?

Concern about inadequate infant growth.

IF YES, *Call pediatric care provider today.*

Are any of the following present?

Diagnosed FTT in a breastfed child.

IF YES, *Referral to growth and nutrition department.*

Are any of the following present?

Continued breastfeeding in a child diagnosed with FTT.

IF YES, *Call lactation care provider today.*

SELF CARE INFORMATION

Practice skin-to-skin contact frequently.

Watch for hunger cues (signs that say "feed me" include hand-to-face or hand-to-mouth movements, lip smacking, seeking with lips, rooting, and head bobbing).

Feed baby at first sign of hunger cues.

Expect 10–12 unscheduled feedings in 24 hours.

Allow baby to end feedings.

IMPORTANT CONDITIONS TO REPORT

Infant disinterest in feeding.

Ongoing problems with milk supply.

Notes

Growth expectations are different in breastfed infants after the first 6 months of age. Because growth charts are based on mixed fed children, breastfeeding babies may appear to fall a few percentiles on the charts sometime between 4 and 12 months of age. This should be individually evaluated; such an occurrence may be an artifact of the charts.

See also Milk supply, inadequate

► Full breastfeeding

DEFINITION   A form of exclusive breastfeeding.

See also Exclusive breastfeeding

► Galactocele

DEFINITION   A milk retention cyst within the breast. Galactoceles are caused by blocked or blind milk ducts. This condition is compatible with breastfeeding. These cysts may be aspirated, but will refill.

Ask about

Onset.

ASSESSMENT

PROMPT CARE NEEDED?
Are any of the following present?
   Suspected galactocele.

IF YES,   *Call obstetric care provider today.*

IMPORTANT CONDITIONS TO REPORT
Recurrence of symptoms.

See also Breast lumps

► Galactogogue

DEFINITION   Foods, herbs, and other substances thought to increase milk production. Requests from mothers for galactogogues indicate concern about milk supply.

Onset.

Age of baby.

ASSESSMENT

EMERGENT CARE NEEDED?

Are any of the following present?

Meconium bowel movements after 5 days of life.

Fewer than 3 bowel movements daily in breastfed newborn after the first two days of life.

No urine in six hours.

Brick dust urine (uric acid crystals) after 2 days of life.

Dark colored urine.

Fewer than 4 urinations daily in the breastfed newborn after day 5.

Noticeably sunken fontanelles (soft spot on top of head).

Decreased activity.

Baby below birthweight at 10–14 days.

Cessation of weight gain.

IF YES, *Seek pediatric care within 2 to 4 hours.*

PROMPT CARE NEEDED?

Are any of the following present?

Scanty or infrequent urination.

IF YES, *Seek pediatric care today.*

Are any of the following present?

Identified milk supply problem.

Concern about milk supply.

IF YES, *Call lactation care provider today.*

SELF CARE INFORMATION

Ensure baby is feeding 10–12 times per 24 hours.

Express milk after feeding and give to baby.

IMPORTANT CONDITIONS TO REPORT

Persistent problems.

Recurrent problems.

SELF CARE INFORMATION

Increasing feeding frequency and milk removal are the keys to increasing milk supply.

Breastfeed your baby at least 10–12 times per 24 hours.

If galactogogues are prescribed, follow instructions carefully.

Report any other medications, herbs, and dietary supplements you are using to everyone who prescribes for you and your baby.

IMPORTANT CONDITIONS TO REPORT

Concerns about milk supply.

Jitteriness.

Insomnia.

Sedation.

Anxiety.

> **Notes**
>
> There are no recommended foods or herbs for increasing milk supply.
>
> Reglan (metoclopramide) may be prescribed for mothers who are pumping for preterm infants. This drug is generally used to increase the muscle tone of the lower esophagus sphincter and is used to treat reflux and nausea. Side effects include cardiac arrhythmias, extrapyramidal signs, jitteriness, insomnia, sedation, and anxiety. Another side effect is the increase in prolactin release that may result in increased milk production. Increased milk production does not happen in all women.
>
> Domperidone, a dopamine agonist drug similar to metoclopramide, is used to control gastrointestinal symptoms. This drug is used in other countries to increase prolactin levels, but is not currently available in the United States. The FDA has warned against use of domperidone.[107]
>
> Herbs should be recommended only by licensed prescibers, certified herbal experts, and other specialists in herb–drug interactions.

See also Domperidone; Increasing milk supply; Milk supply; Milk transfer-estimating; Reglan; Weight loss—baby

Footnotes

[107]U.S. Food and Drug Adminstration. (2004). *FDA talk paper: FDA warns against women using unapproved drug, Domperidone, to increase milk production.* Retrieved March 17, 2005, from http://www.fda.gov/bbs/topics/ANSWERS/2004/ANS01292.html.

Galactopoiesis

DEFINITION   Maintenance of milk production in the breast.

Galactopoiesis is sustained by frequent stimulation of the nipple and frequent removal of milk from the breast.

Galactorrhea

DEFINITION   Production of milk from the breast that is outside normal expectations. This can include production of milk by women who are neither pregnant nor lactating, as well as excessive amounts of milk produced during lactation.

Ask about

Onset.

ASSESSMENT

PROMPT CARE NEEDED?

Are any of the following present?

Production of milk in a nonlactating, nonpregnant woman.

IF YES,   *Seek medical care today.*

Are any of the following present?

Concern about overabundant milk supply.

Excessively large or frequent stools in a breastfed baby.

Recurrent engorgement or mastitis.

Baby has difficulty managing excessive milk flow (sputters at the breast).

IF YES,   *Call lactation care provider today.*

SELF CARE INFORMATION

Frequency of feeding and amount of milk removal drives milk supply.

Worsening of symptoms.
Continuation of symptoms.
Ongoing concerns.

> **Notes**
>
> Because production of milk relies on many different body systems in both mother and baby, any milk supply problem requires consideration of maternal and infant factors. Occasionally medical factors such as endocrine imbalance may require evaluation.

▶ Galactose

DEFINITION A simple sugar that, when combined with glucose, creates **lactose**.

▶ Galactosemia

DEFINITION A congenital inability to metabolize the simple sugar **galactose** due to an enzyme deficiency. This condition is the only *infant* medical contraindication to receiving breastmilk.

▶ GALT

DEFINITION Gut-associated lymphoid tissue. Immunologically active tissue found within the lining of the gastrointestinal tract.

> **Notes**
>
> The breast is thought to act as an extension of gut-associated lymphoid tissue (GALT). When a pathogen enters the gut, GALT tissue responds by triggering the production of an immunoglobulin to attack the pathogen. The breast may also respond to the GALT trigger by manufacturing and releasing appropriate immunoglobulins to fight the organism through the milk.

See also Bioactive components of breastmilk

Gas and gassy foods while breastfeeding

DEFINITION   Referring to foods containing an abundance of indigestible carbohydrates (fiber), and the gas produced by the fermentation of these carbohydrates in the gut.

Foods that adults commonly find gassy include beans, cabbage, broccoli, cauliflower, and whole grain foods.

There is little evidence that any vegetables mothers consume negatively affect their babies.

Notes

Gas and flatulence are normal occurrences in the newborn, as in all humans. An infant's gas may carry the scent of aromatic oils in vegetables and other foods eaten by its mother; however, the oils do not contain fiber, and thus do not cause gastric distress in the infant.

Many mothers will put themselves on unnecessarily restrictive diets, without seeking help for their baby's symptoms.

Clinicians should carefully evaluate mother's concerns and baby's symptoms to distinguish normal gas from colic or digestive difficulty.

See also Colic; Maternal diet

Gastroesophageal (GE) reflux

DEFINITION   Movement of stomach contents up into the esophagus and mouth.

Gastroesophageal (GE) reflux in infants is not common in babies who are exclusively breastfed, except in babies who have been previously tube fed.[108] With GE reflux, the stomach contents move up out of the stomach and back into the esophagus.

With GE reflux, babies vomit after eating. The vomiting happens most of the time and is not projectile.

Ask about

Age of baby.
History of vomiting.
History of weight gain or loss.
History of pneumonia or lung problems.
History of choking.

EMERGENT CARE NEEDED?

Are any of the following present?

Difficulty breathing.

Choking.

Difficulty swallowing.

Rapid progression of symptoms.

IF YES, *Seek emergency care now.*

PROMPT CARE NEEDED?

Are any of the following present?

Decrease in urination.

Decrease in stooling.

Meconium bowel movements after 5 days of life.

Fewer than 3 bowel movements daily in breastfed newborn after the first two days of life.

No urine in six hours.

Brick dust urine (uric acid crystals) after 2 days of life.

Dark colored urine.

Fewer than 4 urinations daily in the breastfed newborn after day 5.

Noticeably sunken fontanelles (soft spot on top of head).

Decreased activity.

Baby below birthweight at 10–14 days.

Cessation of weight gain.

IF YES, *Seek pediatric care within 2 to 4 hours.*

ROUTINE CARE NEEDED?

Are any of the following present?

Baby spits up regularly after nursing.

Weight gain is adequate.

Urination and stooling pattern is adequate.

IF YES, *Call lactation care provider today.*

SELF CARE INFORMATION

Many breastfed babies spit up frequently without any underlying medical cause. A baby who spits up often should be evaluated by his or her health care provider.

IMPORTANT CONDITIONS TO REPORT

Difficulty breathing.
Choking.
Difficulty swallowing.
Rapid progression of symptoms.
Decrease in urination.
Decrease in stooling.
Signs of dehydration.

See also Milk flow—too fast

Footnotes

[108]Heacock, H.J., Jeffery, H.E., Baker, J.L., & Page, M. (1992). Influence of breast versus formula milk on physiological gastroesophageal reflux in healthy, newborn infants. *Journal of Pediatric Gastroenterology and Nutrition, 14,* 41–46.

▶ Gastrointestinal (GI)

DEFINITION   Pertaining to the organs of the digestive tract, including the stomach, small intestine, and large intestine.

▶ Gastrointestinal (GI) infection

DEFINITION   Establishment of virus, bacteria, or other entity in the digestive tract.
Breastfeeding is compatible with GI infection, and offers protection to the infant against common pathogens triggering GI infection.

SELF CARE INFORMATION

Practice careful handwashing, especially when handling baby and changing diapers.

See also Acute infection; Blood in stool; Diarrhea and breastfeeding; Vomiting

► Gastroschisis

DEFINITION   A congenital defect in the abdominal wall, resulting in the protrusion of the intestines through skin. Babies with this condition can be fed breastmilk and go on to breastfeed after surgical repair.

► Gavage feeding

DEFINITION   Delivering food to an infant through a tube that is inserted into the baby's stomach through the nose.

See also Feeding tube devices

► GE (Gastroesophageal) reflux

DEFINITION   Movement of stomach contents up into the esophagus and mouth.
    Gastroesophageal (GE) reflux in infants is not common in babies who are exclusively breastfed, except in babies who have been previously tube fed.[109] With GE reflux, the stomach contents move up out of the stomach and back into the esophagus.
    With GE reflux, babies vomit after eating. The vomiting happens most of the time and is not projectile.

Ask about

Age of baby.
History of vomiting.
History of weight gain or loss.
History of pneumonia or lung problems.
History of choking.

EMERGENT CARE NEEDED?

Are any of the following present?

Difficulty breathing.

Choking.

Difficulty swallowing.

Rapid progression of symptoms.

IF YES, *Seek emergency care now.*

PROMPT CARE NEEDED?

Are any of the following present?

Decrease in urination.

Decrease in stooling.

Signs of dehydration.

IF YES, *Seek pediatric care within 2 to 4 hours.*

ROUTINE CARE NEEDED?

Are any of the following present?

Baby spits up regularly after nursing.

Weight gain is adequate.

Urination and stooling pattern is adequate.

IF YES, *Call lactation care provider today.*

SELF CARE INFORMATION

Many breastfed babies spit up frequently without any underlying medical cause. A baby who spits up often should be evaluated by his or her health care provider.

IMPORTANT CONDITIONS TO REPORT
Difficulty breathing.
Choking.
Difficulty swallowing.
Rapid progression of symptoms.
Decrease in urination.
Decrease in stooling.
Signs of dehydration.

See also Milk flow—too fast

Footnotes
[109] Heacock, H.J., Jeffery, H.E., Baker, J.L., & Page, M. (1992). Influence of breast versus formula milk on physiological gastroesophageal reflux in healthy, newborn infants. *Journal of Pediatric Gastroenterology and Nutrition, 14,* 41–46.

▶ Gel packs

DEFINITION Devices containing gel matrix within a protective covering. Intended to be heated or chilled and worn next to the skin over an inflamed area to provide relief. Care should be taken to use gel packs at a comfortable temperature.

▶ Gel pads

See also Glycerin gel pads; Hydrogel pads

▶ Gentian violet

DEFINITION A chemical dye used in laboratories. Also an antimicrobial and anti-fungal. Use of gentian violet has been reported as a treatment for Candidiasis.

This chemical is a powerful irritant to the skin and can cause tissue necrosis if not used in the proper dilution.

See also Candidiasis; Thrush; Yeast

Footnotes

[110]Hale, T.W. (2004). *Medications and mothers milk*. Amarillo, TX: Pharmasoft Publishing, 375.

▶ # GI

DEFINITION   Gastrointestinal. Pertaining to the organs of the digestive tract, including the stomach, small intestine, and large intestine.

▶ # Gigantomastia

DEFINITION   A rare condition of massive overgrowth of the breasts occurring during pregnancy. The breasts may increase several times their prepregnant size.

Notes

With gigantomastia, serious problems can develop, including hemorrhage within the breast due to rapid change. Surgery may be required to stop hemorrhage.

Gigantomastia generally recedes after delivery, but usually reoccurs with every subsequent pregnancy.

Breastfeeding is not contraindicated, as the condition typically reverses after delivery.

Breastfeeding women who experienced gigantomastia in pregnancy should receive ongoing lactation support.

▶ Glandular tissue, insufficient

DEFINITION A rare condition in which women have an inadequate amount of milk-making tissue in the breast. This may be congenital, or the after effect of trauma or surgery to the chest. Asymmetry between the breasts may be a hallmark of this condition.

Ask about

Onset.
Age of baby.

ASSESSMENT

EMERGENT CARE NEEDED?
Are any of the following present?

Meconium bowel movements after 5 days of life.

Fewer than 3 bowel movements daily in breastfed newborn after the first two days of life.

No urine in six hours.

Brick dust urine (uric acid crystals) after 2 days of life.

Dark colored urine.

Fewer than 4 urinations daily in the breastfed newborn after day 5

Noticeably sunken fontanelles (soft spot on top of head).

Decreased activity.

Baby below birthweight at 10–14 days.

Cessation of weight gain.

IF YES, *Seek pediatric care within 2 to 4 hours.*

PROMPT MEDICAL CARE NEEDED?
Are any of the following present?

Failure of breastfed baby to grow adequately.

IF YES, *Call pediatric care provider today.*

PROMPT LACTATION CARE NEEDED?

Are any of the following present?

Marked asymmetry of the breasts with concerns about milk supply or infant growth.

IF YES, *Call lactation care provider today.*

ROUTINE LACTATION CARE NEEDED?

Are any of the following present?

Reported asymmetry with no concerns about milk supply or infant growth.

IF YES, *Call lactation care provider.*

SELF CARE INFORMATION

Practice skin-to-skin contact frequently.

Feed baby at first sign of hunger cues (signs that say "feed me" include hand-to-face or hand-to-mouth movements, lip smacking, seeking with lips, rooting, and head bobbing).

Feed baby at least 10–12 times per 24 hours.

Listen for signs of baby swallowing.

Allow baby to end feedings.

Expect at least 3–4 infant stools per 24 hours after the first 4 days of life.

Good positioning and attachment are crucial.

If feedings are missed, hand express or pump milk to maintain supply.

IMPORTANT CONDITIONS TO REPORT

Feeding or stooling expectations are not met.

Notes

Growth of baby should be closely followed by a medical care provider.

One sign of possible insufficient glandular tissue is marked asymmetry of the breasts. This may indicate problems with glandular tissue in both breasts. If the mother reports that she had an implant in one breast only, inquire about the reason for this surgery. If the surgery was to correct breast asymmetry, there may be increased concern regarding the mother's ability to make a full milk supply. Marked asymmetry may indicate insufficient glandular tissue in both breasts.

See also Asymmetric breasts; Insufficient milk supply

▶ **Glycerine gel pads**

DEFINITION   Devices designed to give comfort to painful nipples. These gel matrix pads with a cloth backing are intended to be worn over the nipple.

There is little research supporting claims that glycerin gel pads heal trauma to the nipple.

Ask about

Nipple discomfort.

ASSESSMENT

PROMPT CARE NEEDED?

Are any of the following present?

Extreme nipple pain.

Bleeding from nipples.

Unable to breastfeed due to pain.

IF YES, *Call lactation care provider immediately.*

ROUTINE CARE NEEDED?

Are any of the following present?

Feeding discomfort.

Trauma to nipple or breasts.

Misshapen nipple after feedings.

Visible fissures on nipples.

IF YES, *Call lactation care provider today.*

SELF CARE INFORMATION

Any substance that is applied to the nipple area will be consumed by the nursing baby. Do not apply any creams or ointments to the nipple area without getting your medical care provider's approval first.

Report nipple pain to the lactation care provider.

IMPORTANT CONDITIONS TO REPORT

Symptoms worsen or persist.

Signs of infection.

Feeding or stooling expectations are not met.

Notes

Women experiencing **nipple pain** may self-treat with gel pads and other substances rather than seek help to resolve the cause of the pain.

Women experiencing nipple pain should have a breastfeeding evaluation. Face-to-face counseling is effective in assessing and resolving nipple pain.

Any glycerine gel pads used should be approved for use in breastfeeding mothers.

See also Nipple pain; Sore nipples

▶ Goldsmith's sign

DEFINITION   Consistent refusal to breastfeed on one breast without explanation. This indicates the need for routine breast evaluation. Cancer has been diagnosed as late as five years after persistent breast refusal.[111]

Notes

There are many common reasons for breast refusal. Cancer is an unusual, but possible, finding.

See also Breast refusal; Breast cancer; Refusal of infant to breastfeed

Footnotes

[111]Saber, A., Dardik, H., Ibrahim, I.M., & Wolodiger, F. (1996). The milk rejection sign: A natural tumor marker. *The American Surgeon, 62*, 998–999.

▶ Graves' disease

DEFINITION   A type of thyroid disorder resulting in hyperthyroidism.

See also Hyperthyroidism

▶ Growth charts

DEFINITION   A document containing percentile curves showing the comparative height and weight of a population of babies of varying ages. These documents are used to track an individual baby's growth and evaluate that growth against the standards.

> **Notes**
>
> Exclusively breastfed babies have a different growth pattern than mixed fed and formula fed babies. Exclusively breastfed babies grow faster in the the first 4–6 months of age. Because growth charts are based on mixed fed children, breastfeeding babies may appear to fall a few percentiles on the charts beginning sometime between 4 and 12 months of age. Changes in growth percentiles should be individually evaluated; such an occurrence may be an artifact of the charts. (Growth charts for breastfed babies are available from Health Education Associates at www.healthed.cc.)

See also Weight gain—baby

▶ Gut-associated lymphoid tissue (GALT)

DEFINITION   Immunologically active tissue found within the lining of the gastro-intestinal tract.

> **Notes**
>
> The breast is thought to act as an extension of gut-associated lymphoid tissue (GALT). When a pathogen enters the gut, GALT tissue responds by triggering the production of an immunoglobulin to attack the pathogen. The breast may also respond to the GALT trigger by manufacturing and releasing appropriate immunoglobulins to fight the organism through the milk.

See also Bioactive components of breastmilk

▶ Haberman feeder

DEFINITION   A device used to deliver expressed milk or formula to babies with impaired sucking ability. This feeder has a special valve and teat that allow infants to use only positive pressure (compression) to release milk. Babies who are unable to suck effectively are able to obtain milk by compressing the teat.

This feeder is often used for babies with neurologic impairment, Down syndrome, and cleft lip or palate.

See also Down syndrome; Cleft lip and palate; Neurological dysfunction

▶ Hair care products

DEFINITION   Referring to dyes and "permanent" chemical applications to curl or relax curl. No evidence of harm to the breastfeeding infant exists. Application of these products is topical—rarely are chemicals absorbed into the skin.

▶ Hand expression of breastmilk

DEFINITION   A method of removing milk from the lactating breast that does not require any device with the exception of a hand and a bowl or jar to collect milk. Hand expression is a simple skill that should be taught to all breastfeeding mothers.

Ask about

Reason mother plans to express milk.

PROMPT CARE NEEDED?

Are any of the following present?

Imminent separation of mother and baby.

IF YES, *Call lactation care provider today.*

ROUTINE CARE NEEDED?

Are any of the following present?

Desire to learn hand expression.

IF YES, *Call lactation care provider.*

SELF CARE INFORMATION

Wash hands before beginning.

Practice hand expression when baby is latched onto one breast.

Gently massage and then compress the breast.

Your skill will improve with practice.

Store expressed milk in the refrigerator, a cooler with ice packs, or the freezer if it will not be used within 48 hours.

Follow safe milk storage guidelines.

IMPORTANT CONDITIONS TO REPORT

Questions or problems with this technique.

See also Breast pump; Collection and storage of breastmilk

▶ Hand pump

DEFINITION   A device designed to remove milk from the breast. Manual pumps work by hand pressure, squeezing a lever or contracting levers, or pulling out a cylinder to generate pressure to operate the pump.

▶ Headaches and breastfeeding

DEFINITION The occurrence of painful pressure in the head during breastfeeding. Some women experience repeated headaches while breastfeeding. Headache may last only a few minutes and reoccur with subsequent feedings.

Ask about

Onset.
History of headache or migraine.

ASSESSMENT

EMERGENT CARE NEEDED?

Are any of the following present?

Sudden, severe pain.
Sudden weakness, tingling, or numbness on one side of the body.
Confusion.
Difficulty speaking.
Stiff neck and fever.
Persistent vomiting.
High fever.
Eye pain or visual blurring.
Persistent pain.

IF YES, *Seek medical care within 2 to 4 hours.*

ROUTINE CARE NEEDED?

Are any of the following present?

Pain during first minutes of feeding.
No pain between feedings.

IF YES, *Call lactation care provider today.*

SELF CARE INFORMATION

Try a cool compress on the forehead before feedings.
Report any increase in symptoms to a medical care provider.

See also Raynaud's phenomenon

▶ Health Education Associates

DEFINITION "An independent health publishing company, Health Education Associates, Inc. has been leading the patient education field by creating multi-ethnic pamphlets, in various reading levels. Books, modules, monographs, growth charts, breastfeeding assessment forms, and promotional items celebrating breast-feeding are also available."[112]

Notes

Health Education Associates
327 Quaker Meeting House Road
East Sandwich, MA 02537-1300
Phone: 888-888-8077
Web site: www.healthed.cc

Footnotes

[112]Health Education Associates, Inc. (2004). *Health Education Associates, Inc. Home Page.* Retrieved November 7, 2005, from http://www.healthed.cc.

▶ Healthy Children Project

DEFINITION "Healthy Children is defining the field of research based breastfeeding education and ethical, evidence-based breastfeeding practice. Healthy Children is a non-profit 501(c)3 research and educational institution dedicated to improving child health outcomes through partnerships with public, private and non-profit agencies."[113]

Footnotes

[113]Healthy Children's Center for Breastfeeding. (2004). *The Center for Breastfeeding: A major focus of The Healthy Children Project.* Retrieved July 1, 2005, from http://www.healthychildren.cc.

► Heart problems

DEFINITION   Referring to diseases and disorders of the cardiac and circulatory system.

Ask about

Onset.
History of cardiac problems.

ASSESSMENT

EMERGENT CARE NEEDED?

Are any of the following present?

   A bluish tinge to the baby's mouth and lips during feeding.

IF YES,   *Seek emergency care now.*

PROMPT CARE NEEDED?

Are any of the following present?

   Breastfeeding baby diagnosed with cardiac problems.

IF YES,   *Call lactation care provider today.*

IMPORTANT CONDITIONS TO REPORT

Worsening, persistence, or recurrence of symptoms.

Notes

Women with cardiac problems may breastfeed their babies. Any medications taken should be evaluated for their transfer into milk.

Babies with cardiac problems benefit from receiving their mother's milk. They may have problems sustaining attachment to the breast, and suckling may be weak and ineffective.

However, breastfeeding is less physiologically stressful than bottle feeding. Heart, oxygen saturation, and respiratory rates are lower while breastfeeding than while bottle feeding.

Mothers may benefit from pumping or expressing milk after feeding to maintain an adequate milk supply.

Lactation consultation is recommended to evaluate effective positions and techniques.

▶ Heating breastmilk

DEFINITION Techniques used to safely warm milk for consumption by baby.

Notes

Thaw frozen milk in its container.

Warm by:
　　Holding container under lukewarm running tap water.
　　Placing container in lukewarm water.

Hot water is not recommended due to potential nutrient loss.
Milk should never be boiled or microwaved.
Milk does not need to be overly warm before fed to infant.[114]

See also Collection and storage of expressed milk; Storage of breastmilk

Footnotes

[114]Arnold, L.D.W. (2004). *Safe storage of expressed breastmilk for the healthy infant and child.* East Sandwich, MA: Health Education Associates.

▶ Hemorrhage, postpartum

DEFINITION   An abnormally high amount (generally more than 500 ml) of blood loss during or after delivery.

> **Notes**
>
> Postpartum hemorrhage is of concern to breastfeeding because extreme blood loss can cause **Sheehan's syndrome**, an insult to the **pituitary gland**, where the hormones of lactation (**prolactin** and **oxytocin**) are manufactured.
>
> Women affected by Sheehan's syndrome may be unable to make an adequate amount of milk.
>
> Other symptoms of this syndrome include sudden onset of hypothyroidism, diabetes insipidus, and hair loss along with menstrual irregularities. Medical evaluation should include measurement of prolactin levels before and after sucklings. The extent to which women recover from Sheehan's is variable with the degree of infarct.[115]
>
> Babies of mothers who suffered postpartum hemorrhage should be closely monitored for inadequate intake.

See also Sheehan's syndrome

Footnotes

[115]Lawrence, R.A., & Lawrence, R.M. (2005). *Breastfeeding: A guide for the medical profession* (6th ed., p. 573). St. Louis: Mosby.

▶ Hepatitis

DEFINITION   Inflammation of the liver caused by a number of pathogens and substances. Of pertinence here are the common viruses hepatitis A, B, and C.

Breastfeeding is compatible with hepatitis infection in the mother with a few qualifications:

Hepatitis A: breastfeeding may occur after immune globulin and vaccine to the infant.

Hepatitis B: breastfeeding may occur after administering hepatitis B immune globulin (HBIG) and vaccine to infant.

Hepatitis C: breastfeeding may occur, unless mother is co-infected with HIV.[116]

Notes

Seek updates from the Centers for Disease Control and Prevention, as this is a rapidly expanding area of knowledge and research.

See also Acute infection

Footnotes

[116]Lawrence, R.A., & Lawrence, R.M. (2005). *Breastfeeding: A guide for the medical profession* (6th ed., p. 663). St. Louis: Mosby.

▶ # Herbs

DEFINITION   Plants or parts of plants that are valued for their medicinal qualities. Herbs can have powerful effects. As with some drugs taken by breastfeeding mothers, troubling effects have been reported in breastfed babies whose mothers have taken certain herbs.

SELF CARE INFORMATION

Tell all health care providers about any herbs and natural supplements you are taking. Some herbs (such as fenugreek) can decrease the effectiveness of other medications.[117] Investigate medicinal herbs with the same care you would with prescribed and over-the-counter medications.

IMPORTANT CONDITIONS TO REPORT

Any change in the baby's physical condition or behavior such as problems sleeping, vomiting, rash, or irritability.

See also Drugs and breastfeeding; Medications; Over-the-counter medications

Footnotes

[117]Skidmore-Roth, L. (2003). *Mosby's handbook of herbs and natural supplements* (2nd ed.). St. Louis: Mosby.

▶ Herpes simplex virus

DEFINITION   Infection with the herpes simplex 1 or 2 virus, characterized by lesions (blisters) on the skin surface. In the context of breastfeeding, the presence of herpes lesions on the nipple or parts of the breast that the baby's mouth will contact is of great concern, due to the life threatening nature of herpes infection in the newborn.

Herpes lesions elsewhere on the mother's body do not contraindicate breastfeeding; however, mother should be cautioned to cover lesions, avoid touching them, and practice careful handwashing.

Ask about

Onset.
Age of baby.
Known history of herpes lesions or other skin conditions.

ASSESSMENT

EMERGENT CARE NEEDED?

Are any of the following present?

History of herpes lesions on the nipple or breast, or elsewhere on the mother or partner's body, with:

Blisters plus fever and aching.

Baby with blisters, fever, and/or lethargy.

IF YES,   *Seek emergency care now.*

SELF CARE INFORMATION

Wash your hands carefully, especially if you have a herpes outbreak.

Family members with cold sores should refrain from kissing the baby.

IMPORTANT CONDITIONS TO REPORT
Fever.
Signs of infection.

See also Acute infection; Blisters on the nipple or breast

▶ # HHS

DEFINITION   "The Department of Heath and Human Services is the United States government's principal agency for protecting the health of all Americans and providing essential human services, especially for those who are least able to help themselves."[118a]

Notes

U.S. Department of Health and Human Services
200 Independence Avenue SW
Washington, DC 20201
Phone: 202-619-0257 or 877-696-6775
Web site: www.hhs.gov

HHS has several different bureaus and agencies that address maternal/child health issues, including the Centers for Disease Control and Prevention, the Food and Drug Administration, the Center for Food Safety and Applied Nutrition, the Health Resources and Services Administration, the Maternal and Child Health Bureau, Indian Health Services, and the Office on Women's Health.

Footnotes
[118a]Department of Health and Human Services. (2005). *HHS: What We Do.* Retrieved November 15, 2005, from http://www.hhs.gov/about/whatwedo.html.

▶ Higher order multiples (HOM)

DEFINITION   Birth of three or more infants simultaneously.

Mothers can breastfeed higher order multiples. Increased suckling, especially nursing two babies simultaneously, stimulates an increased supply of milk.

Multiples may be born prematurely, spend weeks or months in the hospital before discharge, and not be discharged on the same day.

Mothers may express milk to be fed to hospitalized babies. Expression should start as soon after the babies are born as possible. Mothers should express milk eight or more times per day.

Ask about

Age of babies.
Gestational age of babies at birth.

ASSESSMENT

ROUTINE CARE NEEDED?
Are any of the following present?

Strategies for managing the nursing of multiples.
Strategies for managing milk supply for multiples.
Questions about breastfeeding.
Problems with breastfeeding.

IF YES,   *Call lactation care provider today.*

SELF CARE INFORMATION

Nursing babies simultaneously is helpful for building a milk supply, but may be difficult to manage at first. Ask for help with positioning.

At first, switch the babies from one breast to another. As the babies get older, they may prefer nursing on one breast or another.

Many mothers have found it helpful at first to write down "who nursed when" to ensure that each baby gets enough nourishment.

IMPORTANT CONDITIONS TO REPORT
Lethargy.
Decrease in urine and stools.
Change in breastfeeding behavior.
Problems with feeding.

See also Breast pump; Hospitalization and breastfeeding; NICU, milk storage and handling in; Premature infant; Preterm milk

▶ # Hindmilk

DEFINITION　Refers to the milk that flows from the breast at the end of a feed.

Notes

The belief that hindmilk is always the richest milk is outdated. Fat content in milk varies throughout the day and within each feeding, depending on how full the breast is, as well as how well the baby or pump is eliciting the milk rejection reflex, which flushes fat down through the breast.

There is no scientific evidence to support the common advice that mothers should keep the baby at the breast longer to get more hindmilk.[118b] The baby can regulate its calorie intake when allowed to feed and stop feeding according to its own feeding cues.

The caloric composition of human milk rarely is inadequate. Routine testing of the fat or other content of milk is not recommended, due to diurnal variation and the difficulty of collecting a representative sample.

See also Caloric density of breastmilk; Fat in breastmilk; Foremilk

Footnotes
　[118b]Cregan, M.D., & Hartman, P.E. (1999). Computerized breast measurement from conception to weaning: Clinical implications. *Journal of Human Lactation, 15*, 89.

▶ HIV

DEFINITION   Human immunodeficiency virus. HIV causes the life threatening disease of the immune system, acquired immunodeficiency syndrome (AIDS). People with AIDS have increased susceptibility to infections and rare cancers including Kaposi's sarcoma. HIV is transmitted primarily by exposure to contaminated body fluids, especially blood, semen, and potentially breastmilk.

Ask about

Onset.
Age of baby.

ASSESSMENT

EMERGENT CARE NEEDED?

Are any of the following present?

Breastfeeding mother with concern about possibility of recently contracting HIV.

Breastfeeding mother diagnosed with HIV.

Pregnant woman with concerns about possibility of recently contracting HIV.

Pregnant woman diagnosed with HIV.

Pregnant or breastfeeding woman taking antiretroviral medications.

IF YES,   *Seek medical care within 2 to 4 hours.*

ROUTINE CARE NEEDED?

Are any of the following present?

General questions about HIV.

IF YES,   *Call pediatric or obstetric care provider today.*

SELF CARE INFORMATION

Know your HIV status.
Know your treatment options.
Know the HIV status of all sexual partners.
Practice safe sex.
Avoid intravenous drug use.

IMPORTANT CONDITIONS TO REPORT
Need for testing.

> **Notes**
>
> In the United States, breastfeeding is contraindicated in women diagnosed as HIV positive or with **AIDS**. Women at high risk for HIV (e.g., women who are sex workers, women with an HIV positive sexual partner, women using intravenous drugs, women whose sexual partners use intravenous drugs, and women who are raped or coerced to have sex) should receive ongoing testing and counseling regarding infant feeding.

See also Contraindicated conditions

▶ HMBANA

See also Human Milk Banking Association of North America (HMBANA)

▶ HMHB

See also National Healthy Mothers, Healthy Babies Coalition (HMHB)

▶ HOM

See also Higher order multiples (HOM)

▶ Hormonal contraceptive methods

DEFINITION   Drugs used to reduce fertility.
Progestin-only hormonal methods are considered compatible with breastfeeding.
Combined estrogen/progestin methods are generally not recommended as they may reduce milk supply and affect infant growth.

> **Notes**
>
> Progestin-only injectibles are intended for use in breastfeeding women only at six weeks post-delivery, or when full milk supply is developed. Use prior to that time may decrease milk supply due to high circulating progestin levels, simulating a state of pregnancy.

See also Birth control; Contraception; Progestin-only contraceptives

▶ Hormones

DEFINITION A substance produced by cells that regulates or stimulates other cells and organs. Hormones are produced by several different endocrine glands in the body.

Hormones are crucial to the production and flow of breastmilk. The alveolar cells produce droplets of milk in response to suckling and the resulting spike in the hormone **prolactin**. The hormone **oxytocin** (which is created by nipple stretching, breast massage, and other stimuli) causes the myoepithelial bands around the alveoli to contract, squeezing the milk into the ductules and ducts, propelling it toward the nipple.

Synthetic hormones (e.g., cortisone, progestin, etc.) are used to treat hormone disorders and provide contraception.

See also Birth control; Hyperthyroidism; Hypothyroidism; Progestin-only contraceptives

▶ Hospitalization and breastfeeding

DEFINITION Referring to the effect of separation of mother and baby when required for medical purposes. Mother, baby, or both may be hospitalized. Breastmilk production can be supported during this time if breastfeeding is not possible due to separation. When possible, mothers and babies may be hospitalized together so that breastfeeding can continue.

Ask about

Onset.
Age of baby.
Reason for hospitalization.

PROMPT CARE NEEDED?

Are any of the following present?

Breastfeeding mother planning hospitalization.

IF YES, *Call lactation care provider today.*

SELF CARE INFORMATION

Express milk as much as possible to relieve pressure and maintain milk supply; aim to express milk as often as baby would normally feed (at least eight times daily).

Store milk as appropriate (ask for storage guidelines if baby is premature or ill).

Ask about medication compatibility and side effects.

Arrange for transport and feeding of expressed milk to baby if baby will be separated from the mother.

Ask when skin-to-skin contact and breastfeeding can resume.

IMPORTANT CONDITIONS TO REPORT

Discomfort.

Declining milk production.

See also Abrupt weaning; Breast pump; Hand expression of breastmilk; Separation of mother and baby

---

▶ HTLV-I, HTLV-II

See also Human T-cell lymphotropic virus I and human T-cell lymphotropic virus II (HTLV-I, HTLV-II)

▶ Human immunodeficiency virus (HIV)

DEFINITION Human immunodeficiency virus (HIV) causes the life threatening disease of the immune system, acquired immunodeficiency syndrome (AIDS). People with AIDS have increased susceptibility to infections and rare cancers including Kaposi's sarcoma. HIV is transmitted primarily by exposure to contaminated body fluids, especially blood, semen, and potentially breastmilk.

Onset.

Age of baby.

ASSESSMENT

EMERGENT CARE NEEDED?

Are any of the following present?

Breastfeeding mother with concern about possibility of recently contracting HIV.

Breastfeeding mother diagnosed with HIV.

Pregnant woman with concerns about possibility of recently contracting HIV.

Pregnant woman diagnosed with HIV.

Pregnant or breastfeeding woman taking antiretroviral medications.

IF YES, *Seek medical care within 2 to 4 hours.*

ROUTINE CARE NEEDED?

Are any of the following present?

General questions about HIV.

IF YES, *Call pediatric or obstetric care provider today.*

SELF CARE INFORMATION

Know your HIV status.

Know your treatment options.

Know the HIV status of all sexual partners.

Practice safe sex.

Avoid intravenous drug use.

IMPORTANT CONDITIONS TO REPORT

Need for testing.

See also Contraindicated conditions

▶ Human Milk Banking Association of North America (HMBANA)

DEFINITION "The Human Milk Banking Association of North America (HMBANA) is a multidisciplinary group of health care providers that promotes, protects, and supports donor milk banking. HMBANA is the only professional membership association for milk banks in Canada, Mexico and the United States and as such sets the standards and guidelines for donor milk banking for those areas."[119]

> **Notes**
>
> Human Milk Banking Association of North America (HMBANA)
> 1500 Sunday Drive
> Suite 102
> Raleigh, NC 27607
> Phone: 919-861-4530 ext. 226
> Web site: www.hmbana.org

See also Donor milk; Milk banks

Footnotes

[119]Human Milk Banking Association of North America. (2003). *Human Milk Banking Association of North America*. Retrieved July 12, 2005, from http://www.hmbana.org.

▶ Human milk fortification

DEFINITION The practice of adding minerals, fats, and protein to expressed breast milk to increase its nutrient content. Calcium, phosphorus, zinc, and iron are among the nutrients added. In the United States, commercially available "human" milk fortifiers are made with cow's milk products.

> **Notes**
>
> Human milk fortification is typically used only for very low birthweight infants in neonatal care unit settings.

See also Lactoengineering; Premature infant; Preterm milk

▶ Human T-cell lymphotropic virus I and human T-cell lymphotropic virus II (HTLV-I, HTLV-II)

DEFINITION Infection with the human T-cell lymphotropic virus I or II (HTLV-I, HTLV-II). Breastfeeding is contraindicated in the mother with HTLV infection.

> **Notes**
>
> HTLV infection is not common in the United States, but may be found in intravenous drug users, people with **human immunodeficiency virus (HIV)**, and some Native American, African, and Asian populations.
>
> HTLV testing by enzyme-linked immunosorbent assay, or ELISA (as done by cord blood donation/storage companies), can yield false positives due to cross-reactivity with pregnancy antibodies. Confirmation by Western blot is indicated.

See also Contraindicated conditions

▶ Hydrogel pads

DEFINITION   Devices designed to give comfort to painful nipples. Hydrogel matrix pads with a cloth backing are intended to be worn over the nipple.

There is little research supporting claims that hydrogel pads heal trauma to the nipple.

Ask about

Nipple discomfort.

ASSESSMENT

PROMPT CARE NEEDED?

Are any of the following present?

Extreme nipple pain.

Bleeding from nipples.

Unable to breastfeed due to pain.

IF YES,   *Call lactation care provider now.*

ROUTINE CARE NEEDED?

Are any of the following present?

Feeding discomfort.

Trauma to nipple or breasts.

Misshapen nipple after feedings.

Visible fissures on nipples.

IF YES,   *Call lactation care provider today.*

SELF CARE INFORMATION

Any substance that is applied to the nipple area will be consumed by the nursing baby. Do not apply any creams or ointments to the nipple area without getting your medical care provider's approval first.

Report nipple pain to your lactation care provider.

IMPORTANT CONDITIONS TO REPORT

Symptoms worsen or persist.

Signs of infection.

Feeding or stooling expectations not met.

> **Notes**
>
> Women experiencing **nipple pain** may self-treat with gel pads and other substances rather than seeking help to resolve the cause of the pain.
>
> Women experiencing nipple pain should have a breastfeeding evaluation. Face-to-face counseling is effective in assessing and resolving nipple pain.
>
> Any hydrogel pads used should be approved for use in breastfeeding mothers.

See also Nipple pain; Sore nipples

▶ Hyperadenia

DEFINITION   Breast tissue with no nipples.

> **Notes**
>
> Women can have breast or nipple tissue anywhere along the milk line, which extends from the axilla over the front of the chest and abdomen and into the groin region.

▶ Hyperbilirubinemia

DEFINITION   Presence of an excessive amount of bilirubin (a breakdown product of red blood cells) in the blood.

When bilirubin accumulates in the blood stream a yellow discoloration of the skin and the whites of the eyes called **jaundice** can occur. It is the most common condition requiring medical treatment in the newborn period.

Bilirubin is removed from the blood by the liver.

Although the condition of jaundice may be benign, it can be a symptom of a serious condition called **kernicterus**.

Ask about

Age of baby.
Feeding behavior.
Stooling pattern and color.
Urination pattern.

ASSESSMENT

PROMPT CARE NEEDED?

Are any of the following present?

Severe lethargy (sleepiness).

Poor feeding.

No interest in feeding for more than 6 hours.

Fever.

Meconium bowel movements after 5 days of life.

Fewer than three bowel movements daily in breastfed newborn after the first 2 days of life.

No urine in six hours.

Brick dust urine (uric acid crystals) after 2 days of life.

Dark colored urine.

Fewer than four urinations daily in the breastfed newborn after day 5 of life.

Noticeably sunken fontanelles (soft spot on top of head).

Decreased activity.

Baby below birthweight at 10 to 14 days of life.

Cessation of weight gain.

Any fever in a baby younger than 3 months of age.

Fever higher than 100°F (37.7°C) in a baby younger than 3 months of age.

IF YES, *Seek pediatric care now.*

ROUTINE CARE NEEDED?

Are any of the following present?

Baby sleepy during breastfeedings.

IF YES, *Call lactation care care provider now.*

SELF CARE INFORMATION

Breastfeed as soon as possible after birth.

Encourage the baby to nurse 10–12 times per 24 hours.

Colostrum has laxative properties. Stooling helps to rid the baby's body of bilirubin.

IMPORTANT CONDITIONS TO REPORT

No stool in 24 hours.

Severe lethargy (sleepiness).

Poor feeding.

Fever.

> **Notes**
>
> All jaundiced babies are at risk for kernicterus and should be closely monitored.

See also Bilirubin; Jaundice; Kernicterus; Late onset jaundice

▶ Hypergalactia

DEFINITION   Production of excessive amounts of milk.

> **Notes**
>
> Excess milk production can create problems such as gas and discomfort in the baby, recurrent plugged ducts, mastitis, and sore nipples in the mother. Lactation evaluation is indicated by these symptoms.

▶ Hypermastia

DEFINITION   Refers to two conditions: excessive growth of the breasts, and existence of more than two breasts. Both of these conditions are compatible with breastfeeding.

See also Accessory breast tissue; Gigantomastia

► Hyperthelia

DEFINITION Presence of more than one nipple per breast, or nipples with no breast tissue. These conditions are compatible with breastfeeding.

See also Accessory breast tissue

► Hyperthyroidism

DEFINITION The thyroid gland is the body's master metabolic hormone producer. Hyperthyroidism refers to an overabundance of thyroid hormone.

Breastfeeding is not contraindicated for women who have hyperthyroidism.

A woman whose hyperthyroid problem (thyroiditis) is identified during pregnancy or lactation presents a special problem in the diagnosis and treatment. The mother should tell all health care providers that she is breastfeeding.

Many of the signs and symptoms of thyroid disease can seem "normal" to a postpartum woman. The symptom that is unique to hyperthyroidism is difficulty with initiating and maintaining an adequate milk supply.

Signs and symptoms of hyperthyroidism include:

- Palpitations.
- Heat intolerance.
- Nervousness.
- Insomnia.
- Breathlessness.
- Increased bowel movements.
- Light or absent menstrual periods.
- Fatigue.
- Weight loss.
- Fast heart rate.
- Trembling hands.
- Muscle weakness.
- Warm, moist skin.
- Hair loss.

Both high and low levels of thyroid hormones can affect the mother's milk supply.

Ask about

Age of baby.
Weight gain pattern of baby.

ASSESSMENT

EMERGENT CARE NEEDED?

Are any of the following present?

Meconium bowel movements after 5 days of life.

Fewer than three bowel movements daily in breastfed newborn after the first 2 days of life.

No urine in six hours.

Brick dust urine (uric acid crystals) after 2 days of life.

Dark colored urine.

Fewer than four urinations daily in the breastfed newborn after day 5 of life.

Noticeably sunken fontanelles (soft spot on top of head).

Decreased activity (lethargy).

Baby below birthweight at 10 to 14 days of life.

Cessation of weight gain.

Hard to latch on.

Subtle feeding cues.

Weak suck.

Baby sleepy, difficult to wake.

IF YES, *Seek pediatric care now.*

PROMPT CARE NEEDED?

Are any of the following present?

Inadequate weight gain.

Concern about possible inadequate weight gain.

IF YES, *Call pediatric care provider today.*

ROUTINE CARE NEEDED?

Are any of the following present?

Building up milk supply after medication adjustment.

IF YES, *Call lactation care provider today.*

SELF CARE INFORMATION

Postpartum thyroid problems can initially present as postpartum depression or anxiety. Mothers who struggle with milk supply should have a thorough medical evaluation if the supply does not improve with increased frequency and expression.

IMPORTANT CONDITIONS TO REPORT

Increasing sleepiness in baby.
Increasing fatigue and inability to cope in the mother.
Feelings of hopelessness or depression.
Symptoms of thyroid disease.

See also Hypothyroidism; Maternal fatigue

▶ Hypertonia

DEFINITION   Referring to tight, tense muscle response or stiffness.
Hypertonia can be a symptom of illness and other problems.
Hypertonic babies may arch their bodies away from the breast.
Some of the problems that may be seen with breastfeeding include difficulty latching-on, biting when swallowing (tonic bite reflex), and difficulty sustaining rhythmic suck.

Ask about

Age of baby.
Onset of hypertonia.
Change in feeding behavior.
Change in urination or stooling patterns.

ASSESSMENT

EMERGENT CARE NEEDED?
Are any of the following present?
Sudden onset of change in muscle tone.
Sudden change in feeding behavior.

IF YES,   ***Call pediatric care provider now.***

PROMPT CARE NEEDED?

Are any of the following present?

Feeding problems.

Weight loss or failure to initially gain weight in newborn period.

Constipation.

Decline in milk supply.

IF YES, **Call pediatric care provider today.**

ROUTINE CARE NEEDED?

Are any of the following present?

Feeding problems.

Slow weight gain.

Problems positioning baby at breast.

Nipple discomfort.

Decline in milk supply.

IF YES, **Call pediatric care provider and lactation care provider today.**

SELF CARE INFORMATION

Breastfeeding and breast milk are valuable for babies with high muscle tone.

Pumping may be necessary in order to maintain an adequate milk supply.

"Wearing" the baby in an over-the-shoulder sling can be very helpful to encourage flexion in a hyperextending infant.

IMPORTANT CONDITIONS TO REPORT

Change in feeding behaviors.

Change in urination or stooling patterns.

Declining breastmilk volume.

See also Attachment; Latch-on

▶ Hypoglycemia

DEFINITION   A condition in which an individual's blood glucose (sugar) levels have fallen below a predetermined amount.

Age of baby.
Gestational age of baby.
History of diabetes in mother.
History of labor, especially stress.

ASSESSMENT

EMERGENT CARE NEEDED?

Are any of the following present?

Seizure activity.

Convulsions.

Coma.

Respiratory distress.

Apnea (cessation of breathing).

Cyanosis (blue color).

Thermoregulatory problems.

Jitteriness.

Hypotonia (lack of muscle tone).

Lethargy.

Listnessness.

Poor feeding.

IF YES, *Seek medical care now.*

PROMPT CARE NEEDED?

Are any of the following present?

Feeding problems after treatment for hypoglycemia.

IF YES, *Call lactation care provider today.*

SELF CARE INFORMATION

Establish early and frequent breastfeeding.
Keep the baby warm and dry.
Seek help with breastfeeding if baby feeds poorly.

IMPORTANT CONDITIONS TO REPORT

Seizure activity.

Convulsions.

Coma.

Respiratory distress.

Apnea (cessation of breathing).

Cyanosis (blue color).

Thermoregulatory problems.

Jitteriness.

Hypotonia (lack of muscle tone).

Lethargy.

Listnessness.

Poor feeding.

▶ Hypothyroidism

DEFINITION The thyroid gland is the body's master metabolic hormone producer. Hypothyroidism refers to abnormally low levels of thyroid hormone.

Breastfeeding is not contraindicated for women who have hypothyroidism.

Women with hypothyroidism are prescribed thyroid replacement therapy. These medications are typically compatible with breastfeeding.

Many of the signs and symptoms of thyroid disease can seem "normal" in a postpartum woman. The symptom that is unique to hypothyroidism is difficulty with initiating and maintaining an adequate milk supply.

Ask about

Age of baby.

Weight gain pattern of baby.

ASSESSMENT

EMERGENT CARE NEEDED?

Are any of the following present?

About baby

Baby sleepy, difficult to wake.

Meconium bowel movements after 5 days of life.

Fewer than three bowel movements daily in breastfed newborn after the first 2 days of life.

No urine in six hours.

Brick dust urine (uric acid crystals) after 2 days of life.

Dark colored urine.

Fewer than four urinations daily in the breastfed newborn after day 5 of life.

Noticeably sunken fontanelles (soft spot on top of head).

Decreased activity.

Baby below birthweight at 10 to 14 days of life.

Cessation of weight gain.

Hard to latch on.

Subtle feeding cues.

Weak suck.

IF YES, *Seek pediatric care now.*

PROMPT CARE NEEDED?

Are any of the following present?

About mother

Signs and symptoms of hypothyroidism in the mother include:

Fatigue (may seem to be a "normal" postpartum condition).

Weakness.

Weight gain or difficulty losing weight (difficult to ascertain in postpartum).

Coarse, dry hair.

Dry, rough skin.

Hair loss (difficult to notice in pregnant and postpartum women unless severe).

Inability to tolerate cold as well as others in the same environment.

Muscle cramps and aches.

Constipation.

Depression (may be assumed to be "baby blues").

Irritability.

Memory loss.

Abnormal menstrual periods (normal to not menstruate in the early time postpartum).

Decreased sexual desire (normal in postpartum women).

IF YES, *Seek medical care today.*

PROMPT CARE NEEDED?

Are any of the following present?

About baby

Inadequate weight gain.

Concern about inadequate weight gain in breastfed baby.

IF YES, *Seek pediatric care today.*

ROUTINE CARE NEEDED?

Are any of the following present?

Building up milk supply after medication adjustment.

IF YES, *Call lactation care provider today.*

SELF CARE INFORMATION

Postpartum thyroid problems can initially present as postpartum depression or simply normal tiredness or fatigue. Mothers who struggle with milk supply should have a thorough lactation and medical evaluation if the supply does not improve with increased frequency and expression.

IMPORTANT CONDITIONS TO REPORT

Increasing sleepiness in baby.

Increasing fatigue and inability to cope in the mother.

Feelings of hopelessness or depression.

Symptoms of thyroid disease.

Notes

Hypothyroidism can occur in infants. There are indications that breastfeeding may mask the symptoms of the illness, as breastmilk contains thyroid hormones. There are no contraindications to breastfeeding with thyroid imbalance in the mother or baby.

See also Hyperthyroidism; Maternal fatigue; Milk supply, inadequate

► Hypotonia

DEFINITION   Referring to loose or floppy muscle response. Babies with low muscle tone (also referred to as hypotonia) have relaxed arm and leg joints, like a rag doll. Hypotonia can be a symptom of prematurity and of physical problems or illness. Babies with low muscle tone may have breastfeeding problems such as non-rhythmic suck and weak sucking, and they may tire more easily.

Ask about

Age of baby.
Onset of hypotonia.
Change in feeding behavior.
Change in urination or stooling patterns.
Any identified medical problems for mother or baby.
Any medication use.

ASSESSMENT

EMERGENT CARE NEEDED?

Are any of the following present in infant?

Sudden change in muscle tone.
Sudden change in feeding behavior.
Sudden lethargy.

IF YES,   *Seek emergency care now.*

PROMPT CARE NEEDED?

Are any of the following present?

Weight loss or failure to initially gain in the newborn period.
Meconium bowel movements after 5 days of life.
Fewer than three bowel movements daily in breastfed newborn after the first 2 days of life.
No urine in six hours.
Brick dust urine (uric acid crystals) after 2 days of life.
Dark colored urine.
Fewer than four urinations daily in the breastfed newborn after day 5 of life.

Noticeably sunken fontanelles (soft spot on top of head).

Decreased activity.

Baby below birthweight at 10 to 14 days of life.

Cessation of weight gain or weight loss.

IF YES, *Seek pediatric care now.*

ROUTINE CARE NEEDED?

Are any of the following present?

Breastfeeding baby with diagnosed hypotonia, or a condition that includes hypotonia (such as Down syndrome).

Feeding problems.

Slow weight gain.

Problems positioning baby at breast.

Decline in milk supply.

IF YES, *Call lactation care provider today.*

SELF CARE INFORMATION

Breastfeeding and breast milk are valuable for babies with low muscle tone. Pumping may be necessary in order to maintain an adequate milk supply. Holding the baby skin-to-skin is helpful.

IMPORTANT CONDITIONS TO REPORT

Change in feeding behaviors.

Change in urination or stooling patterns.

Declining breastmilk volume.

See also Down syndrome (DS); Slow weight gain, baby

► Hysterectomy

DEFINITION A surgical procedure that removes the uterus. Women may breastfeed after this surgery.

Date of surgery.
Age of baby.

ASSESSMENT

PROMPT CARE NEEDED?

Are any of the following present?

Breastfeeding mother undergoing hysterectomy.

Breastfeeding problems in a woman who has experienced hysterectomy.

IF YES, *Call lactation care provider today.*

SELF CARE INFORMATION

Express milk as much as possible to relieve pressure and maintain milk supply; aim to express milk as often as baby would normally feed (at least eight times daily).

Store milk as appropriate.

Ask about safety of any medications prescribed (make sure all care providers know you are breastfeeding).

Arrange for transport and feeding of expressed milk to baby.

Ask when skin-to-skin contact and breastfeeding can resume.

IMPORTANT CONDITIONS TO REPORT

Discomfort.

Declining milk production.

Notes

Emergency hysterectomy sometimes occurs immediately after childbirth. Breastfeeding is not contraindicated in these mothers. If mothers hemorrhage severely, milk suply may be impacted by injury to the pituitary gland (**Sheehan's syndrome**).

See also Abrupt weaning; Breast pump; Hand expression of breastmilk; Sheehan's syndrome

▶ IBCLC

DEFINITION International Board Certified Lactation Consultant. An individual who has qualified for and passed the examination administered by the International Board of Lactation Consultant Examiners.

The designations International Board Certified Lactation Consultant (IBCLC) and Registered Lactation Consultant (RLC) are used to denote international board certified lactation care providers in the United States.

▶ IBFAN

See also International Baby Food Action Network (IBFAN)

▶ IBLCE

DEFINITION International Board of Lactation Consultant Examiners.

"The primary purpose of the International Board of Lactation Consultant Examiners (IBLCE) is to benefit the public by setting standards for the lactation care provider profession. The IBLCE is a non-profit organization governed by a Board of Directors. It was established to develop and administer the certification examination for lactation care providers."[120]

Notes

International Board of Lactation Consultant Examiners (IBLCE)
7309 Arlington Boulevard
Suite 300
Falls Church, VA 22042-3215
Phone: 703-560-7330
Fax: 703-560-7332
E-mail: iblce@iblce.org
Web site: www.iblce.org

Footnotes

[120]International Board of Lactation Consultant Examiners. (2004). *The IBLCE organization.* Retrieved July 12, 2005, from http://www.iblce.org/about.htm.

► Ibuprofen

DEFINITION A nonsteroidal anti-inflammatory drug used for pain relief.

> **Notes**
>
> The American Academy of Pediatrics includes ibuprofen on Table 6, "Maternal Medication Usually Compatible with Breastfeeding."[121] Hale rates ibuprofen as an L1 (Safest) drug.[122]

See also Analgesia; Medications; Over-the-counter (OTC) drugs

Footnotes

[121]American Academy of Pediatrics Committee on Drugs. (2001). Transfer of drugs and other chemicals into human milk. *Pediatrics, 108,* 781.

[122]Hale, T.W. (2004). *Medications and mothers milk* (p. 423). Amarillo, TX: Pharmasoft Publishing.

Drug References

Briggs, G.G., Freeman, R.K., & Yaffee, S.J. (Eds.). (2002). *Drugs in pregnancy and lactation* (6th ed.). Philadelphia: Lippincott, Williams, and Wilkins.

Lawrence, R.A., & Lawrence, R.M. (2005). *Breastfeeding: A guide for the medical profession* (6th ed.). St. Louis: Mosby.

► IDDM

DEFINITION Insulin-dependent diabetes mellitus. A chronic disease causing high levels of glucose (sugar) in the blood.

In this form of diabetes, the pancreas makes little or no insulin, requiring daily injections of this hormone that regulates glucose metabolism.

Women with IDDM can breastfeed their babies.

Ask about

Onset.

Type of diabetes.

EMERGENT CARE NEEDED?

Are any of the following present?

Insulin shock in the breastfeeding woman.

IF YES, *Seek emergency care now.*

PROMPT CARE NEEDED?

Are any of the following present?

Difficulty maintaining blood glucose levels during breastfeeding.

IF YES, *Call medical care provider now.*

ROUTINE CARE NEEDED?

Are any of the following present?

Ongoing breastfeeding problems in the diabetic woman.

IF YES, *Call lactation care provider today.*

SELF CARE INFORMATION

Women with diabetes are more prone to infection. Monitor breasts and nipples daily for any red, infected, or painful areas.

If insulin-dependent, be aware that less insulin may be required during breastfeeding—watch for signs of low blood sugar.

IMPORTANT CONDITIONS TO REPORT

Any symptoms of infection.

Difficulty regulating blood sugar.

Notes

Women with diabetes should be encouraged to breastfeed. Breastfeeding is known to reduce the risk of developing diabetes in susceptible individuals (e.g., children of diabetic mothers).

Research suggests that women who have experienced gestational diabetes are less likely to develop diabetes if they breastfeed their babies.

See also Autoimmune diseases

▶ **IgA**

DEFINITION Immunoglobulin A. An immunoglobulin that protects the mucous membranes of the respiratory and digestive tracts from invasion by pathogens.

Human babies are born without IgA. Babies do not produce their own IgA for several months.

Human milk is a rich source of IgA, providing the first level of immune defense until babies develop their own IgA.

SELF CARE INFORMATION

Nursing in the first hours after birth transfers IgA from the mother to the baby.

The IgA coats the baby's intestines, lung surfaces, and other mucous membranes. This helps to protect the baby from bacteria and viruses as soon as possible.

See also Skin-to-skin care

▶ **IgA deficiency and human milk**

DEFINITION Selective deficiency of immunoglobulin A occurs in some adults. Often people with this disorder may be asymptomatic, or they may have recurrent infections, allergies, or autoimmune disorders.

Breastfeeding is still recommended when mother has IgA deficiency.

▶ **IgE**

DEFINITION Immunoglobulin E. An immunoglobulin that combines with antigens in the gut and releases chemicals that cause changes to the permeability of the gut wall.

Human milk contains IgE in lower concentration than IgA.

▶ IGF-I

DEFINITION   Insulin-like growth factor. A beneficial agent found in human milk that triggers growth.

Research suggests that preterm, exclusively breastfed infants have higher serum levels of this growth promoting factor.

▶ ILCA

See also International Lactation Consultant Association (ILCA)

▶ Illegal drugs and breastfeeding

DEFINITION   Use of street drugs, including intoxicants and hallucinogens such as cocaine, heroin, and amphetamines.

Breastfeeding is contraindicated in women with habitual use of illegal drugs.

> **Notes**
>
> See American Academy of Pediatrics Table 2[123] and Hale[124] for review of the specific effects of these drugs.

Footnotes

[123]American Academy of Pediatrics Committee on Drugs. (2001). Transfer of drugs and other chemicals into human milk. *Pediatrics, 108,* 781.

[124]Hale, T.W. (2004). *Medications and mothers milk.* Amarillo, TX: Pharmasoft Publishing.

Drug References

Briggs, G.G., Freeman, R.K., & Yaffee, S.J. (Eds.). (2002). *Drugs in pregnancy and lactation* (6th ed.). Philadelphia: Lippincott, Williams, and Wilkins.

Lawrence, R.A., & Lawrence, R.M. (2005). *Breastfeeding: A guide for the medical profession* (6th ed.). St. Louis: Mosby.

▶ Illicit drugs and breastfeeding

See also Illegal drugs and breastfeeding

▶ Illness, acute

DEFINITION   Sickness in the mother and baby are compatible with breastfeeding, except in rare contraindicated infections in the mother (e.g., HIV, HTLV-1, untreated tuberculosis, and active herpes lesions on the breast).

> **Notes**
>
> An up-to-date drug reference should be consulted to determine the safety and possible side effects of individual drugs taken during acute illness.
>   Newborn and premature babies are at greater risk of side effects due to limited ability to clear drugs from their systems.

See also Acute infection; Contraindicated conditions

▶ Illness, chronic

DEFINITION   Diseases or disorders that last for a long time or reoccur.
    Breastfeeding is known to reduce the severity or risk of developing several chronic illnesses including eczema, asthma, diabetes, multiple sclerosis, and celiac disease.
    Mothers and babies with chronic illnesses may breastfeed, except in rare contraindicated infections in the mother or baby:
    Infant: Classic galactosemia.
    Maternal: Women "who have active untreated tuberculosis disease or are human T-cell lymphotropic virus type I– or II–positive; mothers who are receiving diagnostic or therapeutic radioactive isotopes or have had exposure to radioactive materials (for as long as there is radioactivity in the milk); mothers who are receiving antimetabolites or chemotherapeutic agents or a small number of other medications until they clear the milk; mothers who are using drugs of abuse ('street drugs'); and mothers who have herpes simplex lesions on a

breast (infant may feed from other breast if clear of lesions)." Furthermore, in the United States, the American Academy of Pediatrics indicates that "mothers who are infected with human immunodeficiency virus (HIV) have been advised not to breastfeed their infants."[125]

Notes

An up-to-date drug reference should be consulted to determine the safety and possible side effects of individual drugs taken during acute and chronic illness.

Newborn and premature babies are at greater risk of side effects due to limited ability to clear drugs from their systems.

While breastfeeding is universally recommended, parents with a family history of chronic illness should be strongly encouraged to consider breastfeeding to decrease their child's risk.

Exclusive breastfeeding (offering no food or drink other than breastmilk to the young baby) offers the highest level of protection against chronic diseases.

Footnotes

[125]American Academy of Pediatrics Section on Breastfeeding. (2005). Breastfeeding and the use of human milk. *Pediatrics, 115,* 497.

▶ ## Immune system

DEFINITION   The complex, intricate mechanism through which the body protects itself from invasion by pathogens.

Human milk is a rich source of bioactive factors, including antibodies, antivirals, white blood cells, enzymes, immune-active proteins, fats, and sugars, and numerous growth and immune factors.

Breastfeeding children receive several different types of immunoglobulins as well as live immune cells and factors from their mother's milk.

See also Bioactive components of breastmilk; Bronchus-associated lymphoid tissue (BALT); Gut-associated lymphoid tissue (GALT); Lymphocytes; Macrophages; Mucosa-associated lymphoid tissue (MALT)

▶ Immunization

DEFINITION   The process of becoming protected against a pathogen or disease. This may be naturally acquired through pathogen exposure, or intentionally given by injecting dead or altered pathogens into the body.

Immunizations taken by the mother are generally compatible with breastfeeding, with the exception of the smallpox vaccine and possibly rubella.

Notes

Contact the Centers for Disease Control and Prevention for updates regarding immunizations in the mother, as knowledge about vaccination is constantly updated.

Breastfeeding offers natural immunity to many common pathogens in the family environment.

Breastfeeding during and immediately after infant immunization is recommended to provide pain relief for the baby.

See also Vaccinations and immunizations

▶ Immunoglobulin

DEFINITION   Proteins manufactured by the body to fight infection.

All classes of immunoglobins—Ig, IgG, IgD, IgM, and IgE (*Ig* is an abbreviation for immunoglobulin)—are found in human milk. They are found in higher amounts in colostrum, but continue throughout lactation.

▶ Immunoglobulin A (IgA)

DEFINITION   An immunoglobulin that protects the mucous membranes of the respiratory and digestive tracts from invasion by pathogens.

Human babies are born without IgA. Babies do not produce their own IgA for several months.

Human milk is a rich source of IgA, providing the first level of immune defense until babies develop their own IgA.

SELF CARE INFORMATION

Nursing in the first hours after birth transfers IgA from the mother to the baby.
The IgA coats the baby's intestines, lung surfaces, and other mucous membranes.
This helps to protect the baby from bacteria and viruses as soon as possible.

See also Skin-to-skin care

► Immunoglobulin E (IgE)

DEFINITION   An immunoglobulin that combines with antigens in the gut and releases
chemicals that cause changes to the permeability of the gut wall.
Human milk contains IgE in lower concentration than IgA.

► Impaired mobility, mothers with

DEFINITION   Referring to mothers living with restrictions to physical motion.
Breastfeeding is often an ideal feeding choice for mothers with impaired mobility,
as it requires little preparation for feeding.

Ask about

Type of impairment.
Age of baby.

ASSESSMENT

PROMPT CARE NEEDED?
   Are any of the following present?
         Mother with impaired mobility learning to breastfeed.
         Ongoing breastfeeding support needed.

   IF YES,   *Call lactation care provider today.*

SELF CARE INFORMATION

Set up a feeding station in the home where nonperishable snacks, drinks of water,
baby changing equipment, handwipes, and telephone can be at the ready.

IMPORTANT CONDITIONS TO REPORT

Concern about feeding adequacy or comfort.

▶ Imperforate anus

DEFINITION A defect in the formation of the end of the digestive system where stool exits the body. There may be a total lack of opening of the anus, narrowing of the anus, or misplacement of the opening of the anus.

Breastfeeding is compatible with this condition.

Notes

Children born with this condition require surgery and may have difficulty with stool control. Children with this problem may have associated anomalies such as esophageal atresia and cardiac defects.

▶ Implants, breast

DEFINITION Devices made of saline or gel surgically inserted into the breast to increase its size or to reconstruct the breast after mastectomy or trauma.

Ask about

Onset.
Age of baby.
Location of surgical incision.
Reason for implant.

ASSESSMENT

PROMPT MEDICAL CARE NEEDED?
Are any of the following present?
Meconium bowel movements after 5 days of life.
Fewer than three bowel movements daily in breastfed newborn after the first 2 days of life.

No urine in six hours.

Brick dust urine (uric acid crystals) after 2 days of life.

Dark colored urine.

Fewer than four urinations daily in the breastfed newborn after day 5 of life.

Noticeably sunken fontanelles (soft spot on top of head).

Decreased activity.

Baby below birthweight at 10 to 14 days.

Cessation of weight gain.

IF YES, *Seek medical care within 2 to 4 hours.*

PROMPT LACTATION CARE NEEDED?

Are any of the following present?

Concerns about milk supply.

Slow weight gain in breastfed baby.

IF YES, *Call lactation care provider today.*

SELF CARE INFORMATION

Practice skin-to-skin contact frequently.

Feed baby at first sign of hunger cues (signs that say "feed me" include hand-to-face or hand-to-mouth movements, lip smacking, seeking with lips, rooting, and head bobbing).

Feed baby at least 10–12 times per 24 hours.

Listen for signs of baby swallowing.

Allow baby to end feedings.

Expect at least 3–4 infant stools per 24 hours after the first 4 days of life.

Good positioning and attachment are crucial to reduce nipple pain.

If feedings are missed, hand express or pump milk to maintain supply.

IMPORTANT CONDITIONS TO REPORT

Fewer than four bowel movements daily in newborn time period.

Ongoing concerns or problems with milk supply.

See also Asymmetric breasts; Breast augmentation; Breast surgery

▶ Inadequate milk supply

See also Insufficient milk supply

▶ Inadequate weight gain

See also Insufficient weight gain

▶ Increasing milk supply

DEFINITION   Raising the amount of milk produced by the breast. This is accomplished by increasing stimulation and removal of milk from the breast.

Ask about

Reason for desire to increase milk supply.
Age of baby.

EMERGENT CARE NEEDED?

Are any of the following present?

Meconium bowel movements after 5 days of life.

Fewer than three bowel movements daily in breastfed newborn after the first 2 days of life.

No urine in six hours.

Brick dust urine (uric acid crystals) after 2 days of life.

Dark colored urine.

Fewer than four urinations daily in the breastfed newborn after day 5 of life.

Noticeably sunken fontanelles (soft spot on top of head).

Decreased activity.

Baby below birthweight at 10 to 14 days of life.

Cessation of weight gain or weight loss.

IF YES, *Seek pediatric care now.*

PROMPT CARE NEEDED?

Are any of the following present?

Identified milk supply problem.

Concern about possible milk supply problems.

IF YES, *Call lactation care provider today.*

SELF CARE INFORMATION

Ensure baby is feeding 10–12 times per 24 hours.

Express milk after feeding.

IMPORTANT CONDITIONS TO REPORT

Persistent problems.

Recurrent problems.

See also Decrease in milk supply; Milk supply, inadequate; Relactation

▶ Induced lactation

DEFINITION Induced lactation is the process of establishing a milk supply in a woman who has not given birth.

Ask about

Age of baby.

ASSESSMENT

ROUTINE CARE NEEDED?
Are any of the following present?
Mother wishes to induce lactation for an adopted infant.

IF YES, *Call lactation care provider.*

SELF CARE INFORMATION
Frequent stimulation may increase milk supply.

Practice skin-to-skin contact frequently.

Feed baby at first sign of hunger cues (signs that say "feed me" include hand-to-face or hand-to-mouth movements, lip smacking, seeking with lips, rooting, and head bobbing).

Feed baby at least 10–12 times per 24 hours.

Listen for signs of baby swallowing.

Supplement as needed with milk from an HMBANA milk bank or formula.

Allow baby to end feedings.

Expect at least 3–4 infant stools per 24 hours after the first 4 days of life.

Good positioning and attachment are crucial to reduce nipple pain.

If feedings are missed, hand express or pump milk to maintain supply.

Frequent weight checks to assure adequate nutrition and growth.

IMPORTANT CONDITIONS TO REPORT
Arrival of baby.

First visible milk produced.

Lack of milk production after weeks of attempt.

See also At-breast supplementation

▶ Infant

DEFINITION   A child under 12 months of age.

▶ Infant behavior

DEFINITION   Referring to the interplay of reflexes, levels of awareness, and response of babies to their environment.

Although babies are not able to speak until they are close to the end of the first year, they communicate with their caregivers and their environment through a complex set of behaviors.

Adults can learn to read feeding cues to aid in breastfeeding and the overall development of the parent–child relationship.

SELF CARE INFORMATION
Practice skin-to-skin contact with baby to learn feeding cues.

Infants have a predictable sequence of states of awareness including deep sleep, light sleep (with rapid eye movements), quiet alert, awake, active alert, and crying.

Light sleep, quiet alert, and awake states are the best times to initiate feeding.

Crying is a late feeding cue.

Signs that say "feed me" include hand-to-face or hand-to-mouth movements, lip smacking, seeking with lips, rooting, and head bobbing.

Signs of fullness include removing mouth from nipple with relaxed body tone, falling asleep during feeding, and general bodily relaxation.

▶ Infections, acute

DEFINITION   Invasion and reproduction of microorganisms in the cells or tissues of the body. Infectious microorganisms include bacteria, viruses, fungi, and others. Symptoms of infection may include fever and malaise. Lack of desire to feed can be an additional symptom of infection in the baby.

Ask about

Onset.
Age of baby.
Medications taken.
Known drug allergies.

ASSESSMENT

EMERGENT CARE NEEDED?

Are any of the following present?

About baby

Extreme **lethargy** in baby.

Sudden change in baby's muscle tone—extremely floppy (hypotonic) or extremely stiff (hypertonic).

Baby shows sudden disinterest in feeding.

Unable to wake baby.

IF YES,   *Seek emergency care now.*

PROMPT CARE NEEDED?

Are any of the following present?

About mother

Fever higher than 100°F (37.7°C).

Extreme breast discomfort.

Flu-like aching throughout body.

Extreme exhaustion.

Visible or palpable breast **abscess**.

About baby

Extreme discomfort.

Fever higher than 100°F (37.7°C) in a baby younger than 3 months of age.

Vomiting and diarrhea that last for more than a few hours in a child of any age.

Rash accompanied by a fever.

A cold that gets worse and includes a fever.

Ear pain or drainage from an ear.

Sore throat or problems swallowing.

Sharp or persistent pains in the abdomen or stomach.

Fever and vomiting at the same time.

Not eating for more than a day in the older baby who is eating solid foods.

IF YES, *Seek medical or pediatric care now.*

SELF CARE INFORMATION

Feed baby at least 10–24 times per 24 hours.

Soften breasts between feedings with gentle hand expression.

Finish full course of antibiotics prescribed (unless told to stop by a physician).

Continue non-prescription pain relief as recommended.

Continue to monitor for symptoms of recurring breast infection (redness, heat, fever, chills, pain).

IMPORTANT CONDITIONS TO REPORT

Symptoms worsen or persist.

Signs of infection.

Notes

Rarely, babies experience life threatening infections or events that cause extreme lethargy and disinterest in feeding. They may be suddenly floppy or hypertense. These symptoms indicate a medical emergency, as they may reflect botulism or other life threatening infection.

Many mothers experiencing **mastitis** may mistake symptoms of mastitis for flu. When a mother calls to ask for recommendations of safe flu medications, remember to ask her if she has any red, painful, hot spots on her breasts. See **Mastitis** for more information.

Few infections are incompatible with breastfeeding. Infections in the breastfeeding mother that are not compatible with breastfeeding include **HIV, HTLV-1**, active **herpes** lesion on the nipple and/or other area that will be in contact with baby's mouth.[126]

Mothers with certain infections may breastfeed once a period of treatment is initiated. These infections include tuberculosis, hepatitis, and Lyme disease. The Centers for Disease Control and Prevention and state health departments can provide further information.

See also Breast infection; Fever and breastfeeding

Footnotes

[126]American Academy of Pediatrics Section on Breastfeeding. (2005). Breastfeeding and the use of human milk. *Pediatrics, 115,* 497.

▶ Inflammation, breast

DEFINITION The body's response to injury, infection, or foreign matter that results in pain, redness, swelling, and sometimes impaired function of the affected area.

In this context, inflammation of the breast is assumed.

Mothers with inflammation should continue to breastfeed. There is no reason to cease breastfeeding.

Ask about

Onset.

Extent of redness and involvement.

ASSESSMENT

EMERGENT CARE NEEDED?

Are any of the following present?

Sudden bilateral red streaks on the breasts with fever, aching, or chills.

IF YES, **Seek emergency care now.**

SELF CARE INFORMATION

Feed baby at least 10–12 times per 24 hours.

Soften breasts between feedings with gentle hand expression.

Finish full course of treatment prescribed (unless told to stop by a provider).

Continue non-prescription pain relief as recommended.

Continue to monitor for symptoms of recurring breast infection (redness, heat, fever, chills, pain).

IMPORTANT CONDITIONS TO REPORT

Worsening of symptoms.

Persistence of symptoms.

Reoccurrence of symptoms.

Notes

An up-to-date drug reference should be consulted to determine the safety and possible side effects of medications recommended to treat inflammation.

Newborn and premature babies are at greater risk of drug side effects due to limited ability to clear drugs from their systems.

The symptoms listed previously may also indicate infection.

See also Acute infection; Breast infection; Mastitis

Drug References

American Academy of Pediatrics Committee on Drugs. (2001). Transfer of drugs and other chemicals into human milk. *Pediatrics, 108,* 776–789.

Briggs, G.G., Freeman, R.K., & Yaffee, S.J. (Eds.). (2002). *Drugs in pregnancy and lactation* (6th ed.). Philadelphia: Lippincott, Williams, and Wilkins.

Hale, T.W. (2004). *Medications and mothers milk.* Amarillo, TX: Pharmasoft Publishing.

Lawrence, R.A., & Lawrence, R.M. (2005). *Breastfeeding: A guide for the medical profession* (6th ed.). St. Louis: Mosby.

▶ Innocenti Declaration

DEFINITION   A statement made by a group of participants at a World Health Organization (WHO)/United Nations Children's Fund (UNICEF) policymakers' meeting on "Breastfeeding in the 1990s: A Global Initiative," held in Florence, Italy in 1990, and reaffirmed in 2005.

The declaration sets forth four targets to advance breastfeeding throughout the world, asking each government represented to:

- Appoint a national breastfeeding coordinator and establish a multisectoral national breastfeeding committee.
- Ensure that every facility providing maternity services fully practices all of the Ten Steps to Successful Breastfeeding.
- Take action to give effect to the principles and aim of all Articles of the International Code of Marketing of Breast-Milk Substitutes.
- Enact imaginative legislation protecting the breastfeeding rights of working women.[127]

Footnotes

[127]United Nations Children's Fund. (n.d.). *Innocenti Declaration*. Retrieved July 12, 2005, from http://www.unicef.org/programme/breastfeeding/innocenti.htm.

▶ Insufficient milk supply

DEFINITION   Inadequate production of milk in the breast. Maternal, infant, and environmental factors all have been found to contribute to milk supply problems.

Milk supply can be increased. This is accomplished by increasing stimulation and removal of milk from the breast.

Ask about

Onset.
Age of baby.

EMERGENT CARE NEEDED?

Are any of the following present?

Meconium bowel movements after 5 days of life.

Fewer than three bowel movements daily in breastfed newborn after the first 2 days of life.

No urine in six hours.

Brick dust urine (uric acid crystals) after 2 days of life.

Dark colored urine.

Fewer than four urinations daily in the breastfed newborn after day 5 of life.

Noticeably sunken fontanelles (soft spot on top of head).

Decreased activity.

Baby below birthweight at 10 to 14 days of life.

Cessation of weight gain.

IF YES, *Seek pediatric care now.*

PROMPT CARE NEEDED?

Are any of the following present?

Identified milk supply problem.

Concern about possible milk supply problem.

IF YES, *Call lactation care provider today.*

SELF CARE INFORMATION

Ensure baby is feeding 10–12 times per 24 hours.

Express milk after feeding.

IMPORTANT CONDITIONS TO REPORT

Persistent problems.

Recurrent problems.

See also Milk supply, inadequate

▶ Insufficient weight gain

DEFINITION   Breastfed newborns should gain a minimum of 0.5 oz to 1 oz a day on average after initial weight loss. New studies indicate that breastfed babies gain even faster than was previously believed, probably because breastfeeding used to be done on a schedule and not as frequently as we now know is ideal.

Ask about

Age of baby.
Weight gain pattern.

ASSESSMENT

PROMPT CARE NEEDED?
Are any of the following present?

Lethargy.

Hard to rouse.

Sleeping at the breast without nursing first.

Meconium bowel movements after 5 days of life.

Fewer than three bowel movements daily in breastfed newborn after the first 2 days of life.

No urine in six hours.

Brick dust urine (uric acid crystals) after 2 days of life.

Dark colored urine.

Fewer than four urinations daily in the breastfed newborn after day 5 of life.

Noticeably sunken fontanelles (soft spot on top of head).

Decreased activity.

Baby below birthweight at 10 to 14 days of life.

Cessation of weight gain.

IF YES,   *Seek pediatric care now.*

ROUTINE CARE NEEDED?
Are any of the following present?

Sleeps at the breast after a few sucks.

Hard to latch on.

No audible swallows.

Breastfeeding problem.

Milk supply problem.

Concern about possible milk supply problem.

IF YES, *Call lactation care provider today.*

IMPORTANT CONDITIONS TO REPORT

Decrease in frequency of urination or stools.

Increased sleepiness, hours spent sleeping.

Baby is harder to rouse.

See also Hypotonia; Jaundice

▶ Insulin-dependent diabetes mellitus (IDDM)

DEFINITION   A chronic disease causing high levels of glucose (sugar) in the blood.

In this form of diabetes, the pancreas makes little or no insulin, requiring daily injections of this hormone that regulates glucose metabolism.

Women with IDDM can breastfeed their babies.

Ask about

Onset.

Type of diabetes.

ASSESSMENT

EMERGENT CARE NEEDED?

Are any of the following present?

Insulin shock in the breastfeeding woman.

IF YES, *Seek emergency care now.*

Are any of the following present?

Difficulty maintaining blood glucose levels during breastfeeding.

IF YES, *Call medical care provider now.*

ROUTINE CARE NEEDED?

Are any of the following present?

Ongoing breastfeeding problems in the diabetic woman.

IF YES, *Call lactation care provider today.*

SELF CARE INFORMATION

Women with diabetes are more prone to infection. Monitor breasts and nipples daily for any red, infected, or painful areas.

If insulin-dependent, be aware that less insulin may be required during breastfeeding—watch for signs of low blood sugar.

IMPORTANT CONDITIONS TO REPORT

Any symptoms of infection.

Difficulty regulating blood sugar.

Notes

Women with diabetes should be encouraged to breastfeed. Breastfeeding is known to reduce the risk of developing diabetes in susceptible individuals (e.g., children of diabetic mothers).

Research suggests that women who have experienced gestational diabetes are less likely to develop diabetes if they breastfeed their babies.

See also Autoimmune diseases

▶ Insulin-like growth factor (IGF-I)

DEFINITION   A beneficial agent found in human milk that triggers growth.

Research suggests that preterm, exclusively breastfed infants have higher serum levels of this growth promoting factor.

▶ Intercourse and breastfeeding

DEFINITION   Resumption of sexual activity after childbirth.

Intercourse is compatible with breastfeeding, although the low estrogen level of the breastfeeding mother may contribute to vaginal dryness. There may also be residual discomfort or pain from the birth.

Women may feel differently about sexual relations after the birth of a baby. Many women feel less desire although some women feel more. No one can predict how a woman will feel.

Breastfeeding is an intimate activity that may make the rest of the family feel left out.

In addition, mothers may feel tired and not have the energy for sexual activities.

Ask about

Age of baby.

ASSESSMENT

ROUTINE MEDICAL CARE NEEDED?
Are any of the following present?
> Difficult penetration.
> Pain during intercourse.

IF YES,   *Call obstetric care provider today.*

ROUTINE CARE NEEDED?
Are any of the following present?
> Concern about sexuality in breastfeeding woman.
> Concerns about the normalcy of sensual feelings during breastfeeding.

IF YES,   *Call lactation care provider today.*

SELF CARE INFORMATION

Life changes after the birth of a baby and it is sometimes hard for mothers to know if what they are experiencing is "normal." Many breastfeeding women and their partners may worry about leaking milk, spraying milk, or the appropriateness of breast involvement in sexual activities. Talking about feelings and physical concerns can help couples adjust.

IMPORTANT CONDITIONS TO REPORT
Feelings of extreme worry or anxiety.
Difficult or painful penetration.
Pain during intercourse.

See also Fertility; Menstrual cycle

▶ International Baby Food Action Network (IBFAN)

DEFINITION   The International Baby Food Action Network (IBFAN) is a network of public interest groups working around the world to reduce infant and young child morbidity and mortality.

Notes

International Baby Food Action Network
North American Office
INFACT Canada
P.O. Box 781
10 Trinity Square
Toronto, Ontario M5G 1B1
Canada
Phone: 416-595-9819
Fax: 416-591-9355
E-mail: infact@ftn.net
Web: www.ibfan.org

▶ International Board Certified Lactation Consultant (IBCLC)

DEFINITION An individual who has qualified for and passed the examination administered by the International Board of Lactation Consultant Examiners.

The designations International Board Certified Lactation Consultant (IBCLC) and Registered Lactation Consultant (RLC) are used to denote international board certified lactation care providers.

International Board of Lactation Consultant Examiners (IBLCE)

DEFINITION   "The primary purpose of the International Board of Lactation Consultant Examiners (IBLCE) is to benefit the public by setting standards for the lactation care provider profession. The IBLCE is a non-profit organization governed by a Board of Directors. It was established to develop and administer the certification examination for lactation care providers."[128]

Notes

International Board of Lactation Consultant Examiners (IBLCE)
7309 Arlington Boulevard
Suite 300
Falls Church, VA 22042-3215
Phone: 703-560-7330
Fax: 703-560-7332
E-mail: iblce@iblce.org
Web site: www.iblce.org

Footnotes

[128]International Board of Lactation Consultant Examiners. (2004). *The IBLCE organization.* Retrieved July 12, 2005, from http://www.iblce.org/about.htm.

International Code of Marketing of Breast-milk Substitutes

DEFINITION   A document adopted by the World Health Assembly in 1981 and amended by several subsequent resolutions as a minimum requirement to protect infant health. The International Code of Marketing of Breast-milk Substitutes sets forth a series of expectations about the behavior of the infant formula industry, health care systems, health care providers, governments, and other parties regarding the protection of breastfeeding and ethical marketing of breastmilk substitutes.

> **Notes**
>
> Full text of the International Code of Marketing of Breast-milk Substitutes can be accessed through the World Health Organization's Web site at www.who.int/nut/documents/code_english.PDF.

▶ International Lactation Consultant Association (ILCA)

DEFINITION   "Our vision: A worldwide network of lactation professionals. Our Mission: To advance the profession of lactation consulting worldwide through leadership, advocacy, professional development and research."[129]

> **Notes**
>
> International Lactation Consultant Association (ILCA)
> 1500 Sunday Drive
> Suite 102
> Raleigh, NC 27607
> Phone: 919-861-5577
> Fax: 919-787-4916
> E-mail: info@ilca.org
> Web site: www.ilca.org

Footnotes

[129]International Lactation Consultant Association. (2005). *About ILCA*. Retrieved July 12, 2005, from http://www.ilca.org/about/index.php.

▶ International Society for Research in Human Milk and Lactation (ISRHML)

DEFINITION   "The society is a nonprofit organization dedicated to the promotion of excellence in research and the dissemination of research findings in the field of human milk and lactation."[130a]

Notes

ISRHML
c/o Frank R. Greer, MD
Meriter Hospital, Perinatal Center
202 S. Park Street
Madison, WI 53715
Phone: 608-262-6561
Web site: http://www.isrhml.org.umu.se

Footnotes

[130a]International Society for Research in Human Milk and Lactation. (n.d.). *Home page.* Retrieved November 15, 2005, from http://www.isrhml.org.umu.se.

▶ Intraductal papilloma

DEFINITION   A small, benign (noncancerous) tumor that grows within the milk ducts. It is found within a single milk duct.

Ask about

Age of baby.
Onset of nipple discharge.
Description of nipple discharge.

PROMPT CARE NEEDED?

Are any of the following present?

Appearance of rust colored milk.

Bloody discharge from the nipple.

Any other unusual nipple discharge without nipple pain or abrasion from suboptimal latch.

IF YES, *Call obstetric care provider today.*

SELF CARE INFORMATION

Seek prompt medical evaluation of any unusual discharge from the nipple during breastfeeding and at any other time.

See also Bleeding, breast; Blood in milk; Breast cancer

▶ Intrauterine device (IUD)

DEFINITION A contraceptive device that is placed within the uterus and left there to prevent fertilization.

IUDs are compatible with breastfeeding.

See also Birth control; Contraception

▶ Inverted nipples

DEFINITION Nipples that retreat into the breast when the areola is compressed.

Ask about

Appearance of nipple.

Action of nipple when the areola is compressed.

Nipple changes during pregnancy and lactation.

Diagnosis of inverted nipple.

PROMPT MEDICAL CARE NEEDED?

Are any of the following present?

Meconium bowel movements after 5 days of life.

Fewer than three bowel movements daily in breastfed newborn after the first 2 days of life.

No urine in six hours.

Brick dust urine (uric acid crystals) after 2 days of life.

Dark colored urine.

Fewer than four urinations daily in the breastfed newborn after day 5 of life.

Noticeably sunken fontanelles (soft spot on top of head).

Decreased activity.

Baby below birthweight at 10 to 14 days of life.

Cessation of weight gain.

IF YES, *Seek pediatric care now.*

PROMPT LACTATION CARE NEEDED?

Are any of the following present?

Poor feeding.

Poor milk transfer.

Inadequate weight gain.

IF YES, *Call lactation care provider today.*

SELF CARE INFORMATION

Trying to train inverted nipples to stand out during pregnancy is ineffective.

Mothers with inverted nipples should be encouraged to express milk early and frequently until baby is able to facilitate stretching the nipple deeply into the mouth.

IMPORTANT CONDITIONS TO REPORT

Poor feeding.

Poor milk transfer.

Inadequate weight gain.

Problems with latch-on.

See also Insufficient milk supply

▶ Iron

DEFINITION   A metal that is vital to the process of absorbing oxygen into the blood. Iron deficiency is the most common cause of anemia.

Breastmilk contains iron in a form that is easy for the baby to absorb. Breastmilk also contains lactoferrin, a protein that keeps iron away from microorganisms in the gut that require iron to grow.

> **Notes**
>
> Taking iron supplements is compatible with breastfeeding.
> Women taking high doses of iron may have suffered postpartum hemorrhage, and may be experiencing **Sheehan's syndrome**.

See also Anemia; Sheehan's syndrome

▶ ISRHML

See also International Society for Research in Human Milk and Lactation (ISRHML)

▶ IUD

DEFINITION   Intrauterine device. A contraceptive device that is placed within the uterus and left there to prevent fertilization.

IUDs are compatible with breastfeeding.

See also Birth control; Contraception

▶ Jaundice

DEFINITION   Neonatal jaundice is caused by an excessive amount of bilirubin in the blood. It is the most common condition requiring medical treatment in the newborn period.

Because bilirubin is yellow, the color accumulates in the baby's skin and the sclera (whites) of the eyes. The baby may appear tan, yellow, or light orange in color.

Bilirubin is removed from the blood by the liver.

Although the condition of jaundice may be benign, it can be a symptom of a serious condition called **kernicterus**.

Ask about

Age of baby.
Feeding behavior.
Stooling pattern and color.
Urination pattern.

ASSESSMENT

PROMPT CARE NEEDED?

   Are any of the following present?

   Severe lethargy (sleepiness).

   Poor feeding.

   No interest in feeding for more than 6 hours.

   Fever.

   Meconium bowel movements after 5 days of life.

   Fewer than three bowel movements daily in breastfed newborn after the
      first 2 days of life

   No urine in six hours.

   Brick dust urine (uric acid crystals) after 2 days of life.

   Dark colored urine.

   Fewer than four urinations daily in the breastfed newborn after day 5 of life.

   Noticeably sunken fontanelles (soft spot on top of head).

   Decreased activity.

   Baby below birthweight at 10 to 14 days of life.

Cessation of weight gain.

Any fever in a baby younger than 3 months of age.

Fever higher than 100°F (37.7°C) in a baby younger than 3 months of age.

IF YES, *Seek pediatric care now.*

ROUTINE CARE NEEDED?

Are any of the following present?

Breastfeeding in a jaundiced baby.

Baby sleepy during breastfeedings.

Milk supply problem.

Concern about possible milk supply problem.

IF YES, *Call lactation care provider now.*

SELF CARE INFORMATION

Breastfeed as soon as possible after birth.

Encourage the baby to nurse 10–12 times per 24 hours.

Colostrum has laxative properties. Stooling helps to rid the baby's body of bilirubin.

IMPORTANT CONDITIONS TO REPORT

No stool in 24 hours.

Severe lethargy (sleepiness).

Poor feeding.

Fever.

Notes

All jaundiced infants are at risk for kernicterus and should be closely monitored.

See also Jaundice; Kernicterus; Late onset jaundice

▶ Jogging and breastfeeding

DEFINITION   A form of physical exercise involving running.

Physical exertion is a normal part of the life of lactating women around the world. There is no reason for lactating women to refrain from exercise.

Breastfeeding women may find a supportive sports bra helpful in providing breast comfort while running.

▶ Kangaroo care

DEFINITION   A form of skin contact encouraged between parents and premature babies. Skin contact is beneficial to all parents and babies, but is particularly helpful in establishing breastfeeding and bonding, and in helping the premature baby to regulate body temperature, respiratory rate, and oxygenation.

See also Skin-to-skin (STS) care

▶ Kernicterus

DEFINITION   Damage to the brain, spinal cord, and nerve cells caused by buildup of bilirubin in these tissues.

Any jaundiced baby is at risk for kernicterus. Babies with **jaundice** should be closely monitored.

See also Bilirubin; Hyperbilirubinemia; Jaundice

▶ Kwashiorkor

DEFINITION   A form of malnutrition caused by inadequate protein intake.

Breastmilk is an excellent source of protein. Kwashiorkor is not associated with breastfeeding.

This disorder is rare in the United States, but may occur after weaning in locations where protein rich food is scarce.

▶ Lactational Amenorrhea Method (LAM)

The Lactational Amenorrhea Method (LAM) is a form of natural family planning which is 98% effective in the first 6 months following the birth of a baby, so long as the mother's menses have not returned, her baby is exclusively breastfed, and there are no long periods of time between feedings, day and night. Once the baby is older than 6 months, or any of the above criteria is no longer true, LAM is no longer effective and mothers should utilize other forms of birth control.

Refer mothers with questions about this contraceptive method to a lactation specialist, medical care provider, or family planning counselor.

▶ Lactation care providers, counselors, and specialists

DEFINITION Terminology used to describe individuals who have education and skill in assisting breastfeeding mothers.

Lactation care providers have different professional backgrounds and different levels of training.

> **Notes**
>
> To find a local lactation care provider, contact the **International Board of Lactation Consultant Examiners (IBLCE)**, International Lactation Consultant Association (ILCA), Nursing Mothers' Council, breastfeeding task force, WIC Program, or local hospitals.

▶ Lactation Institute

DEFINITION "The Lactation Institute and Breastfeeding Clinic sets the standard for treatment of breastfeeding problems and our lactation care providers offer options not found anywhere else. Breast pumps, bras, pillows and other breastfeeding products are available. The clinic helps hundreds of mothers every year and is also a research center in the field of lactation. The Lactation Institute has educational programs in lactation for doctors, nurses and other health professions."[130b]

Footnotes

[130b]Lactation Institute. *Home page.* Retrieved August 25, 2005, from http://www.lactationinstitute.org.

▶ Lactiferous duct

DEFINITION   The tube shaped structures in the breast that carry milk from the alveoli to the nipple. There are thought to be roughly nine major ducts in the breast, corresponding with nine pores in the surface of the nipple. Ducts divide into smaller ductules in a branching fashion.

▶ Lactiferous sinus

DEFINITION   A concept suggesting a pooling area behind the areola where milk is stored.

This concept has been challenged by recent ultrasound evidence[131] that showed no presence of a permanent sinus, but rather a temporary widening of the diameter of the ducts under the influence of oxytocin.

Footnotes

[131]Ramsay, D.T., Kent, J.C., Owens, R.A., & Hartmann, P.E. (2004). Ultrasound imaging of milk ejection in the breast of lactating women. *Pediatrics, 113,* 361–367.

► Lactoengineering

DEFINITION   Laboratory techniques used to increase the nutrient content of expressed milk fed to premature infants.

May include concentrating expressed mothers' milk, adding minerals, fat, and protein to expressed milk, or adding cow's milk products to expressed milk.

In the United States, commercially available "human" milk fortifiers are made with cow's milk products.

See also Human milk fortification; Premature infant

► Lactoferrin

DEFINITION   A milk protein that binds to iron, making it easier for the baby to absorb.

Lactoferrin also serves the purpose of keeping iron away from the many microorganisms that require iron for growth.

► Lactose

DEFINITION   A double sugar (disaccharide) made up of the simple sugars glucose and galactose.

Lactose is found only in the milk of mammals.

► Lactose intolerance

DEFINITION   An inability to digest lactose into the simple sugars glucose and galactose.

Lactose intolerance is a common condition in adults. However, lactose intolerance is rarely seen in children prior to 3 years of age.

Lactose intolerance in the mother is compatible with breastfeeding.

Concerns about lactose intolerance in infants should be referred to the medical care provider.

Lactose intolerance arises from lack of adequate production of lactase, an enzyme made in the cells that line the intestinal wall. The role of lactase is to break lactose into the simpler sugars that can be absorbed into the blood stream. Lack of lactase results in
an overload of lactose in the intestine, creating abdominal cramps, gas, diarrhea, and discomfort.

The prevalence of lactose intolerance in many adult populations worldwide is thought to be related to the fact that historically, few populations consumed dairy foods past childhood. Typically, lactase is made by the cells of the gut in response to the amount of lactose in the diet. Thus, when milk is not consumed regularly, the body may lose its ability to digest lactose well.

See also Diarrhea and breastfeeding

La Leche League

DEFINITION "[La Leche League International's] mission is to help mothers worldwide to breastfeed through mother-to-mother support, education, information, and encouragement and to promote a better understanding of breastfeeding as an important element in the healthy development of the baby and mother."[132]

Notes

La Leche League International
P.O. Box 4079
Schaumburg, IL 60168-4079
Phone: 847-519-7730
Web site: www.lalecheleague.org
   La Leche League has numerous documents about breastfeeding on its Web site, as well as research reviews in the newsletter *Breastfeeding Abstracts.*

Footnotes
   [132]La Leche League International. (2005). *Our mission.* Retrieved July 13, 2005, from http://www.lalecheleague.org/whatisLLL.html.

▶ LAM

DEFINITION   Lactational amenorrhea method. A form of natural family planning which is 98% effective in the first 6 months following the birth of a baby, so long as the mother's menses have not returned, her baby is exclusively breastfed, and there are no long periods of time between feedings, day and night. Once the baby is older than 6 months, or any of the above criteria is no longer true, LAM is no longer effective and mothers should utilize other forms of birth control.

Refer mothers with questions about this contraceptive method to a lactation care provider, medical care provider, or family planning counselor.

▶ Lamaze International

DEFINITION   "The mission of Lamaze International is to promote, support and protect normal birth through education and advocacy. We envision for the future a world of confident women choosing normal birth."[133]

Notes

Lamaze International
2025 M Street
Suite 800
Washington, DC 20036-3309
Phone: 800-368-4404
Web site: www.lamaze.org
   Among its other activities promoting childbirth education, Lamaze convenes the Lamaze Institute for Normal Birth.

Footnotes

[133]Lamaze International. (2005). *Mission & vision.* Retrieved July 13, 2005, from http://www.lamaze.org/about/mission.asp?parent=53.

► Lanolin

DEFINITION   A cream containing fatty acids and cholesterol extracted from sheep's wool. Lanolin has been suggested as a topical treatment for maintaining or healing nipple integrity.

Questions about lanolin and other nipple creams suggest that mother may be experiencing nipple pain.

Ask about

Nipple pain.

ASSESSMENT

PROMPT CARE NEEDED?

Are any of the following present?

Extreme nipple pain.

Bleeding from nipples.

Unable to breastfeed due to pain.

IF YES,   *Call lactation care provider now.*

ROUTINE CARE NEEDED?

Are any of the following present?

Feeding discomfort.

Trauma to nipple or breasts.

Misshapen nipple after feedings.

Visible fissures on nipples.

IF YES,   *Call lactation care provider today.*

SELF CARE INFORMATION

Any substance that is applied to the nipple area will be consumed by the nursing baby. Check out the safety of any substance you put on your nipples.

Creams do not cure the causes of nipple pain.

Report nipple pain to your lactation care provider.

IMPORTANT CONDITIONS TO REPORT

Symptoms worsen or persist.

Signs of infection.

Feeding or stooling expectations are not met.

> **Notes**
>
> Women experiencing **nipple pain** may self-treat with this and other substances, some of which may be inappropriate for the baby to consume (which is what happens when creams are applied to the nipple).
>
> Women experiencing nipple pain should have a breastfeeding evaluation. There is no magic fix. Face-to-face counseling is effective in assessing and resolving nipple pain.

See also **Breastfeeding assessment tools; Nipple pain; Sore nipples**

▶ Large for gestational age (LGA)

DEFINITION   This term is used to describe babies whose birth weight is greater than the 90th percentile or greater than two standard deviations from the mean for babies of the same age.

▶ Latch-on

DEFINITION   Refers to the way in which the nursing baby attaches to the breast.

Correct attachment of the baby to the breast is crucial to comfortable breastfeeding, to adequate milk manufacture and transfer, and ultimately to infant growth. When a baby is attached well, mother should feel no pain or discomfort and should hear sounds of swallowing on the part of the baby.

Since concerns about pain and inadequate milk are major reasons mothers stop breastfeeding, mothers should be seen for a feeding evaluation within 24–48 hours of expressing breastfeeding concerns.

Nipple pain.
Weight gain pattern.

ASSESSMENT

PROMPT CARE NEEDED?

Are any of the following present?

Inadequate stooling pattern (less than three stools daily) after the first 2 days of life.

Inadequate weight gain (less than 0.5 oz daily) after the first 2 days of life.

IF YES, *Call pediatric care provider today.*

Are any of the following present?

Extreme nipple pain.

Bleeding from nipples.

Unable to breastfeed due to pain.

IF YES, *Call lactation care provider now.*

Are any of the following present?

Breastfeeding lasting longer than 20 minutes.

Weight gain of less than 0.5 oz per day on average.

No change in suckling rhythm to a suck swallow ratio of 2:1 or 1:1.

Feeding discomfort.

Trauma to nipple or breasts.

Misshapen nipple after feedings.

Visible fissures (cracks) on nipples.

IF YES, *Call lactation care provider today.*

IMPORTANT CONDITIONS TO REPORT

Increased infant lethargy.

Decrease in number of stools and wet diapers.

Weight loss, failure to gain weight after initial weight loss, or slow weight gain in the breastfed baby.

SELF CARE INFORMATION

Any substance that is applied to the nipple area will be consumed by the nursing baby. Check out the safety of any substance you put on your nipples.

Creams do not cure the causes of nipple pain.

Report nipple pain to your lactation specialist.

> **Notes**
>
> Women experiencing nipple pain or infants with slow weight gain should have a breastfeeding evaluation. Face-to-face counseling is effective in assessing and resolving these problems.

See also Asymmetric latch; Nipple pain; Slow weight gain, baby; Sore nipples

▶ Late onset jaundice

DEFINITION A form of jaundice that occurs after the first week of life in breastfed infants. This type of jaundice is unusual and not well understood. It is also called "breastmilk jaundice."

Medical evaluation is indicated to rule out other metabolic reasons for jaundice.

Sometimes the mother is asked to stop breastfeeding for 12 or more hours; the infant's bilirubin levels are checked after this time. If bilirubin levels fall during this time, then the reason for jaundice is assumed to be related to feeding.

Breastfeeding can be resumed once the bilirubin levels have fallen to an acceptable level.

IMPORTANT CONDITIONS TO REPORT

No stool in 24 hours.

Pale or gray stool.

Severe lethargy (sleepiness).

Poor feeding.

Fever higher than 100°F (37.7°C) in a baby younger than 3 months of age.

See also Jaundice; Kernicterus

▶ Laxatives

DEFINITION Drugs taken to relieve constipation.

Occasional laxative use in the breastfeeding mother is not thought to affect the breastfeeding baby.

Questions about giving laxatives to the breastfed infant should be directed to the pediatric care provider. Constipation is not normal in the breastfed infant.

> **Notes**
>
> An up-to-date drug reference should be consulted to determine the safety and possible side effects of individual drugs.
>
> Newborn and premature babies are at greater risk of drug side effects due to limited ability to clear drugs from their systems.

See also Constipation

Drug References

American Academy of Pediatrics Committee on Drugs. (2001). Transfer of drugs and other chemicals into human milk. *Pediatrics, 108,* 776–789.

Briggs, G.G., Freeman, R.K., & Yaffee, S.J. (Eds.). (2002). *Drugs in pregnancy and lactation* (6th ed.). Philadelphia: Lippincott, Williams, and Wilkins.

Hale, T.W. (2004). *Medications and mothers milk.* Amarillo, TX: Pharmasoft Publishing.

Lawrence, R.A., & Lawrence, R.M. (2005). *Breastfeeding: A guide for the medical profession* (6th ed.). St. Louis: Mosby.

▶ LCPUFAs

DEFINITION   Long chain polyunsaturated fatty acids. These fatty acids are present in human milk and known to assist in the development of nerve and brain tissue. LCPUFAs may account for some of the differences between formula-fed and breastfed children in IQ, test scores, and visual acuity.

See also Arachidonic acid (AA); Docosahexanoic acid in breastmilk (DHA); Fat in breastmilk

▶ Lead in breastmilk

DEFINITION   A heavy metal that can damage the nervous system and kidneys. Overdose of lead is known as lead poisoning.

Lead poisoning is of particular concern in babies and children due to the rapid growth of their brains and other organs.

ASSESSMENT

PROMPT CARE NEEDED?

Are any of the following present?

Breastfeeding woman diagnosed with lead poisoning.

Breastfed infant diagnosed with lead poisoning.

IF YES,   *Seek medical care within 2 to 4 hours.*

Notes

The American Academy of Pediatrics lists lead on Table 6, "Food and Environmental Agents: Effects on Breastfeeding," citing possible neurotoxicity as a concern.[134]

Regarding the mother's blood levels, Lawrence states, "A lead level of 40 μg/dL is considered below the level of transfer through the breast milk."[135]

Footnotes

[134]American Academy of Pediatrics Committee on Drugs. (2001). Transfer of drugs and other chemicals into human milk. *Pediatrics, 108,* 782.

[135]Lawrence, R.A., & Lawrence, R.M. (2005). *Breastfeeding: A guide for the medical profession* (6th ed.). St. Louis: Mosby.

▶ Leaking breastmilk

DEFINITION   Phenomenon of milk dripping from the breast between feedings, or from the opposite breast during feedings.

Leaking is a nuisance for many women, but is not associated with breastfeeding problems.

SELF CARE INFORMATION

Choose soft, absorbent breast pads.

Replace damp pads with fresh ones frequently to avoid irritation and softening of nipple.

Avoid waterproof or plastic-lined pads, which can cause irritation.

Breast pads are easily made by cutting appropriately sized circles out of new cloth diapers (edge stitching is recommended to hold the pad together in the wash).

Press the forearms against the nipples to cause temporary cessation of milk.

Wearing shirts or dresses with multi-colored patterns may make leakage less visible.

▶ Let-down reflex

DEFINITION   The neurohormonal response that compresses the myoepithelial cells that surround the alveoli, forcing milk to be squeezed down through the ducts and out the nipple. Also called milk ejection reflex.

This reflex is caused by a spike in the hormone oxytocin, one of the two major hormones of lactation (the other is prolactin). Oxytocin is released from the posterior lobe of the pituitary gland and stimulates the contraction of the smooth muscle of the uterus during labor. This hormone is also responsible for the let-down (ejection) of milk from the breast.

Researchers have found that oxytocin is released in the first hours postpartum by the baby's hand massage of the breast.

Oxytocin is also released by the baby stretching the nipple sufficiently in the mouth. This is why a good latch is so important to milk transfer.

Oxytocin is also released through a conditioned response over time.

SELF CARE INFORMATION

The breastfed newborn should gain well (0.5–1 oz per day on average). If the baby is gaining less than this have a face-to-face breastfeeding evaluation.

At the breast, the baby should have sucking pattern that includes slow, deep sucks. After the first few days, the baby's swallows can be heard, and the baby should have at least six wet diapers and two to five yellow stools each day.

IMPORTANT CONDITIONS TO REPORT

Inadequate weight gain.

Inadequate number of urinations and stools.

See also Milk-ejection reflex; Oxytocin; Overactive let-down reflex

▶ **Lethargy**

DEFINITION A state of sleepiness, sluggishness, or lack of desire to move about and interact.

Lethargy can be a symptom of several diseases and disorders including anemia, botulism, sepsis, infection, meningitis, or other acute illness, dehydration, depression, and thyroid conditions.

In the infant, lethargy is a symptom requiring immediate medical evaluation.

▶ **LGA**

DEFINITION Large for gestational age. This term is used to describe babies whose birth weight is greater than the 90th percentile or greater than two standard deviations from the mean for babies of the same age.

Lobes

DEFINITION   Sections of milk-making tissue in the breast. There are many lobes of milk-making tissue, articulating with the ductal system which carries milk to the nipple pores. Lobes branch into lobules that contain hundreds of alveolar units.

Lochia

DEFINITION   Discharge of blood from the vagina after delivery.

Three types of lochia are recognized, including lochia rubra (red), lochia serosa (pink), and lochia alba (white). Lochia rubra, a red discharge, begins after delivery and continues for two to three days. Lochia serosa, a paler, pinkish discharge, continues for the next week or so. Lochia alba, a whitish discharge, starts around the tenth day postpartum and should be resolved within a month.[136]

Ask about

Onset.
Date of delivery.

ASSESSMENT

EMERGENT CARE NEEDED?

Are any of the following present?

Soaking a sanitary napkin with bright red blood at a rate of one napkin or more per hour.

Clots in the bloody discharge.

Foul odor to the discharge (even if occasional).

Dizziness.

Fever.

Abdominal pain.

IF YES,   *Call obstetric care provider now or seek emergency care now.*

PROMPT CARE NEEDED?

Are any of the following present?

Soaking a sanitary napkin with bright red blood at a rate of one napkin every two to three hours.

Abdominal tenderness.

Lightheadedness.

Sudden resumption of lochia rubra (bright red blood flow).

Continuation of lochia rubra after four days postpartum.

Continuation of lochia serosa after two weeks postpartum.

Signs of infection (fever, chills, pain, malaise, and overall aching).

Milk supply problems coupled with ongoing lochia rubra or serosa.

IF YES, **Call obstetric care provider within 2 to 4 hours.**

SELF CARE INFORMATION

Monitor blood flow.

IMPORTANT CONDITIONS TO REPORT

Continuation of symptoms.

Sudden gushing of blood.

Multiple blood clots passed.

Concerns about milk supply.

Notes

As time progresses, the volume of lochia should also decrease. Sudden return of bright red bleeding is of concern and should be evaluated medically. Retained placental fragments can be indicated by ongoing lochia rubra. In this event, mature milk production may not occur until placental fragments are expelled or removed.

See also Placental fragments, retained

Footnotes

[136]Varney, H., Kriebs, J.M., & Gegor, C.L. (Eds.). (2004). *Varney's midwifery* (4th ed., p. 1043). Sudbury, MA: Jones and Bartlett.

▶ Long chain polyunsaturated fatty acids (LCPUFAs)

DEFINITION   Fatty acids present in human milk known to assist in the development of nerve and brain tissue. LCPUFAs may account for some of the differences between formula-fed and breastfed children in IQ, test scores, and visual acuity.

See also Arachidonic acid (AA); Docosahexanoic acid in breastmilk (DHA); Fat in breastmilk

▶ Low muscle tone

DEFINITION   Referring to loose or floppy muscle response. Babies with low muscle tone (also referred to as hypotonia) have relaxed arm and leg joints, like a rag doll. Hypotonia can be a symptom of prematurity and of physical problems or illness. Babies with low muscle tone may have breastfeeding problems such as non-rhythmic suck and weak sucking, and they may tire more easily.

Ask about

Age of baby.
Onset of hypotonia.
Change in feeding behavior.
Change in urination or stooling patterns.

ASSESSMENT

EMERGENT CARE NEEDED?
Are any of the following present?
Sudden change in muscle tone.
Sudden change in feeding behavior.
Sudden lethargy.

IF YES,   *Seek emergency care now.*

PROMPT CARE NEEDED?

Are any of the following present?

Meconium bowel movements after 5 days of life.

Fewer than three bowel movements daily in breastfed newborn after the first 2 days of life.

No urine in six hours.

Brick dust urine (uric acid crystals) after 2 days of life.

Dark colored urine.

Fewer than four urinations daily in the breastfed newborn after day 5 of life.

Noticeably sunken fontanelles (soft spot on top of head).

Decreased activity.

Baby below birthweight at 10 to 14 days of life.

Cessation of weight gain.

IF YES,   *Seek pediatric care now.*

ROUTINE CARE NEEDED?

Are any of the following present?

Feeding problems.

Slow weight gain.

Problems positioning baby at breast.

Decline in milk supply.

Inadequate milk supply.

Concerns about adequate milk supply.

IF YES,   *Call lactation care provider today.*

SELF CARE INFORMATION

Breastfeeding and breast milk are valuable for babies with low muscle tone. Pumping may be necessary in order to maintain an adequate milk supply.

IMPORTANT CONDITIONS TO REPORT

Change in feeding behaviors.

Change in urination or stooling patterns.

Declining breast milk volume.

See also Slow weight gain, baby

▶ Lyme disease

DEFINITION   An inflammatory response to the bacterium *Borrelia burgdorferi*, received from a deer tick bite.

Symptoms of Lyme disease include a circular rash at the site of the bite, fever, headache, muscle pain, inflammation of the joints, and malaise.

Breastfeeding is compatible with Lyme disease, as soon as treatment has been initiated.[137]

SELF CARE INFORMATION

Make sure that all medical personnel caring for you know that you are breastfeeding. Some drugs used to treat this condition are not recommended while breastfeeding. Ask your medical care provider about safe alternatives to these drugs.

Notes

Antibiotics and anti-inflammatory drugs may be prescribed for Lyme disease. An up-to-date drug reference should be consulted to determine the safety and possible side effects of individual drugs.

See also Acute infection

Footnotes
[137]Lawrence, R.A., & Lawrence, R.M. (2005). *Breastfeeding: A guide for the medical profession* (6th ed.). St. Louis: Mosby.

Drug References
American Academy of Pediatrics Committee on Drugs. (2001). Transfer of drugs and other chemicals into human milk. *Pediatrics, 108,* 776–789.

Briggs, G.G., Freeman, R.K., & Yaffee, S.J. (Eds.). (2002). *Drugs in pregnancy and lactation* (6th ed.). Philadelphia: Lippincott, Williams, and Wilkins.

Hale, T.W. (2004). *Medications and mothers milk.* Amarillo, TX: Pharmasoft Publishing.

Lawrence, R.A., & Lawrence, R.M. (2005). *Breastfeeding: A guide for the medical profession* (6th ed.). St. Louis: Mosby.

▶ Lymphocytes

DEFINITION   White blood cells that are active in defending the body against infection. Some of the lymphocytes in milk are B-cells, so named because they are specialized in the bone marrow. B-cells respond to the presence of antigens by causing the production of the specific antibody to destroy the antigen recognized.

Other lymphocytes are T-cells, named for the thymus where they are specialized. T-cells are sometimes called "helper T-cells" because they either kill infected cells or send out messages to mobilize macrophages and other immune cells.

▶ Lysozyme

DEFINITION   An enzyme that breaks down the cell wall of bacteria. Lysozyme is found in human milk and serves as part of the army of immunologic agents working to benefit the baby's health.

▶ Macrobiotic diet of the mother

DEFINITION   Macrobiotic diets are a particular type of vegetarian diet. A mother on a macrobiotic diet may be eating a diet consisting mostly of grains. Although many vegetarian diets are compatible with breastfeeding, some vegetarian diets (macrobiotic and vegan for example) may not be nutritionally adequate and can put the breastfed infant at risk of malnutrition. The major concerns are deficiencies of vitamins B_{12}, B_2, and D.

Ask about

Type of diet.
Age of baby.
Nutritional supplements taken.

EMERGENT CARE NEEDED?

Are any of the following present?

Infant tetany (a condition characterized by painful muscle spasms and tremors).

Infant seizures.

IF YES, *Seek emergency care now.*

PROMPT CARE NEEDED?

Are any of the following present?

Infant lethargy.

Change in infant feeding behavior.

Infant weight loss after the first week of life.

Slow growth in the breastfed infant of a macrobiotic mother.

IF YES, *Seek pediatric care within 2 to 4 hours.*

ROUTINE CARE NEEDED?

Are any of the following present?

Macrobiotic diet of the breastfeeding mother.

Vegan diet of the breastfeeding mother.

Ovo-lacto vegetarian diet of the breastfeeding mother.

IF YES, *Seek dietary consultation.*

SELF CARE INFORMATION

Nutritional risks of vegetarian diets are especially associated with protein, vitamins B_{12} and B_2, vitamin D, and zinc deficiencies.

IMPORTANT CONDITIONS TO REPORT

Lethargy and poor feeding behavior can be early signs of nutritional inadequacies.

Many people who are vegetarians are knowledgeable about including foods and supplements that balance their diets.

See also Maternal diet; Maternal diet, vegetarian

▶ Macronutrients in human milk

DEFINITION   The three macronutrients in human milk are carbohydrate, fat, and protein. Human milk also contains micronutrients and water as well as immunologic properties, cellular components, and other substances.

▶ Macrophages

DEFINITION   Macrophages are components of both colostrum and mature milk. They are large-complex cells whose functions include phagocytocis (engulfing and destroying) of fungi and bacteria, killing bacteria, and production of other human milk components such as lysozyme and lactoferrin.

▶ Madonna position

DEFINITION   The Madonna position is also called the cradle position or cradle hold. The baby is positioned across the mother's lap and turned toward the mother. In this position, the weight of the baby is often carried on the arm of the mother on the same side as the breast that is being nursed.

   This position is called the "Madonna" position because it is the way the baby Jesus is traditionally held in paintings and sculptures.

See also Cradle hold

▶ Malabsorption syndrome

DEFINITION   Malabsorption syndrome includes any alteration in the ability of the intestine to absorb nutrients adequately.

It is often characterized by two or more weeks of diarrhea that continues even after treatment, as well as bloating, gas, cramping, and weight loss.

▶ Malaise, maternal

DEFINITION   Malaise is a generalized feeling of discomfort, illness, or lack of well-being. Malaise is a nonspecific symptom that can occur along with other specific symptoms of significant disease or illness.

In breastfeeding mothers, malaise may be an early sign of mastitis or abscess as well as a sign of illness. Malaise may be a sign of infection or illness.

Ask about

Onset.
Age of baby.
Medications taken.
Other symptoms.

ASSESSMENT

EMERGENT CARE NEEDED?

Are any of the following present?
Suicidal thoughts.
Thoughts of harming baby.

IF YES,   *Seek emergency care now.*

Are any of the following present?
Visible red areas on breast.
Fever higher than 101°F (38.5°C).
Extreme breast discomfort.

Flu-like aching throughout body.

Extreme anxiety.

IF YES, *Seek medical care now.*

PROMPT CARE NEEDED?

Are any of the following present?

Persistent sadness.

Inability to function.

Fatigue.

Difficulty eating or sleeping.

IF YES, *Call medical care provider today.*

ROUTINE CARE NEEDED?

Are any of the following present?

Feeling of malaise lasting for more than two days without any other symptoms developing.

IF YES, *Call medical care provider.*

SELF CARE INFORMATION

Report new symptoms to your medical care provider.

IMPORTANT CONDITIONS TO REPORT

Watch for any of the following symptoms:

Visible red areas on breast.

Fever higher than 101°F (38.5°C).

Extreme breast discomfort.

Flu-like aching throughout body.

Persistent fatigue, anxiety, or sadness.

Notes

Physical feelings of malaise can be also associated with depression and other postpartum mood disorders.

See also Abscess, breast; Hypothyroidism; Mastitis; Postpartum depression

Malaria

DEFINITION   Malaria is a parasitic disease characterized by fever, chills, headache, and anemia. It is transmitted from one human to another by the bite of an infected mosquito. It is a major health problem in much of the world's tropic and sub-tropic locations. Malaria can also be transmitted congenitally and by blood transfusions.

Breastfeeding does not transmit malaria. Breastfeeding is not contraindicated for mothers who are being treated for malaria. Many of the drugs used to prevent and treat malaria are compatible with breastfeeding.

SELF CARE INFORMATION

Make sure that all medical personnel caring for you know that you are breastfeeding. Some drugs used to treat this condition are not recommended while breastfeeding. Ask your medical care provider about safe alternatives to these drugs.

Notes

More information is available from the Centers for Disease Control and Prevention. Visit www.cdc.gov for the latest information.

Malnourished mother

DEFINITION   Poor nourishment due to inadequate diet or presence of disease or other disorder decreasing absorption and digestion.

Notes

Exercise, hard work, and weight loss do not change the volume of milk produced by nursing mothers. Extremely malnourished women or severely dehydrated women may have a decreased volume of milk.

> Improving the poorly nourished mother's diet may prolong breastfeeding duration as well as the duration of exclusive breastfeeding. Mothers whose diets are improved have more energy and are more interactive with their baby.

See also Macrobiotic diet of the mother; Maternal diet; Maternal diet, vegetarian; Milk production

▶ MALT

DEFINITION   Mucosa-associated lymphoid tissue. Lymphoid tissue in the human body is associated with the mucosal system. Mucosa-associated lymphoid tissue (MALT) is scattered along the body's mucosal linings and serves to protect the body from potentially dangerous antigens that could potentially enter along mucosal surfaces. The direct secretion of secretory immunoglobulin A (IgA) onto mucosal epithelia represents the major mechanism of MALT.

▶ Mammaplasty

DEFINITION   Breast reduction or augmentation surgery may be referred to as mammaplasty.

See also Breast augmentation; Breast reduction; Breast surgery

▶ Mammogenesis

DEFINITION   Mammogenesis is the development of the mammary gland. This development begins early in fetal life and continues through lactation. The mammary gland is one of the few tissues in mammals that can repeatedly undergo growth, functional differentiation, and regression or involution.

▶ Manual expression of breastmilk

DEFINITION   A method of removing milk from the lactating breast that does not require any device with the exception of a hand and a bowl or jar to collect milk. Hand expression is a simple skill that should be taught to all breastfeeding mothers.

Ask about

Reason mother plans to express milk.

ASSESSMENT

PROMPT CARE NEEDED?
Are any of the following present?
Imminent separation of mother and baby.

IF YES,   *Call lactation care provider now.*

ROUTINE CARE NEEDED?
Are any of the following present?
Mother wishes to learn hand expression.

IF YES,   *Call lactation care provider today.*

SELF CARE INFORMATION
Wash hands before beginning.
Practice hand expression when baby is latched onto one breast.
Gently massage and then compress the breast.
Your skill will improve with practice.
Store expressed milk in the refrigerator, a cooler with ice packs, or the freezer if it will not be used within 48 hours.
Follow safe milk storage guidelines.

IMPORTANT CONDITIONS TO REPORT
Problems with hand expression.
Concerns about volume of milk expressed.

See also Breast pump

▶ **Manual pump**

DEFINITION   A device designed to remove milk from the breast. Manual pumps work by hand pressure, squeezing a lever or contracting levers, or pulling out a cylinder to generate pressure to operate the pump.

▶ **Manufactured infant milks**

DEFINITION   May also be called artificial baby milks, manufactured baby milk, infant formula, artificial milks, formulated baby milks, or breast milk substitutes.

See also Formula, infant

▶ **Marijuana**

DEFINITION   Marijuana, although illegal for recreational use in the United States, is commonly used.

Portions of the plant *Cannabis sativa* are dried and, most commonly, smoked.

Marijuana has been placed in the category of drugs that are contraindicated for breastfeeding mothers by the American Academy of Pediatrics Committee on Drugs.

See also Contraindicated medications; Illegal drugs and breastfeeding

▶ **Massage, breast**

DEFINITION   A technique used to encourage milk to flow from the breast. When the suckling baby pauses, the mother gently but firmly massages and compresses the breast to which the baby is attached, thereby increasing the flow of milk and encouraging the suckling again.

See also Alternate breast massage; Premature infant; Slow weight gain, baby

▶ Mastalgia

DEFINITION   Mastalgia is breast pain with no certain cause. There can be many reasons for pain in the breast including breast infection or inflammation, clogs, or cysts.

See also Mastitis; Painful breastfeeding; Plugged ducts; Sore nipples

▶ Mastitis

DEFINITION   Mastitis is breast inflammation. It can be infective or noninfective.

Ask about

Onset.
Prior breast inflammation.
Sore nipples.
Known drug allergies.

EMERGENT CARE NEEDED?

Are any of the following present?

Visible red areas on the breast(s).

Fever higher than 101°F (38.5°C).

Extreme breast discomfort.

Flu-like aching throughout body.

Continuing fever after treatment.

Reaction to antibiotic prescribed.

IF YES, *Seek emergency care urgently if red streaks or red areas are found on both breasts and other symptoms are also present.*

Seek medical care within 2 to 4 hours with other symptoms if red area is on one breast only.

PROMPT MEDICAL CARE NEEDED?

Are any of the following present?

Continuing symptoms after treatment.

IF YES, *Call obstetric care provider now.*

PROMPT LACTATION CARE NEEDED?

Are any of the following present?

Difficulty breastfeeding during mastitis.

IF YES, *Call obstetric care provider now.*

SELF CARE INFORMATION

Breastfeed on both breasts, keeping them as soft as possible.

Start on the unaffected breast.

Take care of yourself as though you have the flu (bed rest, plenty of fluids, help for other children and household chores).

Antibiotics and anti-inflammatory drugs that are used to treat mastitis are generally compatible with breastfeeding. Use an up-to-date drug reference to be sure.

Take medications as they have been prescribed, even after you feel better.

IMPORTANT CONDITIONS TO REPORT

Symptoms that worsen or do not resolve.

> **Notes**
>
> Simultaneous bilateral mastitis may indicate more severe infection.

See also Acute infection; Bilateral mastitis; Breast inflammation; Mastitis

Drug References

American Academy of Pediatrics Committee on Drugs. (2001). Transfer of drugs and other chemicals into human milk. *Pediatrics, 108,* 776–789.

Briggs, G.G., Freeman, R.K., & Yaffee, S.J. (Eds.). (2002). *Drugs in pregnancy and lactation* (6th ed.). Philadelphia: Lippincott, Williams, and Wilkins.

Hale, T.W. (2004). *Medications and mothers milk.* Amarillo, TX: Pharmasoft Publishing.

Lawrence, R.A., & Lawrence, R.M. (2005). *Breastfeeding: A guide for the medical profession* (6th ed.). St. Louis: Mosby.

▶ Maternal and Child Health Bureau (MCHB)

DEFINITION   A branch of the U.S. Department of Health and Human Services, Health Resources, and Services Administration.

"[MCHB's vision is] a future America in which the right to grow to one's full potential is universally assured through attention to the comprehensive physical, psychological and social needs of the maternal and child health population. [MCHB] strive[s] for a society where children are wanted and born with optimal health, receive quality care and are nurtured lovingly and sensitively as they mature into healthy, productive adults. MCHB seeks a nation where there is equal access for all to quality health care in a supportive, culturally competent, family and community setting."[138]

Maternal and Child Health Bureau (MCHB)
Parklawn Building Room 18-05
5600 Fishers Lane
Rockville, MD 20857
Phone: 301-443-2170
Web site: www.mchb.hrsa.gov
   MCHB administers programs and grants to further its mission.

Footnotes

[138]Maternal and Child Health Bureau. (n.d.). *Vision*. Retrieved July 13, 2005, from http://www.mchb.hrsa.gov/about/default.htm.

▶ Maternal diet

DEFINITION   Mothers can produce enough milk, and milk of good quality, even when the mothers' supply of nutrients is limited.[139] Rules about eating or not eating certain foods during lactation are not warranted, may be hard to follow, and may decrease the mother's enjoyment of breastfeeding. However, there may be individual cases where certain foods affect the baby. Most commonly, the mother's drinking of liquid cow's milk has been associated with colic symptoms in some babies. If this is the case, improvement may be seen after the mother eliminates cow's milk from her diet for at least a week. Mothers should seek further information about diet and breastfeeding on an individual basis.

See also Macrobiotic diet of the mother; Maternal diet, vegetarian

Footnotes

[139]Subcommittee on Nutrition, National Academy of Sciences. (1991). *Nutrition during lactation*. Washington, DC: National Academy Press.

▶ Maternal diet, vegetarian

DEFINITION   Although many vegetarian diets are compatible with breastfeeding, some vegetarian diets (macrobiotic and vegan for example) may not be nutritionally adequate and can put the breastfed infant at risk of malnutrition. The major concerns are deficiencies of vitamins B_{12}, B_2, and D.

Ask about

Type of diet.
Age of baby.
Nutritional supplements taken.

ASSESSMENT

EMERGENT CARE NEEDED?

Are any of the following present?

Infant tetany (a condition characterized by painful muscle spasms and tremors).

Infant seizures.

IF YES, *Seek emergency care now.*

PROMPT CARE NEEDED?

Are any of the following present?

Infant lethargy.

Change in infant feeding behavior.

Infant weight loss after the first week of life.

Slow growth in the breastfed infant of a macrobiotic or vegan mother.

IF YES, *Seek pediatric care now.*

ROUTINE CARE NEEDED?

Are any of the following present?

Macrobiotic diet of the mother.

Vegan diet of the mother.

Ovo-lacto vegetarian diet of the mother.

IF YES, *Seek dietary consultation.*

SELF CARE INFORMATION

Dietary risks of vegetarian diets are especially associated with protein, vitamins B_{12} and B_2, vitamin D, and zinc deficiencies.

IMPORTANT CONDITIONS TO REPORT

Lethargy and poor feeding behavior can be early signs of nutritional inadequacies.

> **Notes**
>
> Many people who are vegetarians are knowledgeable about including foods and supplements that balance their diets.

See also Macrobiotic diet of the mother; Maternal diet

▶ Maternal diet and weight loss

DEFINITION   Weight loss of up to 5 lb a month in the first months postpartum has not been associated with poorer growth of the nursing baby. Nursing mothers are likely to be closer to their prepregnancy weight at six months than formula feeding mothers. A pattern of short, frequent feedings has been associated with greater weight loss than a pattern of longer, less frequent feedings.

See also Maternal exercise; Weight loss, mother

▶ Maternal employment

DEFINITION   Mothers who work for pay may do so away from home or in the home. They may be separated from their babies or have their babies nearby. In the United States, more than half of the mothers with babies under the age of 1 are employed.

Ask about

Amount of separation—hours per day, days per week.
Start date of work.

Age of baby.

Mother's plans to continue breastfeeding.

Mother's plans to express milk.

Accommodations at work for expressing and saving milk.

How the baby will be fed away from the mother.

ASSESSMENT

ROUTINE CARE NEEDED?

Are any of the following present?

Information about managing work and breastfeeding.

IF YES, *Call lactation care provider.*

SELF CARE INFORMATION

Stress does not seem to affect milk supply, but frequent milk removal is needed to maintain or improve the milk supply.

Milk can be collected and frozen in the early weeks to supplement milk collected after mother's return to work.

Milk supply is best maintained by using a pump that is intended for that purpose.

Select child care facilities carefully.

Expressed milk is a raw food and should be refrigerated as soon as possible after expression.

The timing of return to work and the number of hours spent away from the baby affect the duration of breastfeeding more than the type of work a woman does.

IMPORTANT CONDITIONS TO REPORT

Problems with expressing milk (check that the equipment is working properly).

Breast problems.

Problems with the infant accepting expressed milk.

Notes

Ongoing support and help with problem solving may be needed after returning to work.

See also Breast pump; Collection and storage of breastmilk; Storage of breastmilk; Working mothers

---

▶ Maternal exercise

DEFINITION   There is usually no reason for healthy women not to exercise in moderation during lactation, even women who have previously been sedentary.

Ask about

Age of baby.
Type and amount of exercise.
Prior cautions against exercise.

SELF CARE INFORMATION

Moderate exercise does not decrease milk production.
Mothers may be more comfortable with a supportive (but not too constricting bra).
Mothers may be more comfortable exercising after nursing, when the breasts are the most soft.
Mothers should be advised to discuss new physical activities with their health care providers.

▶ Maternal fatigue

DEFINITION   Exhaustion, weariness, or lack of energy. May be the result of lack of sleep due to night feedings. May also be associated with anemia, postpartum mood disorder, infection, underactive or overactive thyroid, pain, and the use of some drugs (including prescription drugs).

Ask about

Onset of symptom of fatigue.
Age of baby.
Weight gain of baby.
Medication and/or drugs used.

EMERGENT CARE NEEDED?

Are any of the following present?

Fever.

Confusion.

Dizziness.

Blurred vision.

Swelling, weight gain, and little or no urine.

IF YES, *Seek medical care now.*

PROMPT CARE NEEDED?

Are any of the following present?

Ongoing fatigue.

Sadness or depression.

Intolerance to cold.

Dry skin.

Headache.

Insomnia.

Persistent constipation.

IF YES, *Seek medical care today.*

ROUTINE CARE NEEDED?

Are any of the following present?

Concern about frequency of nighttime and daytime nursings.

Concern about adequacy of milk supply.

IF YES, *Call lactation care provider.*

SELF CARE INFORMATION

Although tiredness is common postpartum, fatigue should be investigated since it can be a nonspecific symptom of other problems.

IMPORTANT CONDITIONS TO REPORT

Fatigue that is not relieved by sleep.

See also Anemia; Postpartum depression; Thyroid disease

▶ Maternal hospitalization

DEFINITION   Breastfeeding mothers may be hospitalized in case of emergency, because of chronic health problems, for psychiatric reasons, for tests, or for elective surgery.

Ask about

Age of baby.
Dependence of baby on mother's milk/exclusivity of breastfeeding.
Drugs the mother may be given.
Ability of mother to express milk in the hospital.
Practicality of breastfeeding baby in the hospital.

ASSESSMENT

PROMPT CARE NEEDED?
Are any of the following present?
Imminent hospitalization of breastfeeding woman.

IF YES, *Call lactation care provider now.*

ROUTINE CARE NEEDED?
Are any of the following present?
Possible hospitalization of a breastfeeding woman.

IF YES, *Call lactation care provider.*

SELF CARE INFORMATION
Tell all of the health care providers that you are nursing and that you want to continue (assuming this is the case).
Make a plan for expressing milk in order to maintain the milk supply and provide milk for the baby.
Ask if it is possible for the baby to visit or stay in the hospital room with you.

See also Abrupt weaning; Breast pump; Hand expression of breastmilk

▶ # Maternal medications

DEFINITION   Many factors influence whether a drug the mother takes will be found in her milk, the amount of the drug that is found in the milk, and the effect of the drug on the baby. Some drugs can also affect the milk supply.

Ask about

Age of baby.
Weight of the baby.
History of taking drug (i.e., was the drug taken during pregnancy?).
How long the drug will be taken.

ASSESSMENT

PROMPT CARE NEEDED?
Are any of the following present?
Questions regarding drug compatibility with lactation.

IF YES, *Consult up-to-date drug references, and seek medical care within 2 to 4 hours regarding safety of medications or possible drug substitutions, and call lactation care provider for assistance with managing milk supply.*

SELF CARE INFORMATION
Do not self medicate while breastfeeding without discussing the drug with your health care provider.
Tell every health care provider that you are breastfeeding.
If you are prescribed a drug that is incompatible with breastfeeding, ask your health care provider about alternative drugs that are compatible.

IMPORTANT CONDITIONS TO REPORT
Any changes in the baby's behavior or appearance.
Any changes in your milk supply.

See also Contraindicated medications; Over-the-counter (OTC) drugs

Drug References
American Academy of Pediatrics Committee on Drugs. (2001). Transfer of drugs and other chemicals into human milk. *Pediatrics, 108*, 776–789.

Briggs, G.G., Freeman, R.K., & Yaffee, S.J. (Eds.). (2002). *Drugs in pregnancy and lactation* (6th ed.). Philadelphia: Lippincott, Williams, and Wilkins.

Hale, T.W. (2004). *Medications and mothers milk.* Amarillo, TX: Pharmasoft Publishing.

Lawrence, R.A., & Lawrence, R.M. (2005). *Breastfeeding: A guide for the medical profession* (6th ed.). St. Louis: Mosby.

▶ Mature milk

DEFINITION   Mature milk is milk that is produced from about 10 days postpartum until the time of weaning.

▶ MCHB

See also Maternal and Child Health Bureau (MCHB)

▶ Meconium

DEFINITION   Thick, sticky, and greenish-black in color, meconium is the first stool (feces) of the newborn. The passage of meconium indicates that the intestines are working properly.

SELF CARE INFORMATION

Passage of meconium is facilitated by frequent nursing in the first days so that the baby receives many colostrum feedings.

Because it is so sticky, meconium may be hard to clean off of the baby's bottom. Putting on a light coating of cream or oil when the diaper is changed can help.

Over the first days, the dark, early stool becomes greener (transitional stool) and then, for the breastfed infant, yellow.

If baby is still passing dark green meconium stools after day 5, call pediatric care provider now.

See also Bowel movements, infant

▶ Medications

DEFINITION Many factors influence whether a drug the mother takes will be found in her milk, the amount of the drug that is found in the milk, and the effect of the drug on the baby. Some drugs can also affect the milk supply.

Ask about

Age of baby.
Weight of the baby.
History of taking drug (i.e., was the drug taken during pregnancy?).
How long the drug will be taken.

ASSESSMENT

PROMPT CARE NEEDED?

Are any of the following present?

Questions regarding drug compatibility with lactation.

IF YES, *Consult up-to-date drug references, and seek medical care within 2 to 4 hours regarding safety of medications or possible drug substitutions, and call lactation care provider for assistance with managing milk supply.*

SELF CARE INFORMATION

Do not self medicate while breastfeeding without discussing the drug with your health care provider.

Tell every health care provider that you are breastfeeding.

If you are prescribed a drug that is incompatible with breastfeeding, ask your health care provider about alternative drugs that are compatible.

Any changes in the baby's behavior or appearance.
Any changes in your milk supply.

See also Contraindicated medications; Over-the-counter (OTC) drugs

Drug References
American Academy of Pediatrics Committee on Drugs. (2001). Transfer of drugs and other chemicals into human milk. *Pediatrics, 108,* 776–789.
Briggs, G.G., Freeman, R.K., & Yaffee, S.J. (Eds.). (2002). *Drugs in pregnancy and lactation* (6th ed.). Philadelphia: Lippincott, Williams, and Wilkins.
Hale, T.W. (2004). *Medications and mothers milk.* Amarillo, TX: Pharmasoft Publishing.
Lawrence, R.A., & Lawrence, R.M. (2005). *Breastfeeding: A guide for the medical profession* (6th ed.). St. Louis: Mosby.

▶ Medicinal herbs

DEFINITION   Medicinal herbs are plants or plant parts that are valued for their medicinal qualities.

Herbs can have powerful effects. As with some drugs taken by breastfeeding mothers, troubling effects have been reported in breastfed babies whose mothers' have taken certain medicinal herbs.

SELF CARE INFORMATION
Tell all health care providers about any herbs and natural supplements you are taking.
Some herbs (such as fenugreek) can decrease the effectiveness of other medications.[140]
Investigate medicinal herbs with the same care you would with prescribed and over-the-counter medications.

IMPORTANT CONDITIONS TO REPORT
Any change in the baby's physical condition or behavior such as problems sleeping, vomiting, rash, or irritability.

See also Fenugreek; Over-the-counter (OTC) drugs

Footnotes

[140]Skidmore-Roth, L. (2003). *Mosby's handbook of herbs and natural supplements* (2nd ed.). St. Louis, MO: Mosby.

▶ Meningitis

DEFINITION Inflammation of the outer membrane of the brain and spinal cord, typically caused by viral or bacterial infection.

> **Notes**
>
> Symptoms of meningitis in an infant include fever, vomiting, stiffness of the neck, lethargy, and irritability that is not calmed by cuddling. If baby has symptoms of meningitis, seek pediatric care now.

See also Lethargy

▶ Menstrual cycle

DEFINITION Research continues in order to better understand the relationship between menstruation, fertility, and breastfeeding. The time after childbirth and before menstruation resumes in nursing mothers is called lactational amenorrhea.

SELF CARE INFORMATION

It is impossible to predict when any woman will get her first period after her baby is born if she is breastfeeding.

Periods can be irregular, or lighter or heavier than when not breastfeeding.

Fertility may return before the first period after childbirth.

The return of menstruation does not mean the end of breastfeeding.

Some mothers report that their nursing babies are less interested in breastfeeding during their periods.

Some mothers experience nipple soreness during menstruation.

Menstruation before four to six weeks postpartum if breastfeeding.

See also Amenorrhea; Birth interval and breastfeeding; Fertility; Lactational Amenorrhea Method (LAM); Placental fragments, retained

▶ Metabolic dysfunction, galactosemia

DEFINITION Galactosemia is a rare genetic metabolic disorder in which the infant must be placed on a galactose-free diet because the liver enzyme needed to break down galactose is missing.

Classic galactosemia is an absolute contraindication to breastfeeding. Duarte galactosemia is a variant in which the baby may tolerate some galactose.

Galactosemia is usually diagnosed in the first week via heel stick screening or the appearance of symptoms including prolonged jaundice, vomiting, and diarrhea.

Ask about

Age of baby.

ASSESSMENT

EMERGENT CARE NEEDED?
   Are any of the following present?
      Jaundice (yellow appearance).
      Vomiting.
      Diarrhea.
      Weight loss.

IF YES,   *Seek pediatric care within 2 to 4 hours.*

PROMPT CARE NEEDED?
   Are any of the following present?
      If the mother has been breastfeeding prior to diagnosis, she may need assistance with finding comfort until milk production ceases.

IF YES,   *Call lactation care provider today.*

SELF CARE INFORMATION

Suddenly stopping breastfeeding or expressing after the baby is diagnosed with galactosemia can lead to breast problems such as mastitis and abscess development.
Milk expression can help to keep the breasts comfortable until milk production
slows and ceases.

IMPORTANT CONDITIONS TO REPORT

Breast inflammation (redness) and painful areas on the breast.
Fever higher than 101°F (38.5°C).
Extreme breast discomfort.
Flu-like aching throughout body.

See also Abrupt weaning; Contraindicated conditions; Weaning

▶ ## Metabolic dysfunction, phenylketonuria

DEFINITION   Phenylketonuria (PKU) is a rare genetic inborn error of metabolism
that is detectable during the first days of life through newborn screening. PKU is
characterized by the absence or deficiency of the enzyme that is necessary to
process the essential amino acid phenylalanine. Babies with PKU may be partially
breastfed together with consumption of a phenylalanine-free formula, per physician's order. These babies must be monitored carefully to protect the central nervous system from high levels of phenylalanine.

ASSESSMENT

PROMPT CARE NEEDED?
Are any of the following present?
Management of breastfeeding after diagnosis of PKU.

IF YES,   *Call lactation care provider today.*

SELF CARE INFORMATION

The physician will prescribe a phenylalanine-free formula and determine how often
the baby's blood levels will be tested for phenylalanine.

Even babies with PKU require some of the amino acid phenylalanine that is found in formula and breastmilk.

Human milk is lower in phenylalanine than standard formulas.

Research indicates that children who had received their mother's milk in addition to the special phenylalanine-free formula during infancy had more than a 10-point IQ advantage compared to children who had received the special formula alone or compared to a standard formula.[141]

IMPORTANT CONDITIONS TO REPORT

Any breastfeeding or formula feeding problems.

Footnotes

[141]Riva, E., Agostoni, C., Biasucci, G., Trojan, S., Luotti, D., Fiori, L., et al. (1996). Early breastfeeding is linked to higher intelligence quotient scores in dietary treated phenylketonuric children. *Acta Paediatrica, 85*, 56.

▶ Metabolism

DEFINITION The processing of a substance by the body, breaking it down into usable fragments.

▶ Metoclopramide (Reglan®)

DEFINITION Metoclopramide (Reglan®) is generally used to increase the muscle tone of the lower esophagus sphincter and is used to treat reflux and nausea. Side effects include cardiac arrhythmias, extrapyramidal signs, jitteriness, insomnia, sedation, and anxiety. Another side effect is the increase in prolactin release that may result in increased milk production. Increased milk production does not happen in all women.

SELF CARE INFORMATION

If prescribed, follow instructions carefully.

IMPORTANT CONDITIONS TO REPORT

Jitteriness.

Insomnia.

Sedation.
Anxiety.

See also Increasing milk supply; Medications; Milk production

▶ MFCI

DEFINITION   Mother-Friendly Childbirth Initiative. A set of ten steps for hospitals, birth centers, and other birth services for provision of mother-friendly care during childbirth. This initiative is a project of the Coalition for Improving Maternity Services.

See also Coalition for Improving Maternity Services (CIMS)

▶ Milk banks

DEFINITION   Donor human milk banks have been in operation since the early 1900s. They collect milk from mothers who have extra milk, beyond what they need for their thriving babies. Mothers are screened by history, and their blood and milk are tested for exposure to bacteria and viruses of concern. In addition, milk is pasteurized. In the United States, milk is distributed only by prescription.

In the U.S., Canada, and Mexico, donor milk should be obtained only from a member milk bank of the Human Milk Banking Association of North America or a state-licensed milk bank.

Ask about

Age of baby.
Does the mother wish to donate?
Does the baby need donor milk?

Mothers who wish to donate milk should be encouraged to contact the Human Milk Banking Association to find a location that is accepting donations. Informal donation of milk from one mother to another cannot be condoned, as it is possible to pass illnesses through unscreened and untreated milk.

Donor milk from a recognized human milk bank will have gone through several different screening processes (history and serology of the donor, bacteriology of the milk before and after heat treatment, etc.) and will be heat-treated to remove most pathogens.

The uses of donor milk are many, including providing nourishment to preterm or chronically ill infants, such as those with feeding intolerance, malabsorption, cardiac problems, metabolic problems, and diarrhea.

Use of donor milk in preterm infants is thought to be preventive of necrotizing enterocolitis.

A prescription is necessary for donor milk to be dispensed from the milk bank.

There is a processing cost associated with obtaining donor milk; this fee may be waived or reduced if cost prohibitive.

Milk banks can be located by contacting the following organization:

Human Milk Banking Association of North America (HMBANA)
1500 Sunday Drive
Suite 102
Raleigh, NC 27607
Phone: 919-861-4530 ext. 226
Web site: www.hmbana.org

▶ Milk blister, bleb

DEFINITION   A tiny, white, milky blockage of a single duct opening on the surface of the nipple. Mothers often describe excruciating, pinpoint pain at the site of the blockage. Blebs may need to be lanced by a medical care provider.

Because of the serious nature of some infectious conditions, including herpes, women reporting rashes or lesions on the breast and nipple should be seen immediately by medical personnel to rule out contraindicated infections.

Ask about

Onset.
Age of baby.
History of herpes lesions or other skin conditions on breast or nipple.

EMERGENT CARE NEEDED?

Are any of the following present?

Lesion on the breast or nipple of a breastfeeding woman with history of herpes lesions in this area.

Active lesion on the nipple or breast of a breastfeeding woman.

IF YES, **Seek medical care now.**

PROMPT CARE NEEDED?

Are any of the following present?

Painful, protruberant bleb on the nipple.

IF YES, **Seek medical care today.**
Call lactation care provider today.

SELF CARE INFORMATION

Follow directions for post-lancing care.

IMPORTANT CONDITIONS TO REPORT

Symptoms of infection (fever, aching, chills, or redness at site).

Notes

Emergency differential diagnosis is crucial in women with history of herpes lesions on the nipple. As herpes can be fatal to the newborn, breastfeeding should be discontinued on the affected nipple until differential diagnosis is obtained.

A bleb "may be 'cured' or disappear when the health professional opens it with a sterile needle. It may reappear and have to be opened again."[142]

See also Blisters on nipple or breast; Nipple pain

Footnotes

[142] Lawrence, R.A., & Lawrence, R.M. (2005). *Breastfeeding: A guide for the medical profession* (6th ed, p. 300). St. Louis: Mosby.

▶ Milk collection and storage

DEFINITION   Procedure by which milk is safely expressed and stored.

SELF CARE INFORMATION

Milk collection may be done by hand or pump expression.

Begin all milk collection by washing hands, pump, and collection device carefully.

Massage breasts prior to expressing.

Label each container with date of expression and name of infant (if it will be used in a multichild setting).

Glass and hard plastic containers with tight lids are recommended. All containers should be food-grade. Plastic bags designed for milk storage may be used, but it may be difficult to prevent spillage and puncture of these bags.

Milk can be safely stored:[143]

Up to four hours at room temperature (lower than 75° F), but should be refrigerated immediately if possible (with frozen gel pack in an insulated lunch bag or cooler if refrigerator is not available).

Up to 72 hours in the refrigerator.

Up to three months in the built-in freezer section of a refrigerator.

Up to six months in a deep freezer.

Milk that will not be used fresh within 72 hours should be frozen as soon as possible. Thaw milk in its container.

Milk can be safely thawed by:

Placing frozen containers in the refrigerator overnight.

Holding frozen containers under lukewarm running tap water.

Placing frozen containers in lukewarm water.

Hot water is not recommended due to potential nutrient loss.

Milk should never be boiled or microwaved.

Milk does not need to be overly warm before being fed to infant.

See also Containers for milk storage; Storage of breastmilk; Thawing and warming frozen milk

Footnotes

[143]Arnold, L.D.W. (2004). *Safe storage of expressed breastmilk for the healthy infant and child.* East Sandwich, MA: Health Education Associates.

▶ Milk-ejection reflex

DEFINITION   The neurohormonal response that compresses the myoepithelial cells that surround the alveoli, forcing milk to be squeezed down through the ducts and out the nipple. Also called let-down reflex.

This reflex is caused by a spike in the hormone oxytocin, one of the two major hormones of lactation (the other is prolactin). Oxytocin is released from the posterior lobe of the pituitary gland and stimulates the contraction of the smooth muscle of the uterus during labor. This hormone is also responsible for the let-down (ejection) of milk from the breast.

Researchers have found that oxytocin is released in the first hours postpartum by the baby's hand massage of the breast.

Oxytocin is also released by the baby stretching the nipple sufficiently in the mouth. This is why a good latch is so important to milk transfer.

Oxytocin is also released through a conditioned response over time.

SELF CARE INFORMATION

The breastfed newborn should gain well (0.5–1 oz per day on average). If the baby is gaining less than this, have a face-to-face breastfeeding evaluation.

At the breast, the baby should have sucking pattern that includes slow, deep sucks. After the first few days, the baby's swallows can be heard, and the baby should have at least six wet diapers and two to five yellow stools each day.

IMPORTANT CONDITIONS TO REPORT

Inadequate weight gain.

Inadequate number of urinations and stools.

See also Oxytocin; Overactive let-down reflex

▶ Milk fed to wrong baby

DEFINITION Accidental feeding of one mother's expressed breastmilk to another baby. This may happen in the hospital or daycare setting. Concern has been raised about the possibility of disease transmission from the milk to the infant. The Centers for Disease Control and Prevention states that this accident should be treated as any other accidental exposure to bodily fluids.

Notes

According to the Centers for Disease Control and Prevention, the following actions should be taken by the provider:

1. "Inform the mother who expressed the breast milk of the bottle switch, and ask
   - When the breast milk was expressed and how it was handled prior to being delivered to the caretaker or facility
   - Whether she has ever had an HIV test and, if so, would she be willing to share the results with the parents of the child given the incorrect milk
   - If she does not know whether she has ever been tested for HIV, would she be willing to contact her physician and find out if she has been tested
   - If she has never been tested for HIV, would she be willing to have one and share the results with the parents of the other child
2. Discuss the mistaken milk with the parents of the child who was given the wrong bottle
   - Inform them that their child was given another child's bottle of expressed breast milk
   - Inform them that the risk of transmission of HIV is very small
   - Encourage the parents to notify the child's physician of the exposure
   - Provide the family with information on when the milk was expressed and how the milk was handled prior to its being delivered to the caretaker so that the parents may inform their own physician
   - Inform the parents that their child should soon undergo a baseline test for HIV"[144]

Footnotes

[144]Centers for Disease Control and Prevention. (2005). *Breastfeeding: Recommendations: What to do if an infant or child is mistakenly fed another woman's expressed breast milk.* Retrieved August 9, 2005, from http://www.cdc.gov/breastfeeding/recommendations/other_mothers_milk.htm.

▶ Milk flow, too fast

DEFINITION   Milk may flow faster than the baby can manage. This may be due to the oversupply of milk, a forceful let-down reflex, or both.

Ask about

Age of baby.
Weight gain of baby.

ASSESSMENT

ROUTINE CARE NEEDED?

Are any of the following present?

Gagging, choking, or coughing at the breast as if the milk is coming too fast.
Baby spits up and is gassy.
Baby pulls off the breast while nursing and milk sprays.
Nipple compressed at the end of the nursing.

IF YES,   *Call lactation care provider today.*

SELF CARE INFORMATION

The too fast let-down is often accompanied by an abundant milk supply.
Positioning the baby in an upright position, with no pressure on the back of the head, may give the baby an opportunity to find the best nursing position.
Try nursing the baby on only one breast at each feeding to decrease the supply.
Some mothers are successful managing the flow by nursing while lying on their backs with the baby positioned flat on top. This technique is known as "posture feeding," "the Australian posture," or "nursing down-under." The baby has complete head control in this position, and the milk is spraying against gravity.

IMPORTANT CONDITIONS TO REPORT

Plugged ducts.
Visible red areas on the breast(s).
Fever higher than 101°F (38.5°C).
Extreme breast discomfort.
Flu-like aching throughout body.

See also Clenching or clamping onto the nipple/areola; Mastitis; Plugged ducts

▶ Milk flow, too slow

DEFINITION   Delayed or slow milk flow may be due to a low milk supply, poor let-down, or both. The nipple may be stretched inadequately due to faulty latch. Rarely, flow may be impeded temporarily by sudden high levels of adrenalin due to extreme stress or crisis.

Ask about

Age of baby.
Weight gain pattern of baby.
History of breast surgery.

ASSESSMENT

PROMPT MEDICAL CARE NEEDED?

Are any of the following present?

Meconium bowel movements after 5 days of life.

Fewer than three bowel movements daily in breastfed newborn after the first 2 days of life.

No urine in six hours.

Brick dust urine (uric acid crystals) after 2 days of life.

Dark colored urine.

Fewer than four urinations daily in the breastfed newborn after day 5 of life.

Noticeably sunken fontanelles (soft spot on top of head).

Decreased activity.

Baby below birthweight at 10 to 14 days of life.

Cessation of weight gain.

IF YES,   *Seek pediatric care now and call lactation care provider today.*

SELF CARE INFORMATION

Some mothers never feel the sensation of let-down or any of the signs of let-down such as thirst and uterine contractions.

Collecting milk by using a breast pump is not the same as breastfeeding; you cannot determine how much a baby is transferring by how much milk is pumped.

IMPORTANT CONDITIONS TO REPORT

Increased infant lethargy.

Decrease in number of stools and wet diapers.

Decrease in infant weight gain.

Notes

Babies with a history of long feedings (more than 20 minutes per breast) should be evaluated by a lactation care provider.

See also Insufficient milk supply; Latch-on; Let-down reflex; Milk-ejection reflex; Slow weight gain, baby

▶ Milk production

DEFINITION   There is a wide variance in the volume of milk intake among healthy breastfed infants but during the first four months, women produce about 750 ml per day.[145] But women can make much more; some women can make more than 4000 ml per day.[146]

See also Increasing milk supply; Milk production; Test weighing

Footnotes

[145]Butte, N.F., Wong, W.W., Garza, C., Stuff, J.E., Smith, E.O., Klein, P.D., et al. (1991). Energy requirements of breast-fed infants. *Journal of the American College of Nutrition, 10,* 190–195.

[146]Saint, L., Maggiore, P., & Hartmann, P.E. (1986). Yield and nutrient content of milk in eight women breast-feeding twins and one woman breast-feeding triplets. *British Journal of Nutrition, 56,* 49–58.

▶ Milk storage bags

DEFINITION   Soft waterproof bags specifically designed to store milk. Some are suitable for collecting milk into directly, refrigerating or freezing the milk, and fitting into a rigid holder for feeding.

SELF CARE INFORMATION

Be sure to read and follow the manufacturer's instructions carefully.

If you are freezing the milk, leave room for expansion (liquids expand when they are frozen).

See also Collection and storage of breastmilk

▶ Milk supply, inadequate

DEFINITION   Insufficient amount of milk produced by the breast. Maternal, infant, and environmental factors all contribute to milk supply problems.

Milk supply can usually be increased by increasing stimulation and removal of milk from the breast.

Ask about

Onset.

Age of baby.

EMERGENT CARE NEEDED?

Are any of the following present?

Exclusively breastfed newborn baby with less than one stool per day.

Meconium bowel movements after 5 days of life.

Fewer than three bowel movements daily in breastfed newborn after the first 2 days of life.

No urine in six hours.

Brick dust urine (uric acid crystals) after 2 days of life.

Dark colored urine.

Fewer than four urinations daily in the breastfed newborn after day 5 of life.

Noticeably sunken fontanelles (soft spot on top of head).

Decreased activity.

Baby below birthweight at 10 to 14 days of life.

Cessation of weight gain.

IF YES, *Seek pediatric care now.*

PROMPT LACTATION CARE NEEDED?

Are any of the following present?

Identified milk supply problem.

Concern about possible milk supply problem.

IF YES, *Call lactation care provider today.*

SELF CARE INFORMATION

Ensure baby is feeding 10–12 times per 24 hours.

Express milk after feeding.

IMPORTANT CONDITIONS TO REPORT

Persistent problems.

Recurrent problems.

See also Increasing milk supply

▶ Milk transfer, estimating

DEFINITION   Milk transfer can be estimated by weighing the baby before and after nursing with an accurate (to 2 grams) digital scale. It is important to realize that the same volume of milk is probably not transferred at each nursing.

The amount of milk a woman pumps may not be related to the amount the baby can transfer.

See also Electronic scales; Increasing milk supply; Milk production

▶ Mixed feeds

DEFINITION   Combining formula or solid foods with breastfeeding is considered mixed feeding.

Full (exclusive) breastfeeding for about the first six months of life is recommended by the American Academy of Pediatrics Committee on Breastfeeding, the World Health Organization, The U.S. Breastfeeding Committee, and other policy groups.

Ask about

Age of baby.
Diet of baby.
Weight gain of baby.

ASSESSMENT

EMERGENT CARE NEEDED?
 Are any of the following present?
   Meconium bowel movements after 5 days of life.
   Fewer than three bowel movements daily in breastfed newborn after the first 2 days of life.
   No urine in six hours.
   Brick dust urine (uric acid crystals) after 2 days of life.
   Dark colored urine.
   Fewer than four urinations daily in the breastfed newborn after day 5 of life.
   Noticeably sunken fontanelles (soft spot on top of head).

Decreased activity.

Difficulty breathing.

Irritability and excessive crying.

IF YES, *Seek pediatric care now.*

PROMPT MEDICAL CARE NEEDED?

Are any of the following present?

Eczema.

Hives.

Vomiting.

Diarrhea.

Blood in the stools.

IF YES, *Seek medical care today.*

PROMPT LACTATION CARE NEEDED?

Are any of the following present?

Identified milk supply problem.

Desire to increase milk supply.

Education needed about combining breast and formula feeding.

IF YES, *Call lactation care provider today.*

SELF CARE INFORMATION

Solid foods do not help babies sleep through the night.

IMPORTANT CONDITIONS TO REPORT

Signs of dehydration (scanty, dark urine).

Difficulty breathing.

Eczema.

Hives.

Vomiting.

Diarrhea.

Blood in the stools.

Irritability and excessive crying.

See also Allergy in the breastfed infant; Formula, infant; Supplemental feeding

► Montgomery glands (Montgomery's tubercles)

DEFINITION   A group of 12–20 tubercles scattered around the areola of the breast that enlarge during pregnancy and lactation. These tubercles are connected to a combination of lactiferous glands and sebaceous glands. The substance secreted is both lubricating and antimicrobial.

SELF CARE INFORMATION
Excessive cleaning of the breast and areola is not necessary and is not recommended.

IMPORTANT CONDITIONS TO REPORT
Blocked or infected Montgomery glands.

> **Notes**
>
> Blocked or infected Montgomery glands look very similar to herpes lesions. Herpes can be deadly to newborns. Because of this, appearance of "blocked" or "infected" Montgomery glands must always be referred immediately to a physician.

See also Breast structure

► Montgomery's tubercles
See also Montgomery glands (Montgomery's tubercles)

► Mother-Friendly Childbirth Initiative (MFCI)

DEFINITION   A set of ten steps for hospitals, birth centers, and other birth services for provision of mother-friendly care during childbirth. This initiative is a project of the Coalition for Improving Maternity Services.

See also Coalition for Improving Maternity Services (CIMS)

► # Mother of preterm infant

DEFINITION Babies are considered preterm if they are born before 37 weeks of gestation.

Ask about

Gestational age of the baby.
Drugs prescribed for the mother.

ASSESSMENT

ROUTINE CARE NEEDED?

Are any of the following present?

Declining milk supply.
Difficulty transitioning baby to breast feeding.
Questions about breast pumps or expressing milk.

IF YES, *Call lactation care provider today.*

SELF CARE INFORMATION

Begin pumping as soon as possible after the baby is born.
Begin skin-to-skin contact with the baby as soon as permitted.
Pump at least eight times a day for best milk supply.
Use a pump designed for pump-dependent mothers (an automatic cycling pump that can remove milk from both breasts at the same time).

IMPORTANT CONDITIONS TO REPORT

Concern about milk supply.

See also Breast pump; Decrease in milk supply; Increasing milk supply; Preterm milk; Transition to breastfeeding

▶ Mother-to-mother counseling

DEFINITION   Delivery of breastfeeding support via trained, knowledgeable women who have breastfed themselves.

See also La Leche League; Peer counseling

▶ MS

DEFINITION   Multiple sclerosis. MS is an autoimmune disease of the central nervous system (CNS). In general, people with MS can experience partial or complete loss of any function that is controlled by or passes through the brain or spinal cord. Breastfeeding is not contraindicated for a woman with MS.

SELF CARE INFORMATION
Breastfeeding may be related to a decreased incidence of MS in later life.[147]

See also Autoimmune diseases

Footnotes
   [147]Pisacane, A., Impagliazzo, N., Russo, M., Valiani, R., Mandarini, A., Florio, C., et al. (1994). Breast feeding and multiple sclerosis. *British Medical Journal, 308,* 1411–1412.

▶ Mucosa-associated lymphoid tissue (MALT)

DEFINITION   Lymphoid tissue in the human body is associated with the mucosal system. Mucosa-associated lymphoid tissue (MALT) is scattered along the body's mucosal linings and serves to protect the body from antigens that could potentially enter along mucosal surfaces. The direct secretion of secretory immunoglobulin A (IgA) onto mucosal epithelia represents the major mechanism of MALT.

▶ Multiple infants (twins, triplets, and higher order multiples)

DEFINITION   Mothers can nurse more than one baby. Increased suckling, especially nursing two babies simultaneously, stimulates an increased supply of milk.

Multiples may be born prematurely, spend weeks or months, in the hospital before discharge, and not be discharged on the same day.

Mothers may express milk to be fed to hospitalized babies. Expression should start as soon after the babies are born as possible. Mothers should express eight or more times per day.

Ask about

Age of babies.

ASSESSMENT

PROMPT CARE NEEDED?

Are any of the following present?

Imminent birth of multiple infants in a woman planning to breastfeed.

Initiation of breastfeeding in a woman with multiple hospitalized babies.

Problems with breastfeeding multiples.

IF YES,   *Call lactation care provider now.*

ROUTINE CARE NEEDED?

Are any of the following present?

Need for strategies for managing the nursing of multiples.

Strategies for managing milk supply for multiples.

IF YES,   *Call lactation care provider today.*

SELF CARE INFORMATION

Nursing babies simultaneously is helpful for building a milk supply, but may be difficult to manage at first. Ask for help with positioning.

At first, switch the babies from one breast to another. As the babies get older, they may prefer nursing on one breast or another.

Many mothers have found it helpful at first to write down "who nursed when" to ensure that each baby gets enough.

IMPORTANT CONDITIONS TO REPORT
Lethargy.
Decrease in urine and stools.
Change in breastfeeding behavior.
Problems with feeding.

> **Notes**
>
> Mothers carrying multiple infants are more likely to deliver prematurely, especially when carrying higher order multiples. Additional time is needed for mothers to recover from multiple pregnancy and birth. Focus on the mother's needs as well as those of the babies.

See also **Breast pump; Higher order multiples (HOM); Premature infant; Triplets; Twins**

▶ Multiple sclerosis (MS)

DEFINITION   Multiple sclerosis (MS) is an autoimmune disease of the central nervous system (CNS). In general, people with MS can experience partial or complete loss of any function that is controlled by or passes through the brain or spinal cord. Breastfeeding is not contraindicated for a woman with MS.

SELF CARE INFORMATION
Breastfeeding may be related to a decreased incidence of MS in later life.[148]

See also **Autoimmune diseases**

Footnotes
[148]Pisacane, A., Impagliazzo, N., Russo, M., Valiani, R., Mandarini, A., Florio, C., et al. (1994). Breast feeding and multiple sclerosis. *British Medical Journal, 308*, 1411–1412.

▶ Muscle tone of infant

DEFINITION   Infant muscle tone can be normal, low, or overreactive. Infants with normal tone have flexed elbows and knees. Low muscle tone is called hypotonia. Overreactive tone is called hypertonia.

Hypotonia and hypertonia can sometimes be symptoms of other problems. Babies who have these symptoms can be more difficult to breastfeed.

Hypotonic babies seem floppy. Their elbows and knees are loosely extended.

Hypertonic babies may arch their bodies away from the breast.

Some of the problems that may be seen with breastfeeding include a nonrhythmic suck, biting when swallowing (tonic bite reflex), weak reflexes for sucking, swallowing, and gagging. Babies also may tire more easily.

Malnourished babies have decreased muscle tone.

Ask about

Age of baby.
Onset of hypotonia or hypertonia.
Change in feeding behavior.
Change in urination or stooling patterns.

ASSESSMENT

EMERGENT CARE NEEDED?

Are any of the following present?

> Sudden change in muscle tone.
> Sudden change in feeding behavior.

IF YES,   *Seek emergency care now and contact pediatric care provider immediately.*

PROMPT CARE NEEDED?

Are any of the following present?

> Feeding problems.
> Weight loss or slow/inadequate weight gain.
> Constipation or decrease in stool output.

IF YES,   *Seek pediatric care today.*

SELF CARE INFORMATION

Breastfeeding and breastmilk are valuable for babies with low or overreactive muscle tone.

Pumping may be necessary to maintain an adequate milk supply.

"Wearing" the baby in an over-the-shoulder sling can be very helpful to encourage flexion in a hyperextending infant.

IMPORTANT CONDITIONS TO REPORT

Change in feeding behaviors.

Change in urination or stooling patterns.

Declining breastmilk volume.

Notes

Because low muscle tone can be a sign of malnutrition, floppy babies should always be evaluated promptly. Similarly, stiffness can be a marker of infection and should be evaluated.

See also Milk production; Premature infant; Test weighing

▶ Myoepithelial cells

DEFINITION   Myoepithelial cells are specialized smooth musclelike cells that surround the milk-making cells. The hormone oxytocin causes these cells to contract. This moves the milk toward the nipple and out of the breast. The action of the myoepithelial cells is called the let-down or milk-ejection reflex.

See also Let-down reflex; Milk-ejection reflex; Oxytocin

► NABA

See also National Alliance for Breastfeeding Advocacy (NABA)

► NAPNAP

See also National Association of Pediatric Nurse Practitioners (NAPNAP)

► National Alliance for Breastfeeding Advocacy (NABA)

DEFINITION "The National Alliance for Breastfeeding Advocacy (NABA) is dedicated to the protection, promotion and support of breastfeeding as an integral part of a vision of wellness for the United States of America. It was formed to be the advocate who endeavors to link and facilitate those involved in national maternal/child health into a cohesive network to this end. This coordination of linkages will provide the synergy to ignite the critical mass of breastfeeding supporters into the force that will move breastfeeding into the public health arena and restore breastfeeding as the cultural norm."[149]

Notes

National Alliance for Breastfeeding Advocacy (NABA)
254 Conant Road
Weston, MA 02493-1756
Web site: www.naba-breastfeeding.org

Footnotes
[149]National Alliance for Breastfeeding Advocacy. (n.d.). *NABA vision.* Retrieved July 13, 2005, from http://www.naba-breastfeeding.org/about.htm.

▶ National Association of Pediatric Nurse Practitioners (NAPNAP)

DEFINITION "National Association of Pediatric Nurse Practitioners (NAPNAP) is the professional organization that advocates for children (infants through young adults) and provides leadership for Pediatric Nurse Practitioners who deliver primary health care in a variety of settings."[150]

Notes

National Association of Pediatric Nurse Practitioners (NAPNAP)
20 Brace Road
Suite 200
Cherry Hill, NJ 08034-2634
Phone: 856-857-9700
Web site: www.napnap.org

Footnotes

[150] National Association of Pediatric Nurse Practitioners. (n.d.). *Welcome to NAPNAP.* Retrieved July 14, 2005, from http://www.napnap.org/index_home.cfm.

▶ National Commission on Donor Milk Banking
See also American Breastfeeding Institute (ABI)

▶ National Healthy Mothers, Healthy Babies Coalition (HMHB)

DEFINITION "The mission of the National Healthy Mothers, Healthy Babies Coalition is to improve the health and safety of mothers, babies and families through education and collaborative partnerships of public and private organizations."[151]

Footnotes

[151a]National Healthy Mothers, Healthy Babies Coalition. (2004). *About us*. Retrieved July 14, 2005, from http://www.hmhb.org/who.html.

▶ National WIC Association (NWA)

DEFINITION   "Our mission is to provide leadership in promoting quality nutrition services; advocating services for all eligible women, infants, and children; and assuring sound, responsive management of the Special Supplemental Nutrition Program for Women, Infants and Children (WIC).

"**Our Breastfeeding Statement:** The National WIC Association (NWA) endorses the American Academy of Pediatrics' Policy Statement on 'Breastfeeding and the Use of Human Milk' (2005), which states, 'Exclusive breastfeeding is the reference or normative model against which all alternative feeding methods must be measured with regard to growth, health, development, and all other short-and long-term outcomes.' NWA promotes exclusive breastfeeding for infant feeding through the first year of life and beyond, with the addition of appropriate complementary foods when the infant is developmentally ready, usually around six months of age. All WIC staff have a role in promoting and providing support for the successful initiation and continuation of breastfeeding."[151b]

See also USDA; WIC program

Footnotes

[151b]National WIC Association. *National WIC Association.* (2003). Retrieved December 12, 2005, from http://www.nwica.org.

▶ Natural family planning

DEFINITION   Natural family planning is focused on planning or preventing pregnancy based on when a woman is fertile. Women may want to use natural family planning methods for religious, medical, or personal reasons. The **Lactational Amenorrhea Method (LAM)** is a type of natural family planning that can be used during the first six months of breastfeeding.

See also Bellagio Consensus; Child spacing; Fertility; Lactational Amenorrhea Method (LAM)

▶ NEC

See also Necrotizing enterocolitis (NEC); Premature infant; Preterm milk

---

▶ Necrotizing enterocolitis (NEC)

DEFINITION   Necrotizing enterocolitis (NEC) is the most common surgical emergency in newborns, especially premature babies. The intestine reacts with an inflammatory response to feedings leading to intestinal necrosis (tissue death). There is no single explanation for why NEC happens, but formula feeding is one factor that has been associated with its incidence.

See also Premature infant; Preterm milk

▶ Neonatal hypoglycemia

DEFINITION   Neonatal hypoglycemia is also called "low blood sugar." It happens because the infant's blood glucose (sugar) levels have fallen below a predetermined amount.

Ask about

Age of baby.
Gestational age of baby.
History of diabetes in mother.
History of labor, especially stress.

ASSESSMENT

EMERGENT CARE NEEDED?
Are any of the following present?

Seizure activity.

Convulsions.

Coma.

Respiratory distress.

Apnea (cessation of breathing).

Cyanosis (blue color of the skin).

Thermoregulatory problems.

Jitteriness.

Hypotonia (floppy or low muscle tone).

Lethargy.

Listlessness.

Poor feeding.

IF YES, *Seek emergency care and call pediatrician immediately.*

SELF CARE INFORMATION

Establish early and frequent breastfeeding.

Keep the baby warm and dry.

Practice frequent skin-to-skin contact at the breast (babies can stay very warm in your arms). To do this, strip baby down to a diaper, remove your bra, and place baby against your skin, inside your shirt. Put a hat on baby's head and cover yourself with a blanket if the room air is cold.

Seek help with breastfeeding if baby feeds poorly.

IMPORTANT CONDITIONS TO REPORT

Seizure activity.

Convulsions.

Coma.

Respiratory distress.

Apnea (cessation of breathing).

Cyanosis (blue color).

Thermoregulatory problems.

Jitteriness.

Hypotonia (floppy muscle tone).

Lethargy.

Listlessness.

Poor feeding.

See also Colostrum; Muscle tone

▶ Neonatal intensive care unit (NICU)

DEFINITION   A special hospital unit providing care for premature and ill infants.

▶ Neonatal jaundice

DEFINITION   Neonatal jaundice is caused by an excessive amount of bilirubin in the blood. It is the most common condition requiring medical treatment in the new-born period.

Because bilirubin is yellow, the color accumulates in the baby's skin and the sclera (whites) of the eyes. The baby may appear tan, yellow, or light orange in color.

Bilirubin is removed from the blood by the liver.

Although the condition of jaundice may be benign, it may be associated with serious conditions such as **kernicterus**, hemolysis, and liver disease.

Ask about

Age of baby.
Feeding behavior.
Stooling pattern and color.
Urination pattern.

ASSESSMENT

EMERGENT CARE NEEDED?
   Are any of the following present?
         No stool in 24 hours.
         Severe lethargy (sleepiness).
         Poor feeding.
         Fever.
         Yellow skin.
         Gray or white stool.

   IF YES,   *Seek emergency care now and call pediatric care provider immediately.*

SELF CARE INFORMATION

Breastfeed as soon as possible after birth.

Encourage the baby to nurse 10–12 times per 24 hours.

Colostrum has laxative properties. Stooling helps to rid the baby's body of bilirubin.

IMPORTANT CONDITIONS TO REPORT

No stool in 24 hours.

Severe lethargy (sleepiness).

Poor feeding.

Fever.

Yellow skin.

Gray or white stool.

Notes

All jaundiced babies are at risk for kernicterus and should be closely monitored. Gray or white stool may indicate biliary atresia, a serious congenital problem with the bile ducts of the liver.

See also Bilirubin; Colostrum; Jaundice; Kernicterus; Late-onset jaundice

▶ Neonate

DEFINITION According to the American Academy of Pediatrics, a neonate is an infant less than 28 days of age.

▶ Neural tube defects

DEFINITION Congenital problems involving the covering of the nervous system are called neural tube defects. The neural tube is part of the baby as it develops in utero that will grow into the spinal cord and brain. Normally bones grow around the brain and spinal cord, and then skin covers the bones. A neural tube defect develops when this does not happen. Spina bifida is the most common neural tube defect. Anencephaly is a neural tube defect in which the brain and spinal cord do not form properly. Anencephaly is always fatal.

SELF CARE INFORMATION
A mother of a baby with spina bifida can express milk for her baby until the baby's condition allows breastfeeding.

IMPORTANT CONDITIONS TO REPORT
Problems expressing milk.
Decreased amount of expressed milk.

See also Breast pump; Hospitalization and breastfeeding; Increasing milk supply; Milk production

▶ Newborn

DEFINITION According to the American Academy of Pediatrics, a newborn is an infant less than 28 days of age.

▶ Nicotine

DEFINITION Chief addictive component of tobacco.
Mothers who smoke tobacco may breastfeed, but they should cut down on smoking and be encouraged to quit if possible. Babies should always be protected from secondhand smoke.

Ask about

Age of baby.
Weight gain pattern of baby.

ROUTINE CARE NEEDED?

Are any of the following present?

Using pacifier to delay, shorten, or eliminate breastfeeding.

More than 12 feedings daily.

Irritable baby.

Smoking in the baby's environment.

Concern about milk supply.

Poor feeding.

Desire to cut down on or stop smoking.

Upper respiratory problems in the baby (coughing, runny nose, etc.).

IF YES, *Report to pediatric care provider and call lactation care provider today.*

SELF CARE INFORMATION

Babies and children should always be protected from second hand smoke.

Research indicates that mothers who smoke may make and secrete less milk, but if they cut down or stop, their milk supply may rebound.

Breastfeeding mothers who smoke should encourage frequent feedings to stimulate milk production and should also avoid pacifier use, as this may decrease milk supply.

Breastfeeding may mitigate the effects to the baby of smoking during pregnancy.[152a]

IMPORTANT CONDITIONS TO REPORT

Weight loss or poor weight gain pattern.

Poor feeding.

Upper respiratory problems in the baby (coughing or runny nose).

Notes

Exposing babies and children to second hand smoke can have serious health consequences and should be avoided.

See also Medications; Smoking and lactation

Footnotes

[152a]Batstra, L., Neeleman, J., & Hadders-Algra, M. (2003). Can breastfeeding modify the adverse effects of smoking during pregnancy on the child's cognitive development? *Journal of Epidemiology and Community Health, 57*(6), 403–404.

▶ NICU

DEFINITION   Neonatal intensive care unit. A special hospital unit providing care for premature and ill infants.

▶ NICU, milk storage and handling in

DEFINITION   Special requirements for milk collection and storage for ill, hospitalized babies.

> **Notes**
>
> Different neonatal care units utilize different requirements for methods and materials used to collect and store milk for ill babies.
>
> Encourage mothers to contact the NICU for specific requirements of the unit where their babies are hospitalized.
>
> Contact the **Human Milk Banking Association of North America (HMBANA)** for recommended milk storage guidelines for NICU settings.

See also Breast pump; Collection and storage of breastmilk; Human Milk Banking Association of North America (HMBANA)

▶ Nifedipine

DEFINITION   Nifedipine (Adalat, Procardia) is a prescription medication (calcium channel blocker) that has been used to treat Raynaud's phenomenon/syndrome (nipple vasospasm) in nursing mothers.

Age of baby.

History of nipple pain.

Triple (white, blue, pink) color sign or Bi (white, pink) color sign of the nipple when cold or wet.

IMPORTANT CONDITIONS TO REPORT

Seek medical help in the case of adverse reactions described in the medication package insert.

Notes

The American Academy of Pediatrics lists Nifedipine on Table 6, "Maternal Medication Usually Compatible with Breastfeeding."[152b] Hale rates Nifedipine as a lactation risk category 2 drug ("Safer").[153]

See also Nipple pain; Raynaud's phenomenon/syndrome; Vasospasm of breast and nipple

Footnotes

[152b]American Academy of Pediatrics Committee on Drugs. (2001). Transfer of drugs and other chemicals into human milk. *Pediatrics, 108,* 781.

[153]Hale, T.W. (2004). *Medications and mothers milk* (p. 599). Amarillo, TX: Pharmasoft Publishing.

▶ Night nursings

DEFINITION   Nighttime nursings are desirable in the early months to ensure that babies are getting enough to eat. Sleeping longer than five hours at a stretch is the operative definition of "sleeping through the night."

Ask about

Age of baby.

Weight gain pattern.

ROUTINE CARE NEEDED?

Are any of the following present?

Baby older than 4 months.

Parents want fewer night feedings.

Call lactation care provider.

SELF CARE INFORMATION

Daytime interventions work best to cut back on nighttime nursings. Babies who sleep a lot during the day and feed infrequently need to make up for the lack of nourishment by nursing frequently at night.

IMPORTANT CONDITIONS TO REPORT

Poor feedings.

Increased wakening.

Weight loss or poor weight gain.

Notes

Many mothers find it more comforting to nurse their babies back to sleep, as compared to "training" baby to go back to sleep. Baby training should never be attempted with babies younger than 4 months, babies who are poor nursers, or babies who are not gaining well.

See also Maternal fatigue

▶ Nipple

DEFINITION The protuberant part of the breast that contains the endings of the lactiferous ducts from which the milk flows.

▶ Nipple creams or ointments

DEFINITION   Topical preparations that have been made for several purposes, such as to protect the skin, to decrease itching, to clean the skin (antiseptics), and to moisturize the skin.

Ask about

Nipple discomfort.

ASSESSMENT

ROUTINE CARE NEEDED?
Are any of the following present?

    Sore nipples.

    Painful breastfeeding.

    Skin rash, breakouts, or itching on the breast, areola, and nipple.

IF YES,   *Report symptoms to obstetric care provider today and call lactation care provider to schedule a feeding evaluation today.*

IMPORTANT CONDITIONS TO REPORT

Symptoms worsen or persist.

Signs of infection.

Feeding or stooling expectations are not met.

SELF CARE INFORMATION

Most ointments and creams are not intended for ingestion. When a mother applies an ointment or cream to her areola or nipple, her baby will be exposed to the ingredients during nursing.

Only use ointments and creams on the breast that are recommended for this purpose. Never use a product that has been prescribed for another problem.

Mothers can have adverse reactions to ointments and creams. Report any changes immediately.

See also Creams and ointments; Breast inflammation; Breast pain; Nipple pain; Sore nipples

Nipple everter

DEFINITION   A device designed to pull out inverted nipples.

See also Nipple, inverted

Nipple, flat

DEFINITION   A nipple that does not change in protuberance when the areola is compressed.

Ask about

Appearance of nipple.
Action of nipple when the areola is compressed.
Nipple changes during pregnancy and lactation.
Diagnosis of flat nipple.

ASSESSMENT

PROMPT CARE NEEDED?
Are any of the following present?
> Poor feeding.
> Poor milk transfer.
> Inadequate weight gain.

IF YES,	Problems with latch-on.
	Concern about milk supply.
	Report symptoms to pediatric care provider and call lactation care provider today.

SELF CARE INFORMATION

Mothers with flat nipples should be encouraged to express milk early and frequently until baby is able to facilitate nipple stretching well into the mouth.

IMPORTANT CONDITIONS TO REPORT

Poor feeding.

Poor milk transfer.

Inadequate weight gain.

Problems with latch-on.

Notes

Training flat nipples to stand out during pregnancy is an ineffective technique.

See also Milk transfer, estimating; Weight gain, baby–low

▶ Nipple, inverted

DEFINITION   The nipple is the protuberant part of the breast that contains the endings of the lactiferous ducts from which the milk flows. With inverted nipples, the nipple retreats into the breast when the areola is compressed.

Ask about

Appearance of nipple.

Action of nipple when the areola is compressed.

Nipple changes during pregnancy and lactation.

Diagnosis of inverted nipple.

PROMPT CARE NEEDED?

Are any of the following present?

Poor feeding.

Poor milk transfer.

Inadequate weight gain.

Problems with latch-on.

IF YES, *Report to pediatric care provider and call lactation care provider today.*

SELF CARE INFORMATION

Training inverted nipples to stand out during pregnancy is an ineffective technique. Mothers with inverted nipples should be encouraged to express milk early and frequently until baby is able to facilitate nipple stretching well into the mouth.

IMPORTANT CONDITIONS TO REPORT

Poor feeding.

Poor milk transfer.

Inadequate weight gain.

Problems with latch-on.

See also Milk transfer, estimating; Weight gain, baby–low

▶ Nipple pain

DEFINITION   Uncomfortable sensation in the tips of the breasts. Pain is not an expected part of breastfeeding and indicates need for feeding evaluation.

There can be many reasons for pain in the breast, including nipple trauma, poor latch and/or positioning and infection.

Ask about

Onset.

Location of pain.

Whether unilateral or bilateral.

PROMPT MEDICAL CARE NEEDED?

Are any of the following present?

Open fissure of nipple with pus.

Maternal fever.

Maternal malaise.

Pain combined with color change of nipple(s).

IF YES, *Call obstetric or primary care provider now.*

PROMPT LACTATION CARE NEEDED?

Are any of the following present?

Persistent pain with feeding.

Persistent pain between feedings.

Constant pain.

Pain combined with color change of nipple(s).

Pain with visible fissure or bleeding of the nipple(s).

IF YES, *Call lactation care provider now to schedule a feeding evaluation.*

ROUTINE CARE NEEDED?

Are any of the following present?

Brief pain at beginning of feeding.

Mild, recurrent pain.

IF YES, *Call lactation care provider today.*

SELF CARE INFORMATION

Practice skin-to-skin contact frequently.

Feed baby at first sign of hunger cues (signs that say "feed me" include hand-to-face or hand-to-mouth movements, lip smacking, seeking with lips, rooting, and head bobbing).

Feed baby at least 10–12 times per 24 hours.

Listen for signs of baby swallowing.

Allow baby to end feedings.

Expect at least 3–4 infant stools per 24 hours after the first 4 days of life.

Good positioning and attachment are crucial to reduce nipple pain.

If feedings are missed, hand express or pump milk to maintain supply.

Notes

Breastfeeding should not be painful. Advise mothers to seek medical or lactation care for breast pain.

See also Latch-on; Mastitis; Raynaud's phenomenon/syndrome; Sore nipples

▶ Nipple shields

DEFINITION   Nipple shields help with latch-on problems by providing a larger surface to fill the baby's mouth.

Modern nipple shields are made of a thin layer of silicone. They come in a variety of sizes and shapes.

Ask about

Age of baby.

History of weight gain.

Stooling pattern.

Urination pattern.

ASSESSMENT

PROMPT CARE NEEDED?

Are any of the following present?

Desire to obtain a nipple shield.

Desire to wean baby off a nipple shield.

Concern about adequacy of milk supply.

IF YES,   *Call lactation care provider today.*

Nipple shields have been associated with decreased milk transfer and poor weight gain in babies whose mothers use them.

Frequent weight checks and milk transfer assessments should be part of the baby's routine care when mother uses a nipple shield for feedings.

IMPORTANT CONDITIONS TO REPORT

Lethargy or poor feeding.

Weight loss or slow weight gain.

Decrease in the stooling or urination pattern.

> **Notes**
>
> Nipple shields have been shown to be helpful for premature babies transitioning to the breast. The mother continues to pump to maintain her milk supply.

See also **Nipple pain**

▶ NNS

See also Nonnutritive suckling (NNS)

▶ Nonnutritive suckling (NNS)

DEFINITION   Nonnutritive suckling (NNS) is the term used to describe the situation in which the baby suckles but there is low milk transfer.

NNS may be intentional, as with a premature infant who may be unable to manage a fast flow of milk. In this case, the mother expresses her milk prior to nursing to facilitate NNS.

It is common and normal for the rate of milk flow to change during a nursing. Some of the sucks will transfer less milk than others.

▶ Nonpuerperal lactation

DEFINITION   Lactation in a woman who has not given birth.

Breast secretions in a nonpuerperal woman, except in the case of induced lactation.

See also **Galactorrhea; Induced lactation**

▶ # Nursing

DEFINITION   A term used in the United States to denote nourishing a child with breastmilk. Also used to indicate the professional care activities of nurses. In other English-speaking cultures, nursing refers to caring for a child.

▶ # Nursing-bottle caries

DEFINITION   Nursing-bottle caries are cavities in the teeth that occur in a distinct pattern and are usually associated with bottle feeding.

SELF CARE INFORMATION
Cavities, though very rare, can occur in the teeth of older breastfeeding babies.
Cavities in nursing children may be associated with eating sticky, gummy, or sugary snacks, drinking sugary beverages, or administering sugary liquid medicines (such as cough medicine) at bedtime. Cavities are also associated with inadequate tooth cleaning.
As soon as a baby erupts a tooth, a tooth cleaning routine should be started. At first, the baby's teeth can be cleaned with a soft, wet facecloth. Later, brush the teeth as instructed by a dental health professional.
Begin visits to the dentist early, especially if there is a family history of caries and problems with the enamel of the teeth.

IMPORTANT CONDITIONS TO REPORT
Discolorations on the teeth.
Toothache.
Any unusual mouth discomfort.

▶ Nursing pads, pillows, and stools

DEFINITION A variety of commonly available items may help the mother position the baby (or babies, in the case of multiples) at the breast in a more optimal way.

Breastfeeding equipment is available from breast pump rental depots, baby product stores, and catalogues such as La Leche League's.

▶ Nursing strike

DEFINITION A nursing strike is the sudden refusal of the baby to nurse. This can happen with a baby of any age.

Ask about

Age of baby.
Nursing history.

ASSESSMENT

PROMPT CARE NEEDED?

Are any of the following present?

Baby refuses to nurse along with any of the following symptoms:

Sudden onset of inconsolable crying.

Change in stooling, urination, or sleep patterns.

Lethargy.

Vomiting.

Breathing difficulties.

Refusal to eat other age appropriate foods.

IF YES,   *Seek emergency care now and call pediatric provider immediately.*

PROMPT LACTATION CARE NEEDED?

Are any of the following present?

Baby refuses to nurse but otherwise seems normal.

Baby feeds well on one breast and not on the other.

Concerns about adequacy of milk supply.

IF YES,   *Call lactation care provider today.*

SELF CARE INFORMATION

Mothers whose babies go on strike need to express milk for comfort and to maintain supply.

Many babies who have gone on strike return to the breast once the problem has been resolved.

Do not "starve" the baby back to the breast. Babies need to be fed.

Babies go on strike when something is wrong in their lives. Some of the reasons reported for strikes include:

Teething.

Stuffy nose.

Ear infection.

Baby has bitten the mother who yelled; this frightened the baby.

Reaction to being left unattended to "cry it out."

Family stress.

Recent separation of mother and baby, such as mother's return to work.

To end a nursing strike:

Find out and correct what started the strike.

Give the baby lots of skin-to-skin contact, such as snuggling.

Do not force the baby to the breast. Try offering the breast just before bedtime, a nap, or first thing in the morning when baby is drowsy.

Avoid feeding the baby via a bottle. Try cup feeding.

Offer the breast to sleeping baby.

Try "peer pressure." Attend a breastfeeding support meeting with baby, or bring baby to visit with a nursing friend.

IMPORTANT CONDITIONS TO REPORT

Change in stooling or urination patterns.

Sleepiness, lethargy.

Breathing difficulties.

Vomiting.

Inconsolable crying.

See also Abrupt weaning; Breast refusal; Goldsmith's sign

Nutritional values of breastmilk

DEFINITION   At more than 87% water, human milk is the most dilute of mammal milks and is easily digested by human babies. That means that babies should nurse frequently—10–12 times per 24 hours at first.

Lactose (the primary carbohydrate in human milk) constitutes about 7% of human milk's volume. Fat constitutes about 3.8%, protein constitutes about 0.9%, and the ash (mineral) content constitutes about 0.2%.

Mother's milk has approximately 22 calories per ounce (75 kcal per 100 mL).

Milk composition is dynamic, changing in composition throughout each feeding, throughout the day, and throughout the months of breastfeeding.

SELF CARE INFORMATION

Eat in moderation from a wide variety of healthy foods.

There are no forbidden foods.

Consult a dietitian if you are following a strict diet for any reason.

Notes

Humans make human milk. Women on excessively restrictive diets (complete vegetarian diets such as vegan or macrobiotic, and women who avoid all dairy foods) should seek dietary counseling because certain important components (such as vitamins B_{12} and D) may be transferring into their milk in lowered amounts. These women may be advised to add nutritional supplements to their routine.

Health care providers should avoid telling women that they must have perfect diets to breastfeed. There is little difference in the composition of milk of well-nourished women and mal-nourished women. Women should be encouraged to eat well to protect their own health and energy.

See also Macrobiotic diet of the mother; Maternal diet; Maternal diet, vegetarian; Vitamin supplements

NWA

See also National WIC Association (NWA)

Obesity and breastfeeding

DEFINITION Breastfeeding has been identified as one of several strategies to reduce childhood obesity by both the Centers for Disease Control and Prevention and the American Academy of Pediatrics. Other strategies include eating more healthful foods such as fruits and vegetables, increasing exercise, and spending less time watching television or engaging in other sedentary activities. Mothers should be encouraged to breastfeed and supported in their decision.

Researchers have found that a longer duration of breastfeeding may result in a lower incidence of obesity within a population of people.

Breastfed infants normally gain weight faster in the first months of life as compared to formula fed infants. Their weight gain slows around 4–6 months and continues throughout the first year.

Some studies have shown that obese mothers may encounter more problems with breastfeeding. However, the likely cause of these breastfeeding problems is thought to be the underlying reason(s) for the mother's excess weight that may impact breastfeeding. Conditions such as hypo- or hyperthyroidism and Polycystic Ovarian Syndrome (PCOS), which both affect weight, may also have a direct impact on milk volume. The symptom of obesity alone generally will not cause problems for the breastfeeding mother.

> **Notes**
>
> Ensure that the baby's growth is compared to the normal growth pattern of breastfed infants.
>
> Advise overweight mothers with milk supply problems to have a complete medical evaluation.

See also Hyperthyroidism; Hypothyroidism; Growth charts; Maternal diet; Polycystic Ovarian Syndrome (PCOS); Weight loss, mother

Obturator, palatal

DEFINITION A palatal obturator is a device that is fitted individually for the baby with a cleft palate. The obturator blocks the cleft opening and allows for easier suckling. Modern obturators are made from the same material as athletic mouth guards and take only a few minutes to fit. As the baby grows, new obturators must be made. After the palatal repair, the obturator will no longer be needed.

Notes

For babies with cleft palates, nipple shields have been used to improve breastfeeding before the obturator is fitted.

Advise the mother to follow cleaning instructions for the obturator that has been provided to her, and return to her child's pediatric dentist for scheduled re-fittings.

See also Cleft lip and palate

▶ Occupational therapy

DEFINITION Occupational therapy is skilled treatment that helps individuals achieve the skills for living that they need. An occupational therapist can help develop feeding skills in babies with physical and developmental challenges.

Notes

The American Occupational Therapy Association
4720 Montgomery Lane
P.O. Box 31220
Bethesda, MD 20824
Phone: 301-652-2682
Web site: www.aota.org

▶ Office on Women's Health (OWH)

DEFINITION "The Office on Women's Health within the Department of Health and Human Services (OWH DHHS) [is] the government's champion and focal point for women's health issues, and works to redress inequities in research, health care services, and education that have historically placed the health of women at risk. The Office on Women's Health coordinates women's health efforts in HHS to eliminate disparities in health status and supports culturally sensitive educational programs that encourage women to take personal responsibility for their own health and wellness."[154]

Footnotes

[154]Office on Women's Health. (n.d.). *Welcome*. Retrieved August 4, 2005, from http://www.womenshealth.gov/owh/about.

▶ Ointments and creams

DEFINITION   Topical preparations that have been made for several purposes, such as to protect the skin, to decrease itching, to clean the skin (antiseptics), and to moisturize the skin.

Ask about

Nipple discomfort.

ROUTINE CARE NEEDED?

Are any of the following present?

Sore nipples.

Painful breastfeeding.

Skin rash, breakouts, or itching on the breast, areola, and nipple.

IF YES, *Report symptoms to obstetric care provider today and call lactation care provider to schedule a feeding evaluation today.*

IMPORTANT CONDITIONS TO REPORT

Symptoms worsen or persist.

Signs of infection.

Feeding or stooling expectations are not met.

SELF CARE INFORMATION

Most ointments and creams are not intended for ingestion. When a mother puts an ointment or cream on her areola or nipple, her baby will be exposed to the ingredients during nursing.

Only use ointments and creams on the breast that are recommended for this purpose. Never use a product that has been prescribed for another problem.

Mothers can have reactions to ointments and creams. Report any changes immediately.

Notes

Women experiencing **nipple pain** may self-treat with this and other inappropriate substances.

Women experiencing nipple pain should have a breastfeeding evaluation. Face-to-face counseling is effective in assessing and resolving nipple pain.

See also Breast pain; Nipple pain; Sore nipples

▶ Oligosaccharides in breastmilk

DEFINITION Oligosaccharides are short chains of sugar molecules. Researchers have found that some of the oligosaccharides in human milk have a protective effect against pathogens, especially in the urinary tract. Oligosaccharides are unique to human milk.

See also Bioactive components of breastmilk

▶ One-sided nursing

DEFINITION A baby who prefers one breast over the other. The nipples may be different from one side to the other, the flow of milk or the volume of milk may be greater or less, or the baby may be more comfortable positioned at one breast compared to the other.

Ask about

Age of baby.

ASSESSMENT

PROMPT CARE NEEDED?

Are any of the following present?

About mother

Fever higher than 101° F (38.5° C).

Reddened area on the breast.

Flulike symptoms.

About baby

Sudden refusal of one breast.

Inconsolable crying.

Decrease in stooling or urination.

IF YES, *Call medical care provider now and call lactation care provider now.*

SELF CARE INFORMATION

Sudden refusal of the breast, or refusal of one breast from birth can be a symptom of a medical problem in the baby or the mother. Common reasons include mastitis in the mother or nasal stuffiness in the baby.

There can be more serious medical problems that should be investigated when a baby refuses to nurse. Breast refusal has been associated with undetected breast cancer, for example.

If the baby is nursing less because of a stuffy nose or ear infection, the mother should express her milk in order to maintain lactation and stay comfortable.

IMPORTANT CONDITIONS TO REPORT

Decrease in baby's stooling or urination.

Fever or flulike feelings in mother.

Fever or inconsolable crying in baby.

See also Breast refusal; Goldmith's sign

► Oral contraceptives

DEFINITION Oral contraceptives have been studied in relation to breastfeeding. Some oral contraceptives are a combination of estrogen and progestin. Others are progestin-only.

Ask about

Age of baby.

Duration of oral contraceptive use.

PROMPT CARE NEEDED?

Are any of the following present?

Inadequate weight gain.

Perception of decreased milk supply.

IF YES, *Call lactation care provider today.*

ROUTINE CARE NEEDED?

Are any of the following present?

More information desired about oral contraception and breastfeeding.

More information desired about breastfeeding and family planning or birth control.

IF YES, *Consult up-to-date drug references, call obstetric care provider, and call lactation care provider.*

SELF CARE INFORMATION

Consider the **Lactational Amenorrhea Method (LAM)**, other natural family planning methods, and barrier methods of contraception if hormonal contraceptives are not acceptable. They are all compatible with breastfeeding.

IMPORTANT CONDITIONS TO REPORT

Decreased milk supply.

Decreased stooling or urination in baby.

Notes

Hale states that the health care provider should "suggest that the mother establish a good flow (60–90 days) prior to beginning oral contraceptives. If necessary, use only LOW DOSE combination oral contraceptives with 30–50 μg of estrogen, or better, progestin-only mini pills."[155] Hale rates oral contraceptives as L3 (moderately safe) drugs.

The AAP lists oral contraceptives on Table 6 (maternal medication usually compatible with breastfeeding).[156]

See also Birth control; Depo-Provera® contraceptive (Medroxyprogesterone); Fertility; Hormonal contraceptive methods; Lactational Amenorrhea Method (LAM); Progestin-only contraceptives

Footnotes

[155]Hale, T.W. (2004). *Medications and mothers milk* (p. 626). Amarillo, TX: Pharmasoft Publishing.

[156]American Academy of Pediatrics Committee on Drugs. (2001). Transfer of drugs and other chemicals into human milk. *Pediatrics, 108*, 780.

▶ Oral rehydration therapy (ORT)

DEFINITION   Oral rehydration therapy (ORT) is promoted by the World Health Organization (WHO) to reduce the number of infant deaths from dehydration due to diarrhea. Research confirms that rehydration solution made from inexpensive ingredients (glucose and electrolytes) is advantageous. Breastfed infants receiving ORT should continue breastfeeding.

See also Diarrhea and breastfeeding

▶ ORT
See also Oral rehydration therapy (ORT)

▶ Osteoporosis

DEFINITION   A disease in which the bones become extremely porous, often causing fracture. This is typically a problem of women after menopause.
Breastfeeding is thought to provide some protection against osteoporosis.

See also Bone loss; Bone mineral density (BMD)

▶ OTC drugs
See also Over-the-counter (OTC) drugs

▶ Otitis media

DEFINITION Otitis media is an infection or inflammation of the middle ear. The inflammation may begin with an infection that causes a sore throat, cold, or other respiratory or breathing problem. Babies who are breastfed have a lower incidence of otitis media compared to babies who are not. Pacifier use increases the incidence of otitis media.

Ask about

Age of baby.
History of sore throat, cold, or respiratory problem.
Change in breastfeeding behavior.

ASSESSMENT

PROMPT CARE NEEDED?

Are any of the following present?

Unusual irritability.
Difficulty sleeping.
Tugging or pulling at one or both ears.
Fever.
Fluid draining from one or both ears.
Difficulty breastfeeding.
Crying at the breast or pulling away and crying after a few sucks.

IF YES, *Seek pediatric care within 2 to 4 hours and call lactation care provider today.*

ROUTINE CARE NEEDED?

Are any of the following present?

Baby has been treated for ear infection but continues to fret or cry at the breast.

IF YES, *Call lactation care provider.*

SELF CARE INFORMATION

Even after the otitis media has resolved, the baby may be uncomfortable nursing, or may remember the pain of nursing with the ear infection. Changing positions may help. If the problem persists, have the baby's ears checked again by the health care provider.

Keep the breasts soft and express excess milk during the time the baby is not nursing well.

IMPORTANT CONDITIONS TO REPORT

Less urination or stooling.

Continued symptoms of otitis media after treatment.

Continued problems with breastfeeding after treatment is initiated.

Notes

Pacifier use has been associated with ear infection[157] and should be reexamined in babies with recurrent ear infection.

See also Ear infection; Nursing strike; Weaning

Footnotes

[157]Niemela, M., Pihakari, O., & Pokka, T. (2000). Pacifier as a risk factor for acute otitis media: A randomized, controlled trial of parental counseling. *Pediatrics, 106*(3), 483–488.

▶ Overactive let-down reflex

DEFINITION Milk may flow faster than the baby can manage. This may be due to the oversupply of milk, a forceful let-down reflex, or both.

Ask about

Age of baby.

Weight gain of baby.

ROUTINE CARE NEEDED?

Are any of the following present?

Gagging, choking, or coughing at the breast as if the milk is coming too fast.

Baby spits up and is gassy.

Baby pulls off the breast while nursing and milk sprays.

Nipple compressed at the end of the nursing.

IF YES, *Call lactation care provider today.*

SELF CARE INFORMATION

The overactive let-down is often accompanied by an abundant milk supply.

Positioning the baby in an upright position, with no pressure on the back of the head, may give the baby an opportunity to find the best nursing position.

Try nursing the baby on only one breast at each feeding to decrease the supply of milk.

IMPORTANT CONDITIONS TO REPORT

Symptoms of mastitis, including:

Plugged ducts.

Visible red areas on the breast(s).

Fever higher than 101°F (38.5°C).

Extreme breast discomfort.

Flulike aching throughout body.

See also Mastitis; Milk flow, too fast; Plugged ducts

▶ ## Oversupply

DEFINITION   An excessively abundant milk supply.

PROMPT CARE NEEDED?

Are any of the following present?

Perception of overabundant milk supply.

Excessively large or frequent stools in a breastfed baby.

Recurrent engorgement or mastitis.

Baby has difficulty managing excessive milk flow (sputters at the breast).

IF YES, *Call lactation care provider today.*

SELF CARE INFORMATION

Frequency of feeding and amount of milk removal drives milk supply. Many women with oversupply may need to gradually decrease breast stimulation by nursing on only one side per feed, and decreasing milk expression, if practiced.

IMPORTANT CONDITIONS TO REPORT

Worsening of symptoms.

Continuation of symptoms.

Ongoing concerns.

Any symptoms of mastitis, including:

Plugged ducts.

Visible red areas on the breast(s).

Fever higher than 101°F (38.5°C).

Extreme breast discomfort.

Flu-like aching throughout body.

Notes

Because production of milk relies on many different body systems in both mother and baby, any milk supply problem requires consideration of maternal and infant factors.

Occasionally medical factors such as endocrine imbalance and the use of some medications may require evaluation.

See also Mastitis; Milk flow, too fast; Plugged ducts

Over-the-counter (OTC) drugs

DEFINITION   Over-the-counter (OTC) drugs are medications that are available to the public without a prescription. However, their convenient availability does not guarantee they are compatible with breastfeeding.

SELF CARE INFORMATION

Use up-to-date drug references to determine compatibility of OTC drugs with breastfeeding.

IMPORTANT CONDITIONS TO REPORT

Report any changes in the baby as soon as they are noticed.

Report any changes in milk supply as soon as they are noticed.

See also Medications; Medicinal herbs

Drug References

American Academy of Pediatrics Committee on Drugs. (2001). Transfer of drugs and other chemicals into human milk. *Pediatrics, 108,* 776–789.

Briggs, G.G., Freeman, R.K., & Yaffee, S.J. (Eds.). (2002). *Drugs in pregnancy and lactation* (6th ed.). Philadelphia: Lippincott, Williams, and Wilkins.

Hale, T.W. (2004). *Medications and mothers milk.* Amarillo, TX: Pharmasoft Publishing.

Lawrence, R.A., & Lawrence, R.M. (2005). *Breastfeeding: A guide for the medical profession* (6th ed.). St. Louis: Mosby.

Ovulation and lactation

DEFINITION   Research continues to help health care providers better understand the relationship between menstruation, fertility, and breastfeeding. The time after childbirth and before menstruation resumes in nursing mothers is called Lactational Amenorrhea. Ovulation may happen before the first menstrual period after childbirth.

SELF CARE INFORMATION

It is impossible to predict when any woman will ovulate or get her first period after her baby is born if she is breastfeeding.

Fertility may return before the first menstrual period after childbirth.

Home care products and natural methods can be used to detect ovulation.

Periods can be lighter, heavier, or more irregular than when not breastfeeding.

The return of menstruation does not mean the end of breastfeeding.

Some mothers report that their nursing babies are less interested in breastfeeding during their periods.

Some mothers experience nipple soreness during menstruation.

IMPORTANT CONDITIONS TO REPORT

Menstruation before four to six weeks postpartum if breastfeeding.

See also Amenorrhea; Fertility; Lactational Amenorrhea Method (LAM); Menstrual cycle

▶ **OWH**

See also Office on Women's Health (OWH)

▶ **Oxytocin**

DEFINITION   Oxytocin is one of the two major hormones of lactation (the other is prolactin). Oxytocin is released from the posterior lobe of the pituitary gland and stimulates the contraction of the smooth muscle of the uterus during labor. Oxytocin is responsible for the let-down (ejection) of milk.

Researchers have found that oxytocin is released in the first hours postpartum by the baby's hand massage of the breast, as well as by suckling.

Oxytocin is also released by the baby stretching the nipple sufficiently in the mouth. This is why a good latch is so important to milk transfer.

Oxytocin is also released through a conditioned response over time.

SELF CARE INFORMATION

The breastfed baby should gain well (0.5 oz to 1 oz per day on average). If the baby is gaining less than this, have a face-to-face breastfeeding evaluation.

At the breast, the baby should have sucking pattern that includes slow deep sucks. After the first few days, the baby's swallows can be heard, and the baby should have at least six wet diapers and two to five yellow stools each day.

IMPORTANT CONDITIONS TO REPORT
Meconium bowel movements after 5 days of life.
Fewer than three bowel movements daily in breastfed newborn after the first 2 days of life.
No urine in six hours.
Brick dust urine (uric acid crystals) after 2 days of life.
Dark colored urine.
Fewer than four urinations daily in the breastfed newborn after day 5 of life.
Noticeably sunken fontanelles (soft spot on top of head).
Decreased activity.
Baby below birthweight at 10 to 14 days of life.
Cessation of weight gain.

See also Hormones; Let-down reflex; Milk-ejection reflex

▶ # Pacifier

DEFINITION An artificial nipple, usually connected to a ring or solid backing. Pacifiers are sometimes called dummies.
   Pacifiers are used to calm babies, but their use may result in underfeeding.

SELF CARE INFORMATION
Pacifiers have been controversial in relation to breastfeeding. Research indicates that breastfed babies who use pacifiers spend less time nursing, are more likely to be given formula supplements, and are weaned from the breast at a younger age.[158]
Babies who are given pacifiers have a higher risk of ear infection (otitis media).[159]
Premature babies who cannot suck during feedings because they are being tube fed grow better if they can suck on a pacifier during the feeding.

Footnotes
[158]Howard, C.R., Howard, F.M., Lanphear, B., deBlieck, E.A., Eberly, S., & Lawrence, R.A. (1999). The effects of early pacifier use on breastfeeding duration. *Pediatrics, 103*(3), E33.

[159]Jackson, J.M., Mourino, A.P. (1999). Pacifier use and otitis media in infants twelve months of age or younger. *Pediatric Dentistry, 21*(4), 255–260.

▶ ## Paget's disease

DEFINITION   Paget's disease is a form of breast cancer affecting the nipple and the areola.

▶ ## Painful breastfeeding

DEFINITION   Uncomfortable sensations in the breast. Pain is not an expected part of breastfeeding and indicates the need for a feeding evaluation.

There can be many reasons for pain in the breast including breast infection or inflammation, clogs, or cysts. Poor latch-on or positioning can also cause pain.

Ask about

Onset.
Location of pain.
Whether unilateral or bilateral.

ASSESSMENT

PROMPT MEDICAL CARE NEEDED?
  Are any of the following present?
        Visible red areas on the breast(s).
        Fever higher than 101°F (38.5°C).
        Extreme breast discomfort.
        Flu-like aching throughout body.
        Continuing fever after treatment.
        Reaction to antibiotic prescribed.

IF YES,	*Seek emergency care if red streaks are found on both breasts and other symptoms are also present.* *Seek medical care within 2 to 4 hours with other symptoms in the absence of red areas on both breasts.*

PROMPT LACTATION CARE NEEDED?

Are any of the following present?

Persistent pain during nursing.

Persistent pain between feedings.

Constant pain.

Pain combined with color change of nipple(s).

Pain with visible fissure or bleeding of the nipple.

IF YES, *Call lactation care provider now.*

ROUTINE CARE NEEDED?

Are any of the following present?

Brief pain at beginning of feeding.

Mild recurrent pain.

IF YES, *Call lactation care provider today.*

SELF CARE INFORMATION

Practice skin-to-skin contact frequently.

Feed baby at first sign of hunger cues (signs that say "feed me" include hand-to-face or hand-to-mouth movements, lip smacking, seeking with lips, rooting, and head bobbing).

Feed baby at least 10–12 times per 24 hours.

Listen for signs of baby swallowing.

Allow baby to end feedings.

Expect at least 3–4 infant stools per 24 hours after the first 4 days of life.

Good positioning and attachment are crucial to reduce nipple pain.

If feedings are missed, hand express or pump milk to maintain supply.

Notes

Breastfeeding should not be painful. Advise mothers to seek medical or lactation care for breast pain.

See also Latch-on; Mastitis; Plugged breasts; Sore nipples

▶ Paladai

DEFINITION   A paladai is a South Indian feeding device shaped like a miniature gravy boat. The infant sips from the paladai when he or she is separated from the mother and is unable to breastfeed. Research comparing behavior of babies feeding from cups, bottles, and paladai shows that babies feed better and sleep longer between feedings when they are fed from the paladai.[160]

See also Cup-feeding; Feeding methods, alternate; Supplemental feeding

Footnotes
[160]Malhotra, N., Vishwambaran, L., Sundaram, K.R., Narayanan, I. (1999). A controlled trial of alternative methods of oral feeding in neonates. *Early Human Development, 54,* 29–38.

▶ Palatal obturator

DEFINITION   A palatal obturator is a device that is fitted individually for the baby with a cleft palate. The obturator blocks the cleft opening and allows for easier suckling. Modern obturators are made from the same material as athletic mouth guards and take only a few minutes to fit. As the baby grows, new obturators must be made. After the palatal repair, the obturator will no longer be needed.

SELF CARE INFORMATION

For babies with cleft palates, nipple shields have been used to improve breastfeeding before the obturator is fitted.

Advise the mother to follow cleaning instructions for the obturator that has been provided to her, and return to her child's pediatric dentist for scheduled re-fittings.

See also Cleft lip and palate

▶ Palate, abnormal

DEFINITION   The palate is the roof of the mouth. Both the hard and soft palate play an important role in suckling. One in 700 babies is born with a cleft of the lip or palate.

Intact palates may have a high arch, making placement of the nipple and effective suckling difficult.

Notes

Babies with abnormal palates can breastfeed or be fed expressed breastmilk. Pediatric occupational speech therapists or speech/language pathologists should be considered.

See also Cleft lip and palate; Haberman feeder; Palatal obturator

▶ Papilloma, intraductal

DEFINITION An intraductal papilloma is a small, benign (noncancerous) tumor that grows within a single milk duct.

Ask about

Age of baby.
Onset of nipple discharge.
Description of nipple discharge.

ASSESSMENT

PROMPT CARE NEEDED?
Are any of the following present?
Appearance of rust colored milk.
Bloody discharge from the nipple.
Any other unusual nipple discharge without nipple pain or abrasion from suboptimal latch.

IF YES, *Call obstetric care provider today.*

SELF CARE INFORMATION
Seek prompt medical evaluation of any unusual discharge from the nipple during breastfeeding and at any other time.

See also Bleeding, breast; Blood in milk; Breast cancer

▶ **Parlodel®**

DEFINITION   Parlodel®, also called bromocriptine, is a medication once used to dry up the milk of women who did not wish to breastfeed. Several deaths were attributed to bromocriptine use. This drug is no longer approved for this use.

> **Notes**
>
> The American Academy of Pediatrics lists bromocriptine in Table 5 (drugs associated with significant side effects and should be given with caution).[161] Hale lists bromocriptine as a category L5 (contraindicated) drug.[162]

See also Medications; Weaning

Footnotes

[161]American Academy of Pediatrics Committee on Drugs. (2001). Transfer of drugs and other chemicals into human milk. *Pediatrics, 108*, 779.

[162]Hale, T.W. (2004). *Medications and mothers milk* (pp. 98–99). Amarillo, TX: Pharmasoft Publishing.

▶ **Pasteurization**

DEFINITION   The process of pasteurization was named after Louis Pasteur who discovered that organisms that could spoil wine were inactivated by heating to temperatures below the boiling point.

This process was later applied to milk. Pasteurization of human milk has been studied at a variety of temperatures and times.

Some of the components of human milk are lost with heat treatment along with the target microorganisms, but the composition of human milk remains essentially the same.

The Food and Drug Administration and the Centers for Disease Control and Prevention do not recommend the use of donor milk without heat treatment. Milk from milk banks has been pasteurized.

See also Donor milk; Milk banks

▶ Pathogen

DEFINITION   An invading microorganism or toxin.

▶ PCOS

See also Polycystic Ovarian Syndrome (PCOS)

▶ Pedicle technique for breast reduction

DEFINITION   With the pedicle technique for breast reduction surgery, the nipple and areola remain attached while excess breast tissue is removed.

Breastfeeding women who have had breast reduction surgery will need careful evaluation and close monitoring.

See also Breast reduction; Breast surgery

▶ Peer counseling

DEFINITION   Delivery of breastfeeding support via trained peers.

See also La Leche League; Special Supplemental Food Program for Women, Infants, and Children (WIC)

▶ Pesticides and pollutants in breastmilk

DEFINITION   Breastmilk is one of the easiest and least painful body tissues to sample. For this reason, it is used to monitor population exposure to chemicals.

> **Notes**
>
> Women who know they had high level exposure to specific chemicals or pollutants should consult with their physician regarding analysis of the contaminant content of their milk.
>
>   Many researchers have looked for negative effects of toxin exposure via breastmilk and have found only benefits for breastfed babies, as compared with formula fed babies.
>
>   Adult body fat has approximately 30 times the concentration of environmental contaminants compared to the concentration of contaminants in human milk.[163]

See also Chemical contaminants in breastmilk; DDT in breastmilk

Footnotes
   [163]Lawrence, R.A., & Lawrence, R.M. (2005). *Breastfeeding: A guide for the medical profession* (6th ed.). St. Louis: Mosby, p. 415.

▶ Phenylketonuria (PKU) and breastfeeding

DEFINITION   Phenylketonuria (PKU) is the congenital absence or deficiency of the enzyme that is necessary to process the essential amino acid phenylalanine. It is a genetic inborn error of metabolism that is detectable during the first days of life through newborn screening. The baby will need to be fed a phenylalanine-free formula but may continue to be breastfed with careful monitoring.

PROMPT CARE NEEDED?

Are any of the following present?

Questions about management of breastfeeding after diagnosis of PKU.

IF YES, *Call lactation care provider today.*

SELF CARE INFORMATION

The physician will prescribe a phenylalanine-free formula and determine how often the baby's blood levels will be tested for phenylalanine.

Even babies with PKU require some phenylalanine, which is found in formula and breastmilk.

Human milk is lower in phenylalanine than standard formulas.

Research indicates that children who have received their mother's milk in addition to the special phenylalanine-free formula have more than a 10-point IQ advantage compared to children who had received the special formula alone.[164]

Footnotes

[164]Riva, E., Agostoni, C., Biasucci, G., Trojan, S., Luotti, D., Fiori, L., et al. (1996). Early breastfeeding is linked to higher intelligence quotient scores in dietary treated phenylketonuric children. *Acta Paediatrica, 85,* 56.

▶ Phototherapy

DEFINITION Phototherapy is the process of using light to treat certain medical conditions. In infants, phototherapy is commonly used to treat jaundice (hyperbilirubinemia).

The baby is exposed to a fluorescent light that is absorbed by the skin. During this process, the bilirubin is changed and is more easily moved out of the baby's body.

As much of the baby's skin as possible is exposed to the light.

The baby's eyes are covered to protect them.

There is no need to stop breastfeeding, although the baby may be sleepy and need coaxing as well as shorter, more frequent feedings.

The baby's bilirubin will be monitored and when it is low enough, the lights will no longer be required.

SELF CARE INFORMATION

If the baby is too sleepy to nurse effectively, the mother should express her milk frequently to encourage her supply.

See also Bilirubin; Hyperbilirubinemia; Jaundice

▶ Pierre Robin sequence

DEFINITION   Pierre Robin sequence is also called Pierre Robin complex or syndrome. Many children with this syndrome have difficulty with feeding and/or breathing. It is a condition present at birth that is characterized by the co-existence of two or more of the following conditions:

A very small jaw with a receding chin.

A tongue that appears large (due to the size of the jaw) and is placed unusually far back in the mouth.

High arched palate.

Cleft soft palate.

Choking on tongue.

Presence of teeth at birth.

Ask about

Diagnosis of Pierre Robin sequence in baby.

ASSESSMENT

PROMPT CARE NEEDED?

Diagnosis of Pierre Robin sequence in a breastfed baby.

IF YES, *Call lactation care provider today.*

SELF CARE INFORMATION

Begin expressing milk as soon as possible after birth. Breastmilk may be fed to the baby even before breastfeeding can begin.

Babies with Pierre Robin sequence often have swallowing problems. At-breast feeding devices such as the Lactaid, Supplemental Nursing System (SNS), and Supply Line can be helpful.

See also At-breast supplementation; Breast pump; Cleft lip and palate; Haberman feeder; Palate, abnormal

▶ PKU

DEFINITION   Phenylketonuria (PKU) is the congenital absence or deficiency of the enzyme that is necessary to process the essential amino acid phenylalanine. It is a genetic inborn error of metabolism that is detectable during the first days of life through newborn screening. The baby will need to be fed a phenylalanine-free formula but may continue to be breastfed with careful monitoring.

ASSESSMENT

PROMPT CARE NEEDED?

Are any of the following present?

Questions about management of breastfeeding after diagnosis of PKU.

IF YES,   *Call lactation care provider today.*

SELF CARE INFORMATION

The physician will prescribe a phenylalanine-free formula and determine how often the baby's blood levels will be tested for phenylalanine.

Even babies with PKU require some phenylalanine, which is found in formula and breastmilk.

Human milk is lower in phenylalanine than standard formulas.

Research indicates that children who have received their mother's milk in addition to the special phenylalanine-free formula have more than a 10-point IQ advantage compared to children who had received the special formula alone.[165]

Footnotes

[165]Riva, E., Agostoni, C., Biasucci, G., Trojan, S., Luotti, D., Fiori, L., et al. (1996). Early breastfeeding is linked to higher intelligence quotient scores in dietary treated phenylketonuric children. *Acta Paediatrica, 85,* 56.

▶ Placental fragments, retained

DEFINITION   Small pieces of placenta (fragments) can be retained in the uterus after the placenta is delivered. The fragment continues to be supported, but may subsequently break away. When this happens, the area of the uterus continues to bleed. The mother may hemorrhage and lose a considerable amount of blood.

A sign of retained placental fragments is the continued flow of red blood after the early days postpartum.

Retained placental fragments are associated with failure to produce sufficient milk due to hormonal influence of progesterone, a hormone of pregnancy that is produced by the placenta.

Ask about

Age of baby.
Current vaginal bleeding.
Breastfeeding difficulties.

ASSESSMENT

EMERGENT CARE NEEDED?
  Are any of the following present?
        Soaking a sanitary napkin with bright red blood at a rate of one napkin or
          more per hour.
        Clots in the bloody discharge.
        Foul odor to the discharge (even if occasional).
        Dizziness.
        Fever.
        Abdominal pain.

  IF YES,   *Call obstetric care provider now or seek emergency care now.*

PROMPT MEDICAL CARE NEEDED?

Are any of the following present?

Soaking a sanitary napkin with bright red blood at a rate of one napkin every two to three hours.

Abdominal tenderness.

Low-grade fever.

Lightheadedness.

IF YES,   *Call obstetric care provider within 2 to 4 hours.*

PROMPT LACTATION CARE NEEDED?

Are any of the following present?

Problems with milk supply in a woman diagnosed with retained placental fragments.

IF YES,   *Call lactation care provider today.*

ROUTINE CARE NEEDED?

Are any of the following present?

Soaking a sanitary napkin with bright red blood at a rate of one napkin every three or more hours.

Abdominal tenderness.

IF YES,   *Call obstetric care provider today.*

SELF CARE INFORMATION

Rapid soaking of a sanitary napkin with bright red blood after the early days postpartum may be associated with retained placental fragments and can be the first sign of hemorrhage.

Retained placental fragments have been associated with the failure to establish an adequate milk supply.

IMPORTANT CONDITIONS TO REPORT

Increase in bright red blood flow.

Bright red blood after two weeks postpartum.

See also Bleeding, postpartum vaginal; Lochia; Retained placental fragments; Slow weight gain, baby

▶ Plugged ducts

DEFINITION　The milk ducts of the breast can become plugged. The mother may experience tenderness and feel a lump at the site of the plug.

Ask about

Age of baby.
Location of the lump.
Tenderness around the lump.
When lump was first noted.

ASSESSMENT

PROMPT CARE NEEDED?

Are any of the following present?

Temperature higher than 101° F (38.5° C).
Reddened area on the breast.
Identified lump or lumps on the breast that persist for more than 24–48 hours.

IF YES, *Call obstetric care provider now and call lactation care provider now.*

ROUTINE CARE NEEDED?

Are any of the following present?

Identified lump or lumps on the breast which persist for more than 24–48 hours with no other symptoms.

IF YES, *Call obstetric care provider and call lactation care provider today.*

SELF CARE INFORMATION

Plugged ducts in the breast should move and disappear within 24–48 hours. If not, consult a physician for further evaluation.

Some mothers find manual massage of the area helps the plug to dislodge and move out of the breast. Others prefer warmth, such as a warm, wet towel.

Nursing the baby frequently on the affected breast will help to drain it.

Changing the baby's position can help to move the plug.

Try to understand why the plug happened. Could it be caused by an underwire bra or car seat belt applying pressure on the breast? Then, avoid the cause so that plugs do not reoccur.

IMPORTANT CONDITIONS TO REPORT
Temperature higher than 101° F (38.5° C).
Reddened area on the breast.

> **Notes**
>
> New mothers are not protected from breast cancer. Prompt evaluation is warranted if a lump does not move in 24–48 hours.

See also **Breast infection; Breast inflammation; Breast lumps; Breast pain; Mastitis**

▶ Polycystic Ovarian Syndrome (PCOS)

DEFINITION   Polycystic Ovarian Syndrome (PCOS) is caused by hormonal imbalances. Cysts form on the ovaries' surface due to high levels of androgen, and ovulation does not occur. The menstrual cycle may not occur, the uterine lining is not released, and abnormal uterine growths may form.

PCOS is also associated with glucose intolerance and insulin resistance.

Symptoms of PCOS include irregular menstrual periods, elevated male hormone levels in the blood (which can cause excessive facial and body hair), obesity, acne, cystic ovaries, or enlarged ovaries.

SELF CARE INFORMATION
Some mothers with PCOS struggle to achieve and maintain an adequate milk supply for their babies.[166]

IMPORTANT CONDITIONS TO REPORT
Indequate urination or stooling.
Poor weight gain.

See also Hormones; Obesity and breastfeeding; Slow weight gain, baby; Thyroid disease

Footnotes

[166]Marasco, L., Marmet, C., & Shell, E. (2000). Polycystic ovary syndrome: A connection to insufficient milk supply? *Journal of Human Lactation, 16*(2), 143–148.

▶ # Poor weight gain in the breastfed baby

DEFINITION   Breastfed newborns should gain a minimum of 0.5 oz to 1 oz a day on average. New studies indicate that breastfed babies gain even faster than was previously believed, most likely due to the fact that in the past, breastfeeding was done on a schedule (and not as frequently as we now know is ideal).

Ask about

Age of baby.
Weight gain pattern.

ASSESSMENT

PROMPT CARE NEEDED?
Are any of the following present?
Meconium bowel movements after 5 days of life.
Fewer than three bowel movements daily in breastfed newborn after the first 2 days of life.
No urine in six hours.
Brick dust urine (uric acid crystals) after 2 days of life.
Dark colored urine.
Fewer than four urinations daily in the breastfed newborn after day 5 of life.
Noticeably sunken fontanelles (soft spot on top of head).
Decreased activity.
Baby below birthweight at 10 to 14 days of life.
Cessation of weight gain.
Sleeping at the breast.

IF YES,   *Seek pediatric care now.*

IMPORTANT CONDITIONS TO REPORT

Decrease in number of urinations or stools.

Increased sleepiness, or many hours spent sleeping.

Baby is harder to rouse.

See also Hypotonia; Jaundice

▶ Positioning

DEFINITION   Properly positioning the baby at the breast should allow for the nipple to stretch, the milk to flow, and the mother and the baby to feed in comfort. The mother should feel gentle tugging at the most. She should certainly not feel pain. Pain is a reason to seek help.

SELF CARE INFORMATION

Proper positioning allows the baby to transfer milk and breathe at the breast without pain for the mother.

If the mother feels pain, the baby has trouble coordinating suck-swallow-breathe, or there is not enough milk transfer, the mother should have an evaluation of breastfeeding by a skilled observer.

IMPORTANT CONDITIONS TO REPORT

Breast or nipple pain.

Poor weight gain.

Baby struggling to breathe while nursing (this may not be due to positioning, but may indicate an anatomical issue in the baby).

See also Asymmetric latch; Attachment; Clutch hold; Cradle hold; Sore nipples; Weight gain, baby–high; Weight gain, baby–low

▶ Postmature baby

DEFINITION   A postmature baby is one who has stayed in utero beyond the capacity of its placenta. Instead of continuing to grow in utero, the baby has begun to lose weight before it is born. These babies often have trouble maintaining their blood sugar and temperature at first. Postmature babies also may need extra encouragement to nurse, so they should nurse as soon as possible after birth and then very frequently.

▶ Postpartum depression

DEFINITION   Symptoms of depression are not unusual for women during the early days postpartum. More than 50% of women experience some form of mood disorder during this period.

Ask about

Onset.
Age of baby.
Past history of depression.

ASSESSMENT

EMERGENT CARE NEEDED?
Are any of the following present?
Suicidal thoughts.
Thoughts of harming baby.

IF YES,   *Seek emergency care now.*

SELF CARE INFORMATION

Mood swings are normal in the postpartum period, but may become more severe. Seek support.

Practice skin-to-skin contact frequently.

Feed baby at first sign of hunger cues (signs that say "feed me" include hand-to-face or hand-to-mouth movements, lip smacking, seeking with lips, rooting, and head bobbing).

Feed baby at least 10–12 times per 24 hours.

Listen for signs of baby swallowing.

Allow baby to end feedings.

Expect at least 3–4 infant stools per 24 hours after the first 4 days of life.

Good positioning and attachment are crucial to reduce nipple pain.

If feedings are missed, hand express or pump milk to maintain supply.

IMPORTANT CONDITIONS TO REPORT

Exacerbation of symptoms.

Nonresolution of symptoms.

Past history of depression, mood disorders, premenstrual syndrome, or thyroid disorders.

Notes

Symptoms of depression can progress to other postpartum mood disorders. It is important to encourage mothers to report any worsening of symptoms.

Women who experienced depression during pregnancy and those with a prior history of depression, mood disorders, or premenstrual syndrome are at greater risk for postpartum depression.

Hypothyroidism, anemia, and other physical disorders share many symptoms with postpartum depression.

> Many breastfeeding women resist reporting depression as they fear that medication may be incompatible with breastfeeding. There are many antidepressant medications that are considered safe for use in breastfeeding women.

See also Anemia; Baby blues; Drugs and breastfeeding; Hypothyroidism; Postpartum mood disorders

▶ Postpartum mood disorders

DEFINITION A spectrum of emotional difficulties occurring in the period after birth, including anxiety, baby blues, depression, obsessive-compulsive behavior, panic, post-traumatic stress, and psychosis.

Notes

It is important to encourage mothers to report any unusual or aggravated emotional distress.

Women who experienced depression during pregnancy and those with a prior history of depression, mood disorders, or premenstrual syndrome are at greater risk for postpartum mood disorders.

Many breastfeeding women resist reporting emotional distress as they fear that medication may be incompatible with breastfeeding. There are many antidepressant medications that are considered safe for use in breastfeeding women.

See also Baby blues; Drugs and breastfeeding; Postpartum depression

▶ Pregnancy, breastfeeding during

DEFINITION If a mother becomes pregnant while she is breastfeeding a baby from a prior pregnancy, she may experience extremely sore nipples and a decrease in her milk supply. It is possible to continue breastfeeding through the pregnancy and then continue nursing the two babies together. This is called tandem nursing.

Deciding to nurse during pregnancy and to practice tandem nursing is an individual choice that the mother makes for herself and her family.

Although there are no reported problems with nursing during pregnancy and no reports of nursing causing premature labor, mothers with a prior history of premature birth or threatened premature labor should consider the risk as they make their decision.

Mothers should seek lactation help for sore nipples and other discomforts of pregnancy.

See also Tandem nursing

▶ Prelacteal feeds

DEFINITION   Feedings that are given to babies before they go to the breast for the first time are called prelacteal feeds.

▶ Premature infant

DEFINITION   Any infant born before 37 weeks of gestation. Due to increased use of fertility treatment, multiple pregnancies (e.g., twins) account for an increased percentage of all premature births. The problems of prematurity are related to the immaturity of the organ systems.

The infant requires specialized care in a nursery until his or her organ systems have developed enough to sustain life without specialized support, usually around the original due date. Depending on the extent of prematurity, this may take weeks or months.

SELF CARE INFORMATION
Mothers of premature infants should begin expressing milk as soon as possible and do so regularly in order to increase the supply for the growing baby.

The hospital nursery will have instructions available for the collection and storage of milk.

For about the first 30 days after she gives birth, the mother of the premature baby will produce milk that is higher in some of the components the baby needs.

Premature babies can learn to breastfeed. Mothers should seek skilled lactation help.

See also Academy of Breastfeeding Medicine (ABM); NICU, milk storage and handling in; Preterm milk

▶ Preterm milk

DEFINITION For about the first 30 days after she gives birth, the mother of the premature baby will produce milk that is higher in some of the components the baby needs. This breastmilk is called preterm milk.

Notes

The volume and calorie amounts of preterm milk are similar to that of the milk of mothers who have delivered at term. Lactose and fat amounts are comparable.

The components of preterm mothers' milk that are higher than term mothers' milk include protein and nonprotein nitrogen, long-, short- and medium-chain fatty acids, sodium, chloride, and iron.

Preterm babies may require nutrition beyond their mother's milk in order to achieve adequate growth.

See also Bioactive components in breastmilk; Human milk fortification; Lactoengineering; Premature infant

▶ Proctocolitis

DEFINITION Inflammation of the colon and rectum, typically caused by allergy or disease process.

Notes

Proctocolitis often results in blood in the stool. This finding requires immediate medical evaluation.

This disorder occasionally occurs in breastfed infants.

If the infant is reacting to a protein in its mother's diet, the problem may be improved by an avoidance diet. In this case, mother may benefit from consultation with a dietitian or nutritionist.

See also Allergy in the breastfed infant; Blood in stool

▶ Progestin-only contraceptives

DEFINITION   Oral contraceptives have been studied in relation to breastfeeding. The recommendation is that hormonal contraceptives used by nursing mothers should contain only progestin. Intrauterine devices (IUDs) can be injected with progestin. Depo-Provera® is an injectable progestin-only contraceptive.

Ask about

Age of baby.
Duration of contraceptive use.

ASSESSMENT

PROMPT CARE NEEDED?
Are any of the following present?
Inadequate weight gain in baby.
Perception of decreased milk supply.

IF YES,   *Call lactation care provider today.*

ROUTINE CARE NEEDED?
Are any of the following present?
More information desired about contraception and breastfeeding.
More information desired about breastfeeding and family planning or birth control.

IF YES,   *Consult up-to-date drug references, call lactation care provider, and call obstetric care provider.*

SELF CARE INFORMATION
Consider the **Lactational Amenorrhea Method (LAM)**, other natural family planning methods, and barrier methods of contraception if hormonal contraceptives are not acceptable or if milk supply drops.

Decreased milk supply.
Less stooling or urination in the baby.

See also Birth control; Depo-Provera® contraceptive (Medroxyprogesterone); Fertility; Hormonal contraceptive methods; Lactational Amenorrhea Method (LAM); Natural family planning

▶ Projectile vomiting

DEFINITION   Projectile vomiting in the infant can be differentiated from vomiting or spitting up by the distance it travels. Projectile vomit clears the chin of the infant. It may travel several feet. Occasional projectile vomiting in an otherwise well infant is not uncommon, although persistent projectile vomiting can indicate the presence of an underlying problem, such as pyloric stenosis, that requires treatment.

SELF CARE INFORMATION
Occasional projectile vomiting in an otherwise well infant is not uncommon.
Projectile vomiting even in a baby with no other symptoms can indicate the presence of an underlying problem, such as pyloric stenosis, that requires treatment if persistent.

IMPORTANT CONDITIONS TO REPORT
Persistent projectile vomiting.
Signs that the baby is unwell in combination with projectile vomiting.
Decrease in stools and urinations.
Poor feeding behavior.
Weight loss or failure to gain weight adequately.

See also Pyloric stenosis and breastfeeding; Spitting up; Vomiting

▶ Prolactin

DEFINITION   Prolactin is the hormone that stimulates the synthesis and secretion of milk. It works to prepare the milk cells to make milk during pregnancy. Male and female humans both have prolactin.

See also Hormones; Milk production

▶ Protuberance

DEFINITION   The degree to which something (in the context of breastfeeding, the nipple or tongue) sticks or stands out.

▶ Pump

DEFINITION   A device designed to remove milk from the lactating breast.

SELF CARE INFORMATION

A breast pump cannot tell you how much milk you are making. If you have concerns about milk supply, please call or see a lactation care provider.

Problems with pumps should be reported to the manufacturer and to the Food and Drug Administration (FDA). The FDA's Manufacturer and User Facility Device Experience Database (MAUDE) database contains prior complaints filed about pumps. Visit www.fda.gov/cdrh/maude.html for more information.

Notes

A plethora of breast pumps are available. Styles, intended uses, and costs vary widely. There is no one pump that works best for all mothers.

It is never appropriate to recommend mixing one manufacturer's pump kits with another manufacturer's pump.

Pumps can be rented or purchased from representatives of various companies.

Most pumps (with the exception of rental grade models) are not intended for sharing between women. It is possible for the interior part of these pump motors to be contaminated with microorganisms.

Women will sometimes request a breast pump when they have doubts about their milk supply. Pumps should not be used to quantify or provide reassurance about a woman's milk supply.

See also **Automatic electric breast pumps; Battery operated breast pump; Hand expression of breastmilk; Manual pump**

▶ Pyloric stenosis and breastfeeding

DEFINITION   Pyloric stenosis happens when the pyloric sphincter (located at the outlet of the stomach) becomes thickened. The food in the stomach is prevented from moving into the small intestine as it should. Vigorous contractions of the stomach begin in an effort to force the stomach contents through the obstruction. As the sphincter tightens, projectile vomiting occurs, usually within 30–60 minutes after a feeding.

SELF CARE INFORMATION

Babies can resume nursing after surgery for pyloric stenosis.

During the surgery, the mother should express her milk to keep her breasts comfortable.

Notes

Pyloric stenosis happens more frequently in boy babies. Only about 1% of babies are diagnosed with pyloric stenosis. The babies are otherwise healthy. Pyloric stenosis is diagnosed less frequently among exclusively breastfed babies. Pyloric stenosis typically presents at 3–6 weeks of age, but may be seen as early as 1 week and as late as 5 months.

Pyloric stenosis is a serious condition that can result in severe dehydration, weakness, and weight loss. Surgery is usually recommended.

See also **Projectile vomiting**

Quadruplets and quintuplets

DEFINITION   Quadruplets ("quads") are four babies and quintuplets ("quints") are five babies born from the same pregnancy.

Mothers can produce enough milk to support quints and quads, usually with a combination of expressing and nursing.

ASSESSMENT

ROUTINE CARE NEEDED?

Are any of the following present?

Need for strategies for managing nursing quadruplets or quintuplets.

Need for strategies for managing milk supply for quadruplets or quintuplets.

IF YES,   *Call lactation care provider today.*

SELF CARE INFORMATION

Pumping should start as soon as possible after the babies are born.

Many mothers of multiples have found it helpful to keep a journal of "who nursed when," number of wet and dirty diapers, and weight gain for each baby, to ensure that none of the babies is being overlooked.

Mothers of **higher order multiples (HOM)** may have been on bed rest during their pregnancies and can become easily fatigued. Advise them to ask for help.

Suggest easy ways for mothers to snack and drink while caring for multiple babies.

Help mothers to connect to any parent support groups for families with multiples.

See also **Higher order multiples (HOM); Multiple infants (twins, triplets, and higher order multiples)**

Radioactive agents

DEFINITION   Refers to chemicals such as iodine, gallium, and technetium that are used in diagnostic tests and therapeutically in treatment of some conditions (e.g., thyroid ablation). Use of these agents in the lactating woman may require a temporary cessation of breastfeeding until the radioactive material is removed from her milk.

Age of baby.

Specific name of radioactive agent being used.

ASSESSMENT

ROUTINE CARE NEEDED?

Are any of the following present?

Use of a radioactive chemical in a lactating woman.

IF YES, *Consult up-to-date drug references and refer mother back to health care provider for consultation.*

SELF CARE INFORMATION

Express or pump and discard milk during the time of cessation of feeding to maintain breast comfort.

Ask your radiologist for recommendations about how close you can safely be to the baby during the period of cessation of feeding.

Notes

There is a broad range of radioactive agents in use for these purposes. Each agent requires a different length of cessation of breastfeeding. It is essential to know the specific agents(s) involved.

X-rays do not have this same effect and may be used safely in the breastfeeding woman. Computed tomography, magnetic resonance, and ultrasound imaging are also compatible with breastfeeding.

▶ Rancid odor of frozen breastmilk

DEFINITION   Human milk contains digestive properties. When the baby nurses, these components of milk go right into the baby with the milk. It is one of the reasons breastmilk is so easy for babies to digest. When milk is collected and stored, these active components still work.

For some women, the milk takes on a soapy or rancid odor that they notice when the milk is defrosted. The milk is not spoiled. Rather, the odor is the result of the continued activity of digestive enzymes in the milk.

Women who want to stop this digestive activity can gently heat the milk to scalding after collecting it and before freezing. This process usually stops the digestive components.

See also Collection and storage of breastmilk

▶ Rapid weight gain

DEFINITION Well fed breastfed babies gain weight more rapidly in the early months compared to standard growth charts and to formula fed babies. However, some breastfed babies can be uncomfortable when getting too much milk, and rapid weight gain may be a sign of oversupply.

Ask about

Age of baby.
Weight gain pattern of baby.

ASSESSMENT

ROUTINE CARE NEEDED?

Are any of the following present?

About mother

Persistent sore nipples.

Nipples often compressed at the end of nursing.

About baby

Weight gain of more than 1 lb per week consistently.

Frequent, explosive, large stools.

Gassy, often unhappy baby.

IF YES, *Call lactation care provider today.*

SELF CARE INFORMATION

Oversupply can cause discomfort for mother and baby.

Careful management of the mother's milk supply can increase the baby's comfort.

IMPORTANT CONDITIONS TO REPORT

Symptoms of mastitis, including:

Plugged ducts.

Visible red areas on the breast(s).

Fever higher than 101°F (38.5°C).

Extreme breast discomfort.

Flu-like aching throughout body.

See also Milk flow, too fast

▶ Raynaud's phenomenon/syndrome

DEFINITION   Nipple pain may occur because of Raynaud's phenomenon/syndrome.[167] This is a condition in which blood flow to the extremities is temporarily reduced. It has also been called nipple vasospasm. The affected extremity becomes cold and numb and turns white. As the blood flow returns, it may quickly turn blue and then reddish pink. This is the tri-color sign of Raynaud's. There is also a bi-color sign (white and pink). As the color returns, the pain increases. The pain can be brief, lasting for just a few minutes, or it can be prolonged, lasting up to an hour.

The reaction occurs in response to cold, wetness, stress, and certain medications.

Usually the fingers and toes are affected, but the nipples are also extremities and can therefore be affected.

Ask about

Age of baby.

History of nipple pain.

ROUTINE CARE NEEDED?

Are any of the following present?

Persistent nipple pain.

Breast pain in reaction to cold, wet, and nursing.

Tri-color sign (white, blue, pink) or bi-color sign (white, pink) of the nipple when cold or wet.

IF YES, *Call obstetric care provider today and call lactation care provider.*

IMPORTANT CONDITIONS TO REPORT

If Nifedipine is prescribed, seek medical help in the case of adverse reactions described in the package insert.

SELF CARE INFORMATION

Nifedipine (Adalat, Procardia) is a prescription medication (calcium channel blocker) that has been used to treat Raynaud's phenomenon/syndrome in nursing mothers.

Mothers with Raynaud's syndrome are usually advised also to avoid caffeine and nicotine.

See also Nifedipine; Painful breastfeeding; Sore nipples

Footnotes

[167]Lawlor-Smith, L., & Lawlor-Smith, C. (1997). Vasospasm of the nipple—a manifestation of Raynaud's phenomenon: Case reports. *British Medical Journal, 314*(7081), 644–645.

▶ Reaction to foods in the mother's diet

DEFINITION   Rules about eating or not eating certain foods during lactation are not warranted, may be hard to follow, and may decrease the mother's enjoyment of breastfeeding.

Gassy foods do not make babies gassy. However, there may be individual cases where certain foods affect the baby.

Flavors from foods in the mother's diet do pass into amniotic fluid prenatally and into the milk after birth. This exposure to flavors of the mother's diet may help the child to accept family foods later in childhood.

Ask about

Age of baby.
Description and onset of symptom.

ASSESSMENT

ROUTINE CARE NEEDED?

Are any of the following present?

Colic after mother eats of certain foods.
Inconsolable crying after mother eats certain foods.
Other baby reactions that the mother attributes to foods she eats.

IF YES, *Call lactation care provider.*

SELF CARE INFORMATION

The mother's drinking of liquid cow's milk has been associated with colic symptoms in some babies. If this is the case, improvement may be seen after the mother eliminates cow's milk from her diet for at least a week.

If a mother thinks that her baby is reacting to a food in her diet, she should try eliminating it for a period of a week or longer. Keeping a record of foods eaten each day and baby's temperament may help to identify any potential problem foods.

Mothers should seek further information about diet and breastfeeding on an individual basis.

IMPORTANT CONDITIONS TO REPORT

Difficulty breathing.
Difficulty swallowing.
Rapid progression of symptoms.

See also Allergy in the breastfed infant; Cabbage; Colic, infantile; Maternal diet

▶ Readiness for solid foods

DEFINITION The American Academy of Pediatrics (AAP), The United States Breastfeeding Committee (USBC), The United Nations Children's Fund (UNICEF), and The World Health Organization (WHO) recommend exclusive breastfeeding for about the first six months of life.

Researchers have shown that flavors from the foods the mother eats in pregnancy and during lactation pass into the milk. When family foods taste familiar, baby is more accepting.

In addition to age, signs of readiness may include:

Increased interest in table foods.

Ability to sit up.

Ability to pick up objects and put them in the mouth.

Decreased tongue thrusting (automatically pushing foods out of the mouth with the tongue).

Ask about

Age of baby.

Reason for wanting to start solid foods.

ASSESSMENT

PROMPT CARE NEEDED?

Are any of the following present?

Breastfed baby under 5 months of age with one or more of the following:

Mother concerned about baby's weight gain.

Decreased stooling or urination.

IF YES, *Call pediatric care provider today and call lactation care provider today.*

ROUTINE CARE NEEDED?

Are any of the following present?

Breastfed baby around 6 months of age, with maternal questions about starting solids.

IF YES, *Call lactation care provider.*

SELF CARE INFORMATION

Babies are not equally interested in starting solid foods. If the baby is not interested, wait a few days and try again.

When babies start solid foods around 6 months, they do not usually have a prolonged time on the semi-liquid foods that were popular years ago when starting solids was recommended at younger ages.

Move the baby onto family foods as appropriate.

IMPORTANT CONDITIONS TO REPORT

Difficulty breathing.

Difficulty swallowing.

Rapid progression of symptoms.

See also Allergy in the breastfed infant; Mixed feeds; Solid foods for breastfed babies

▶ Reduction surgery, breast

DEFINITION A procedure that decreases the size of the breast by removing fat and glandular tissue. Reduction surgery is likely to affect a woman's ability to produce milk.

Ask about

Date of surgery.

Type of procedure.

ASSESSMENT

PROMPT CARE NEEDED?

Are any of the following present?

Meconium bowel movements after 5 days of life.

Fewer than three bowel movements daily in breastfed newborn after the first 2 days of life.

No urine in six hours.

Brick dust urine (uric acid crystals) after 2 days of life.

Dark colored urine.

Fewer than four urinations daily in the breastfed newborn after day 5 of life.

IF YES, *Seek pediatric care now.*

PROMPT CARE NEEDED?

Are any of the following present?

Concerns about milk supply.

Concerns about infant weight gain without symptoms above.

IF YES, *Call lactation care provider today.*

SELF CARE INFORMATION

Monitor baby's feeding, stooling, and urination patterns daily.

Practice skin-to-skin contact frequently.

Feed baby at first sign of hunger cues (signs that say "feed me" include hand-to-face or hand-to-mouth movements, lip smacking, seeking with lips, rooting, and head bobbing).

Feed baby at least 10–12 times per 24 hours.

Listen for signs of baby swallowing.

Allow baby to end feedings.

Expect at least 3–4 infant stools per 24 hours after the first 4 days of life.

Good positioning and attachment are crucial to reduce nipple pain.

If feedings are missed, hand express or pump milk to maintain supply.

IMPORTANT CONDITIONS TO REPORT

Inadequate feeding (less than 10 feedings daily in the newborn).

Inadequate stooling pattern (less than three stools daily in the newborn after day 4).

Ongoing concerns.

Notes

It is not possible to predict the degree of lactation success before giving birth. Women who are interested in breastfeeding should be encouraged to do so with ongoing, proactive monitoring of baby's growth.

Surgical techniques that include complete removal of the nipple are more likely to impact innervation of the nipple (and thus the production of appropriate hormones through neuroendocrine pathways). Post-surgical nipple sensation may indicate the extent to which innervation has been altered.

> Pedicle techniques which preserve nipple attachment may have a lesser impact on potential for milk production.

See also Breast surgery; Insufficient milk supply; Pedicle technique for breast reduction

▶ Reflux, gastroesophageal (GE)

DEFINITION   Gastroesophageal (GE) reflux in infants is not common in babies who are exclusively breastfed, except in those who have been previously tube fed.[168] With GE reflux, the stomach contents move up and out of the stomach and back into the esophagus.

Babies with GE reflux vomit after eating. The vomiting happens regularly and is not projectile.

Ask about

Age of baby.
History of vomiting.
History of weight gain or loss.
History of pneumonia or lung problems.
History of choking.

ASSESSMENT

EMERGENT CARE NEEDED?
> *Are any of the following present?*
>> Difficulty breathing.

IF YES,   *Seek emergency care now.*

PROMPT CARE NEEDED?
> *Are any of the following present?*
>> Choking.
>> Difficulty swallowing.
>> Rapid progression of symptoms.

Decrease in urination.

Decrease in stooling.

Signs of dehydration.

IF YES, *Seek pediatric care now.*

ROUTINE CARE NEEDED?

Are any of the following present?

Baby spits up regularly after nursing.

Weight gain is adequate.

Urination and stooling pattern is adequate.

IF YES, *Report to pediatric care provider and call lactation care provider.*

SELF CARE INFORMATION

Many breastfed babies spit up frequently without any underlying medical cause. A baby who spits up often should be evaluated by his or her health care provider.

IMPORTANT CONDITIONS TO REPORT

Difficulty breathing.

Choking.

Difficulty swallowing.

Rapid progression of symptoms.

Decrease in urination.

Decrease in stooling.

Signs of dehydration.

See also Gastroesophageal (GE) reflux; Milk flow, too fast

Footnotes

[168]Heacock, H.J., Jeffery, H.E., Baker, J.L., & Page, M. (1992). Influence of breast versus formula milk on physiological gastroesophageal reflux in healthy, newborn infants. *Journal of Pediatric Gastroenterology and Nutrition, 14,* 41–46.

▶ Refusal of infant to breastfeed

DEFINITION   Babies can refuse to breastfeed even from the first nursing, although this is rare. A nursing strike is a sudden refusal of the baby to nurse. This can happen with a baby of any age.

A young baby who is refusing to breastfeed is telling us that there is something wrong. Careful evaluation of the baby and the mother's breasts, and observation of breastfeeding is important.

Ask about

Age of baby.
Nursing history.
History of any recent mother–baby separation.

ASSESSMENT

PROMPT CARE NEEDED?

Are any of the following present?

Baby refuses to nurse.
Onset of inconsolable crying.
Baby refuses other age appropriate foods.
Change in stooling, urination, or sleep patterns.
Lethargy.

IF YES,   *Call pediatric care provider today and call lactation care provider today.*

ROUTINE CARE NEEDED?

Are any of the following present?

Baby refuses to nurse but otherwise seems normal.

IF YES,   *Call lactation care provider today and report to pediatric care provider if no change in 48 hours.*

SELF CARE INFORMATION

Mothers whose babies refuse to nurse should express milk for comfort and to maintain the milk supply.

Many babies who have gone on strike return to the breast once the problem has been resolved.

Do not starve the baby to the breast. Babies need to be fed.

Babies refuse to nurse when something is wrong in their lives. Some of the reasons
   reported for newborns refusing to nurse include:
   Birth injury.
   Low milk volume.
   Poor positioning technique.
   Baby has an undiagnosed medical problem.
   Mother has undiagnosed breast cancer.

Some of the reasons reported for older babies refusing to nurse include:
   Teething.
   Stuffy nose.
   Ear infection.
   Baby has bitten the mother who yelled; this frightened the baby.
   Reaction to being left unattended to "cry it out."
   Family stress.
   Recent separation of mother and baby, such as mother's return to work.

IMPORTANT CONDITIONS TO REPORT
   Change in stooling or urination patterns.
   Sleepiness, lethargy.
   Breathing difficulties.
   Vomiting.
   Inconsolable crying.

See also Breast refusal; Goldsmith's sign; Nursing strike; One-sided nursing

▶ Reglan® (metoclopramide)

DEFINITION   Reglan® (generic name metoclopramide) is generally used to increase
   the muscle tone of the lower esophagus sphincter and is used to treat reflux and
   nausea. Side effects include cardiac arrhythmias, extrapyramidal signs (tremors,
   rigidity, drooling, rolling eyes, and a mask-like expression), jitteriness, insomnia,
   sedation, and anxiety. Another side effect is the increase in prolactin release that
   may result in increased milk production. Increased milk production does not happen in all women.

SELF CARE INFORMATION

If prescribed, follow instructions carefully.

IMPORTANT CONDITIONS TO REPORT

Jitteriness.
Insomnia.
Sedation.
Anxiety.

See also Increasing milk supply; Medications; Premature infant

▶ Relactation

DEFINITION   Relactation is the bringing back of lactation. A woman who has given birth has been in the state of lactation even if she did not breastfeed. A woman can relactate weeks or months after giving birth.

Ask about

Lactation history.
Age of baby.
Duration of time since last breastfeeding (if there was any breastfeeding).
Reason for wanting to relactate (baby's tolerance of other foods).

ASSESSMENT

ROUTINE CARE NEEDED?

Are any of the following present?

Mother desires information about relactation.
Mother desires to relactate.

IF YES,   *Call lactation care provider today and report this plan to pediatric care provider.*

SELF CARE INFORMATION

The infant's willingness to nurse is an important consideration in whether breast-feeding can be possible.

If the reason the mother did not breastfeed or did not lactate after birth (severe breast reduction for example) is still present, relactation may be very difficult. Pumping or hand expression are excellent ways to collect milk and build up the milk supply in relactating mothers.

Notes

Mothers may be successful at bringing in a full supply of milk via pumping. Transitioning the baby to the breast may take longer.

See also Decrease in milk supply; Increasing milk supply; Milk production; Pump

► Retained placental fragments

DEFINITION Small pieces of placenta (fragments) can be retained in the uterus after the placenta is delivered. The fragment continues to be supported, but may subsequently break away. When this happens, the area of the uterus continues to bleed. The mother may hemorrhage and lose a considerable amount of blood.

A sign of retained placental fragments is the continued flow of red blood after the early days postpartum.

Retained placental fragments are associated with failure to produce sufficient milk due to the influence of the hormone progesterone, which is manufactured by the placenta.

Ask about

Age of baby.
Current vaginal bleeding.
Breastfeeding difficulties.

EMERGENT CARE NEEDED?

Are any of the following present?

Soaking a sanitary napkin with bright red blood at a rate of one napkin or more per hour.

Clots in the bloody discharge.

Foul odor to the discharge (even if occasional).

Dizziness.

Fever.

Abdominal pain.

IF YES, *Seek emergency care now or call obstetric care provider immediately.*

PROMPT CARE NEEDED?

Are any of the following present?

Soaking a sanitary napkin with bright red blood at a rate of one napkin every two to three hours.

Abdominal tenderness.

Low-grade fever.

Lightheadedness.

IF YES, *Seek obstetric care within 2 to 4 hours.*

ROUTINE CARE NEEDED?

Are any of the following present?

Soaking a sanitary napkin with bright red blood at a rate of one napkin every three or more hours.

Abdominal tenderness.

IF YES, *Seek obstetric care today.*

PROMPT LACTATION CARE NEEDED

Are any of the following present?

Problems with milk supply in a woman diagnosed with retained placental fragments.

IF YES, *Call lactation care provider today.*

SELF CARE INFORMATION

Rapid soaking of a sanitary napkin with bright red blood after the early days post-partum may be associated with retained placental fragments and can be the first sign of hemorrhage.

Retained placental fragments have been associated with the failure to establish an adequate milk supply.

IMPORTANT CONDITIONS TO REPORT

Increase in bright red blood flow.

Bright red blood after two weeks postpartum.

See also Bleeding, postpartum vaginal; Lochia

▶ Reverse cycle breastfeeding

DEFINITION   A nursing style where the working mother nurses when she is with the baby, giving the baby the majority of calories while they are together. Then, when she is away from the baby, the baby needs less expressed milk or other foods.

Ask about

Age of baby.

ASSESSMENT

ROUTINE CARE NEEDED?

Are any of the following present?

Mother is going to work and will be separated from her baby.

IF YES,   *Call lactation care provider.*

IMPORTANT CONDITIONS TO REPORT

Change in baby's weight gain pattern.

See also Co-sleeping; Feeding pattern of breastfed infants; Maternal employment; Night nursings

---

▶ Rooming-in

DEFINITION   Rooming-in is a hospital arrangement in which the baby stays in the mother's hospital room. The expectation of the UNICEF/WHO Baby-Friendly Hospital Initiative is that in Baby-Friendly hospitals, babies will room-in with their mothers most of 24 hours a day.

SELF CARE INFORMATION

Rooming-in offers the opportunity for mothers and babies to get to know each other, for observation of feeding cues, and for frequent nursing.

According to research studies, mothers who room-in with their babies get off to a better start at breastfeeding.

See also Baby-Friendly Hospital Initiative (BFHI); Ten Steps to Successful Breastfeeding

▶ Rusty-pipe syndrome (Rusty-pipe milk)

DEFINITION   Pumped milk with small bloody streaks, or small amounts of rust colored milk, may be called rusty-pipe milk. When examined, the milk is positive for the mother's blood. The condition is temporary (lasts only a few days) and babies accept the milk.

Ask about

Age of baby.
History of pumping.

ASSESSMENT

ROUTINE CARE NEEDED?
Are any of the following present?
Orange or blood streaked pumped milk that does not improve over the course of a week.

IF YES, *Call lactation care provider today and report to obstetric care provider (rusty-pipe milk could also be a sign of intraductal papilloma).*

IMPORTANT CONDITIONS TO REPORT

Recurrence.

Ongoing rusty color in milk.

See also Blood in milk; Papilloma, intraductal; Sore nipples

▶ Salty taste of breastmilk

DEFINITION   Human milk can taste salty if the mother has mastitis, if the milk supply is very low, or in some cases during weaning. The sodium in human milk is never as high as it is in formula.

Ask about

Age of baby.

Onset of salty taste.

Any symptoms in baby.

ASSESSMENT

EMERGENT CARE NEEDED?

Are any of the following present?

About baby

Seizures or convulsions.

Lethargy.

Inadequate urine or stool output.

Rapid progression of symptoms.

IF YES,   *Seek pediatric care now.*

PROMPT CARE NEEDED?

Are any of the following present?

About mother

Visible red areas on the breast(s).

Fever higher than 101° F (38.5° C).

Extreme breast discomfort.

Flu-like aching throughout body.

Continued fever after treatment.

Reaction to antibiotic prescribed.

IF YES, **Seek obstetric care within 2 to 4 hours.**

ROUTINE CARE NEEDED?

Are any of the following present?

Weaning.

IF YES, **Call lactation care provider.**

SELF CARE INFORMATION

Breast milk sodium can increase naturally during gradual weaning and the milk will taste salty.

See also Failure to thrive (FTT); Mastitis; Weaning

▶ **SCU**

See also Neonatal Intensive Care Unit (NICU); Special care unit (SCU)

▶ **Secretory IgA**

DEFINITION The "Ig" in IgA stands for immunoglobulin. All classes of immunoglobins (including IgG, IgD, IgM, and IgE) are found in human milk. They are found in higher amounts in colostrum.

Human babies are born without IgA, which coats all of the mucous membranes in adult humans forming a protective barrier to viruses and bacteria.

SELF CARE INFORMATION

Nursing in the first hours after birth transfers IgA from the mother to the baby. The IgA coats the baby's intestines, lung surfaces, and other mucous membranes. This helps to protect the baby from bacteria and viruses as soon as possible.

See also Bioactive components in breastmilk; Immunoglobulin

▶ Seizures and breastfeeding

DEFINITION   A sudden change in behavior caused by temporary changes in activity of the brain and nerves. Seizures may be characterized by jerking in the limbs, eyes rolling up, eyelids fluttering, incontinence, twitching, breathing difficulty, and many other symptoms. Seizure is a medical emergency in an infant. Seizure disorder in the breastfeeding mother calls for careful evaluation, including her medications.

Ask about

Age of baby.
Onset of seizure.
History of seizure in mother.

ASSESSMENT

EMERGENT CARE NEEDED?
Are any of the following present?

Symptoms of seizure in an infant, including:

Excessive drooling.

Turning blue.

Rolling back eyes.

Uncontrollable shaking in the arms and legs.

IF YES,   *Seek emergency care now.*

PROMPT CARE NEEDED?
Are any of the following present?

Questions about breastfeeding in a woman with history of epilepsy or seizure disorder.

Questions about compatibility of seizure control medications with breastfeeding.

IF YES,   *Call lactation care provider today and consult up-to-date drug references.*

See also Epilepsy and breastfeeding

Drug References

American Academy of Pediatrics Committee on Drugs. (2001). Transfer of drugs and other chemicals into human milk. *Pediatrics, 108,* 776–789.

Briggs, G.G., Freeman, R.K., & Yaffee, S.J. (Eds.). (2002). *Drugs in pregnancy and lactation* (6th ed.). Philadelphia: Lippincott, Williams, and Wilkins.

Hale, T.W. (2004). *Medications and mothers milk.* Amarillo, TX: Pharmasoft Publishing.

Lawrence, R.A., & Lawrence, R.M. (2005). *Breastfeeding: A guide for the medical profession* (6th ed.). St. Louis: Mosby.

▶ # Separation of mother and baby

DEFINITION   Referring to occasions where mother and baby are not in close contact with one another. Ideally, mothers and babies can maintain close contact from the moment of birth throughout the newborn period. Unless there are medical problems for mother and/or baby, there is no need for mother–baby separation in the early postpartum period.

Ask about

Age of baby.
Reason for separation.
Duration of separation.

ASSESSMENT

PROMPT LACTATION CARE NEEDED?
Are any of the following present?

Immediate need to express milk due to hospitalization or surgery.

Drug questions related to maternal hospitalization or surgery.

IF YES,   *Call lactation care provider now and consult up-to-date drug references.*

ROUTINE LACTATION CARE NEEDED?
Are any of the following present?

Questions about facilitating milk expression for future separation for reasons of medical procedure, or return to work/school.

IF YES,   *Call lactation care provider.*

During long periods of separation, express milk frequently via hand expression or pumping.

Seek to replicate baby's normal breastfeeding pattern, expressing milk 10–12 times per 24 hours.

See also Expression of mothers' milk; Hand expression of breastmilk; Pump

▶ Sepsis

DEFINITION   Refers to serious infection in the bloodstream. Sepsis is a life threatening condition in infants.

See also Fever and breastfeeding; Lethargy; Uncoordinated suckling; Weak suck

▶ Sexuality and breastfeeding

DEFINITION   Sexual intercourse is compatible with breastfeeding, although the low estrogen level of the breastfeeding mother may contribute to vaginal dryness. She may also experience residual discomfort or pain from the birth or episiotomy.

Women may feel differently about sexual relations after the birth of a baby. Many women feel less desire although some women feel more. No one can predict how a woman will feel.

Breastfeeding is an intimate activity that may make the rest of the family feel left out.

In addition, mothers may feel tired and not have the energy for sexual activities.

Ask about

Age of baby.

ROUTINE MEDICAL CARE NEEDED?

Are any of the following present?

Difficult penetration.

Pain during intercourse.

IF YES, *Call obstetric care provider.*

ROUTINE LACTATION CARE NEEDED?

Are any of the following present?

Questions about normalcy of feelings.

IF YES, *Call lactation care provider.*

SELF CARE INFORMATION

Life changes after the birth of a baby and it is sometimes hard for mothers to know if what they are experiencing is "normal." Talking about feelings and physical concerns can help a mother with the adjustment.

IMPORTANT CONDITIONS TO REPORT

Feelings of extreme worry or anxiety.

Difficult or painful penetration.

Pain during intercourse.

See also Fertility; Menstrual cycle

▶ SGA

See also Small for gestational age (SGA)

▶ Sheehan's syndrome

DEFINITION   Sheehan's syndrome is a condition that may develop when the pituitary gland is deprived of blood and oxygen because of a severe postpartum hemorrhage. Sheehan's syndrome is a condition that is uncommon with modern obstetric care and blood transfusions.

Because of the pituitary damage from the blood loss, the mother may have failure to lactate.

Transient cases of Sheehan's syndrome have been reported.

The amount of damage to the pituitary gland is variable and there may be no other symptoms besides insufficient milk and insufficient milk transfer until the mother is stressed later in life. Some women go undiagnosed for a long time.

Other symptoms include:

Diabetes insipidus.

Hair loss (especially from the armpit and pubic area).

Hypothyroidism.

Infertility or amenorrhea.

Ask about

Age of baby.

Weight gain pattern of baby.

History of hemorrhage.

ASSESSMENT

EMERGENT CARE NEEDED?

Are any of the following present?

Soaking a sanitary napkin with bright red blood at a rate of one napkin or more per hour.

Clots in the bloody discharge.

Foul odor to the discharge (even if occasional).

Dizziness.

Fever.

Abdominal pain.

IF YES, *Call obstetric care provider now and seek emergency care now.*

PROMPT MEDICAL CARE NEEDED?

Are any of the following present?

Soaking a sanitary napkin with bright red blood at a rate of one napkin every two to three hours.

Abdominal tenderness.

Low-grade fever.

Lightheadedness.

IF YES, *Call obstetric care provider within 2 to 4 hours.*

PROMPT LACTATION CARE NEEDED?

Are any of the following present?

Problems with milk supply in a woman diagnosed with retained placental fragments.

IF YES, *Call lactation care provider today.*

ROUTINE CARE NEEDED?

Are any of the following present?

Soaking a sanitary napkin with bright red blood at a rate of one napkin every three or more hours.

Abdominal tenderness.

IF YES, *Call obstetric care provider today.*

IMPORTANT CONDITIONS TO REPORT

Frequent urination and excessive thirst.

Feeling cold frequently.

Feeling dizzy or lightheaded.

See also Hemorrhage, postpartum; Lochia; Retained placental fragments; Thyroid disease

▶ SIDS

DEFINITION   Sudden Infant Death Syndrome. SIDS is the unexpected death of a healthy appearing baby under the age of 1.

SIDS is rare in the first month of life and most cases of SIDS occur before 6 months of age.

In the United States there are more SIDS cases in the fall and winter seasons as compared to the spring and summer months.

The National "Back to Sleep" Campaign encourages parents to put their babies to sleep on their backs. Since the initiation of this campaign, the number of babies to die from SIDS per year has been reduced by 50%.

About 2200 babies die per year from SIDS in the United States.

SIDS is sudden and silent. The baby shows no signs of suffering.

The risk of SIDS increases if babies are not put to sleep on their backs, if they are overheated, if they are exposed to secondhand smoke, and if they have unsafe bedding.

Babies who are using pacifiers to help regulate their breathing should not be put to bed without their pacifiers until a physician gives the okay.

SELF CARE INFORMATION

Learn about safe sleeping practices for babies.

Protect the baby from secondhand smoke.

See also Co-sleeping; Crib death; Smoking and lactation

▶ Silicone breast implants

DEFINITION   Inserts surgically added to the breast to increase its size.

Implants can affect milk making ability to some extent.

Ask about

Date of implant surgery.

Age of baby.

Location of surgical incision.

ASSESSMENT

PROMPT CARE NEEDED?

Are any of the following present?

Presence of implants with:

Concerns about milk supply.

Poor weight gain in breastfed baby.

IF YES,   *Call lactation care provider now and report to pediatric care provider.*

SELF CARE INFORMATION

Practice skin-to-skin contact frequently.

Feed baby at first sign of hunger cues (signs that say "feed me" include hand-to-face or hand-to-mouth movements, lip smacking, seeking with lips, rooting, and head bobbing).

Feed baby at least 10–12 times per 24 hours.

Listen for signs of baby swallowing.

Allow baby to end feedings.

Expect at least 3–4 infant stools per 24 hours after the first 4 days of life.

Good positioning and attachment are crucial to reduce nipple pain.

If feedings are missed, hand express or pump milk to maintain supply.

IMPORTANT CONDITIONS TO REPORT

Fewer than four bowel movements daily after day 4 of life.

Ongoing concerns or problems with milk supply.

Notes

The location and extent of the incision may impact the sensation of the nerves in the nipple area. Loss of or decreased sensation may decrease milk-making potential. Trauma to the nerves may hinder the stimulation of the brain to release prolactin (the milk-making hormone) in response to suckling. Periareolar incisions suggest more potential nerve injury than do incisions underneath the breast.

Babies of women who have had breast augmentation surgery should be followed closely to ensure proper growth.

If the mother reports that she had an implant in one breast only, inquire about the reason for this surgery. If augmentation corrected breast asymmetry, there may be increased concern regarding the mother's ability to make a full milk supply. Marked asymmetry may indicate insufficient glandular tissue in both breasts. Baby and mother should be closely followed.

Concern has been expressed about the possibility of silicon entering the breastmilk, but research has not indicated negative effects.

See also Breast asymmetry; Breast surgery; Weight gain, baby–low

▶ Skin-to-skin (STS) care

DEFINITION   Skin-to-skin care (STS care or Kangaroo care) is a special kind of holding where the baby is skin-to-skin with the mother. Skin-to-skin can start right after birth for mothers of term babies and whenever the NICU staff say that a premature baby is ready.

Research indicates that premature babies maintain their temperature, heart rates, and oxygenation when held skin-to-skin, and breathing rates are more stable than in standard NICU care.[169]

Term babies who have been held skin-to-skin breastfeed better[170] and are more likely to sleep more soundly and peacefully in the night.[171]

SELF CARE INFORMATION

Pregnant women should discuss skin-to-skin care with their providers so that the provider knows that it is important to the mother.

Do not just think about skin-to-skin care as something to do for the first few minutes after the baby is born. Hold the baby skin-to-skin often. The baby can hear your heartbeat, and feel comforted and warm.

See also Kangaroo care

Footnotes

[169]Ludington-Hoe, S.M., Anderson, G.C., Swinth, J.Y., Thompson, C., & Hadeed, A.J. (2004). Randomized controlled trial of kangaroo care: Cardiorespiratory and thermal effects on healthy preterm infants. *Neonatal Network, 23*(3), 39–48.

[170]Anderson, G.C., Moore, F., Hepworth, J., & Bergman, N. (2003). Early skin-to-skin contact for mothers and their healthy newborn infants. *The Cochrane Database of Systematic Reviews, 2,* CD003519.

[171]Ferber, S.G., & Makhoul, I.R. (2004). The effect of skin-to-skin contact (kangaroo care) shortly after birth on the neurobehavioral responses of the term newborn: A randomized, controlled trial. *Pediatrics, 113*(4), 858–865.

▶ Sleep patterns

DEFINITION   Newborn babies have no idea what time it is. They do not have a pattern to their sleep and waking. They do not know if it is night or day, and they are not manipulating their parents.

Night feedings are expected for the first four months or so and then babies might sleep one five-hour stretch at night. Night waking is normal well into the toddler years.

Many babies continue to nap during the day well into their second year. Preschools and daycare centers structure naps into their day.

Ask about

Age of baby.
Weight gain pattern.

ASSESSMENT

PROMPT CARE NEEDED?
  Are any of the following present?
      Sleep deprivation in the parent.
      Anger or other strong reaction to baby waking at night.

IF YES, *Call medical care provider today.*

ROUTINE CARE NEEDED?
  Are any of the following present?
      Concern about:
        Night wakening.
        Night feedings.
        Night crying.

IF YES, *Call lactation care provider.*

SELF CARE INFORMATION

Keeping baby close at night can minimize sleep loss. In addition babies may transfer more milk.

Try daytime interventions for nighttime wakening problems. Nurse the baby more often during the daytime, and watch out for long naps in the car seat.

IMPORTANT CONDITIONS TO REPORT
Anger at baby wakening in the night.

See also Co-sleeping; Feeding pattern of breastfed infants; Maternal fatigue; Night nursings; Reverse cycle breastfeeding

▶ Sleepy baby

DEFINITION   Some babies are sleepy at first, making it difficult to accomplish 10–12 effective feedings per day after the first day of life.

There can be many reasons for this temporary condition such as sepsis (severe infection in the bloodstream), jaundice (which may cause lethargy), drug effects from labor analgesia, and a difficult labor and birth.

Ask about

Age of baby.
History of sleepiness.
History of weight gain or loss.

ASSESSMENT

EMERGENT CARE NEEDED?
Are any of the following present?

Cannot rouse baby.

Baby sleeps more than 3 hours between feedings consistently.

Shallow breathing or breathing difficult to observe. (Observe the newborns breathing for at least 1–2 minutes. Sleeping newborns often exhibit periodic breathing which may include rapid shallow breaths interspersed with brief pauses in breathing.)

Meconium bowel movements after 5 days of life.

Fewer than three bowel movements daily in breastfed newborn after the first 2 days of life.

No urine in six hours.

Brick dust urine (uric acid crystals) after 2 days of life.

Dark colored urine.

Fewer than four urinations daily in the breastfed newborn after day 5 of life.
Low muscle tone or floppiness.

IF YES, *Seek pediatric care now.*

PROMPT CARE NEEDED?
Are any of the following present?
Baby nurses fewer than 10 times in 24 hours.
Baby consistently falls asleep after sucking briefly at the breast.
Baby is not gaining at least 0.5 oz a day.

IF YES, *Call lactation care provider today.*

SELF CARE INFORMATION
Parents who observe the baby for feeding cues—hand-to-face or hand-to-mouth movements, lip smacking, seeking with lips, rooting, and head bobbing—may find it easier to feed the baby at the baby's best time.
Young babies tend to cluster their feedings. Nurse the baby again when baby gives the next feeding cue (i.e., watch the baby, not the clock to determine the timing of the next feeding). The baby never completely empties the breast.

IMPORTANT CONDITIONS TO REPORT
Babies that are hard to rouse and sleep longer than three hours between nursings should be evaluated.
Babies who fall asleep after a minute or two at the breast should be evaluated.

See also Feeding cues; Hyperbilirubinemia; Hypotonia; Lethargy

▶ Sling/baby carrier

DEFINITION There are many types of slings and baby carriers, from simple cloths to complex packs. Babies and mothers often have a preference based on their comfort and need. Slings that allow breastfeeding may facilitate cue-based breastfeeding for mothers who are simultaneously working or caring for other children.
Some slings and baby carriers allow the mother to have two hands free. Others require the mother to use her arm to support the baby. Some allow the baby to

nurse while being carried. Slings that cradle the baby in a flexed position are especially good for babies who are hypertonic or hypotonic.

SELF CARE INFORMATION

Use the sling or carrier the first few times when the baby is in a good mood to get the baby used to it.

See also Hypertonia; Muscle tone of infant

▶ # Slow weight gain, baby

DEFINITION Breastfed babies should gain a minimum of 0.5 oz to 1 oz a day on average in the early weeks. New studies indicate that breastfed babies gain even faster than was previously believed, probably because breastfeeding used to be done on a schedule and not as frequently as we now know is ideal. New growth charts for exclusively breastfed babies are forthcoming from the World Health Organization. Rates of growth change throughout the first year. Babies are thought to generally double their birthweight by 6 months and triple it by 12 months.

Ask about

Age of baby.
Weight gain pattern.

ASSESSMENT

PROMPT CARE NEEDED?

Are any of the following present?

Lethargy.
Hard to rouse.
Meconium bowel movements after 5 days of life.
Fewer than three bowel movements daily in breastfed newborn after the first 2 days of life.
No urine in six hours.
Brick dust urine (uric acid crystals) after 2 days of life.

Dark colored urine.

Fewer than four urinations daily in the breastfed newborn after day 5 of life.

Noticeably sunken fontanelles (soft spot on top of head).

Decreased activity.

Baby below birthweight at 10 to 14 days of life.

Cessation of weight gain.

Poor feedings.

Sleeping at the breast.

IF YES, *Seek pediatric care now.*

ROUTINE CARE NEEDED?

Are any of the following present?

Sleeps at the breast after a few sucks.

Hard to latch-on.

No audible swallows.

Pediatric referral for breastfeeding evaluation.

IF YES, *Call lactation care provider today.*

IMPORTANT CONDITIONS TO REPORT

Decrease in number of urinations or stools.

Increased sleepiness, hours spent sleeping.

Baby is harder to rouse.

See also Hypotonia; Jaundice; Muscle tone of infant

▶ **Small for gestational age (SGA)**

DEFINITION   Meaning smaller in weight or length than expected for newborns at this gestational age.

▶ **Smoking and lactation**

DEFINITION   Mothers who smoke may breastfeed. However, all babies should be protected from secondhand smoke.

Age of baby.

Weight gain pattern of baby.

ASSESSMENT

ROUTINE CARE NEEDED?

Are any of the following present?

Baby using pacifier.

Frequent feedings.

Smoking in the baby's environment.

Low milk supply.

Poor feeding.

Poor weight gain.

Desire to cut down or stop smoking.

IF YES, *Call lactation care provider today and report to pediatric care provider today.*

SELF CARE INFORMATION

Research indicates that mothers who smoke may make and secrete less milk, but if they cut down or stop, their milk supply may rebound.

Babies and children should always be protected from secondhand smoke.

Breastfeeding may mitigate the effects of smoking during pregnancy.

IMPORTANT CONDITIONS TO REPORT

Poor weight gain pattern or weight loss.

Poor feeding.

Upper respiratory problems in baby (e.g., coughing or runny nose).

See also Nicotine

▶ Soapy odor in frozen milk

DEFINITION   Human milk contains digestive properties. When the baby nurses, these components of milk go right into the baby with the milk. It is one of the reasons breastmilk is so easy for babies to digest. When milk is collected and stored, these active components still work.

See also Rancid odor of frozen breastmilk; Salty taste of breastmilk

▶ Sodium in breastmilk

DEFINITION   Human milk can increase in sodium if the mother has mastitis, if the milk supply is very low, or in some cases during weaning. The sodium in human milk is never as high as it is in formula.

Ask about

Age of baby.
Presence of symptoms.

ASSESSMENT

PROMPT CARE NEEDED?
  Are any of the following present?
    Breastfeeding infant hospitalized for dehydration, jaundice, or hypernatremia associated with poor milk intake.

IF YES,   *Call lactation care provider now for feeding assessment.*

SELF CARE INFORMATION
   Breast milk sodium can increase naturally during gradual weaning and the milk will taste salty.

See also Failure to thrive (FTT); Mastitis; Weaning

▶ Solid foods for breastfed babies

DEFINITION   The American Academy of Pediatrics (AAP), the United States Breastfeeding Committee (USBC), the United Nations Children's Fund (UNICEF) and the World Health Organization (WHO) recommend exclusive breastfeeding for about the first six months of life.

Researchers have shown that flavors from the foods the mother eats in pregnancy and during lactation pass into the milk. When foods taste familiar, baby is more accepting of family foods.

In addition to age, signs of readiness may include:

Increased interest in table foods.

Ability to sit up.

Ability to pick up objects and put them in the mouth.

Decreased tongue thrusting (automatically pushing foods out of the mouth with the tongue).

Ask about

Age of baby.

Reason for wanting to start solid foods.

PROMPT CARE NEEDED?

Are any of the following present?

Breastfed baby under 5 months of age.

Mother concerned about baby's weight gain.

Decreased stooling or urination.

IF YES, *Report to pediatric care provider today and call lactation care provider today.*

ROUTINE CARE NEEDED?

Are any of the following present?

Breastfed baby around 6 months of age.

Questions about starting solids.

IF YES, *Call lactation care provider or nutritionist.*

SELF CARE INFORMATION

Babies are not equally interested in starting solid foods. If the baby is not interested, wait a few days and try again.

When babies start solid foods around 6 months, they do not usually have a prolonged time on the semi-liquid foods that were popular years ago when starting solids was recommended at younger ages.

Move the baby onto family foods as appropriate.

IMPORTANT CONDITIONS TO REPORT

Difficulty breathing.

Difficulty swallowing.

Rapid progression of symptoms.

See also Allergy in the breastfed infant; Solid foods for breastfed babies

▶ Sore nipples

DEFINITION Uncomfortable sensations in the tips of the breasts. Pain is not an expected part of breastfeeding and indicates the need for feeding evaluation.

There can be many reasons for pain in the breast including nipple trauma and infection. Poor latch-on or positioning can also cause pain.

Ask about

Onset.
Location of pain.
Whether unilateral or bilateral.

ASSESSMENT

PROMPT CARE NEEDED?

Are any of the following present?

Persistent pain with feeding.
Persistent pain between feedings.
Constant pain.
Pain combined with color change of nipple(s).
Pain with visible fissure or bleeding of the nipple.

IF YES, *Call lactation care provider now.*

ROUTINE CARE NEEDED?

Are any of the following present?

Brief pain at beginning of feeding.
Mild recurrent pain.

IF YES, *Report to lactation care provider.*

SELF CARE INFORMATION

Practice skin-to-skin contact frequently.
Feed baby at first sign of hunger cues (signs that say "feed me" include hand-to-face or hand-to-mouth movements, lip smacking, seeking with lips, rooting, and head bobbing).
Feed baby at least 10–12 times per 24 hours.
Listen for signs of baby swallowing.
Allow baby to end feedings.
Expect at least 3–4 infant stools per 24 hours after the first 4 days of life.
Good positioning and attachment are crucial to reduce nipple pain.

See also Latch-on; Mastitis; Raynaud's phenomenon/syndrome

▶ Special care unit (SCU)

See also Neonatal Intensive Care Unit (NICU)

▶ Special needs baby

DEFINITION   Babies with special needs such as inborn errors of metabolism, congenital anomalies, and prematurity can all benefit from breastmilk. The only exception is the baby who has been diagnosed with galactosemia.

Ask about

Age of baby.
Special need of baby.
Weight gain.
Milk transfer.

ASSESSMENT

PROMPT CARE NEEDED?

Are any of the following present?

Baby does not latch onto the breast.
Baby does not stay on the breast.
Baby is not gaining adequately.
Baby does not seem to transfer milk.

IF YES,   *Call lactation care provider now.*

As soon after birth as a mother knows that her baby will have special needs, she should begin expressing her milk. When the baby is capable of stimulating the hormones, transfering the milk, and maintaining the milk supply, the mother can reduce the amount of milk expression.

▶ Special Supplemental Food Program for Women, Infants, and Children (WIC)

DEFINITION   WIC is a supplemental food program for women, infants, and children that is administered through the United States Department of Agriculture (USDA).

"The mission of WIC is to safeguard the health of low-income women, infants, and children up to age 5 who are at nutritional risk by providing nutritional foods to supplement diets, information on healthy eating, and referrals to health care."[172]

Breastfeeding rates among WIC participants are rising. The percentage of WIC participants who initiated breastfeeding increased by 69% over a 10-year period. The percentage of women who breastfed at 6 months increased by 145% during the same time period.[173]

Notes

WIC at FNS Headquarters:
Supplemental Food Programs Division
Food and Nutrition Service - USDA
3101 Park Center Drive
Alexandria, VA 22302
Phone: 703-305-2746
Fax: 703-305-2196
Web site: www.fns.usda.gov/wic

Footnotes

[172]The Special Supplemental Nutrition Program for Women, Infants, and Children. (2003). *WIC's mission*. Retrieved August 4, 2005, from http://www.fns.usda.gov/wic/aboutwic/mission. htm.

[173]United States Department of Agriculture. (2003). *WIC and breastfeeding rates* (Food and Nutrition Research Report, Number 34-2). Washington, DC.

▶ Spitting up

DEFINITION   Spitting up or vomiting in the infant can be differentiated from projectile vomiting by the distance it travels. Projectile vomiting vomit clears the chin of the infant. It may travel several feet. Spitting up does not clear the chin on its way out.

Spitting up, even after every feeding, may not be an indication that there is anything wrong with the baby. The mother may have a very powerful let-down reflex for example. Also, a baby's lower esophageal sphincter is normally lower in tone than that of an older child or adult.

SELF CARE INFORMATION

Occasional spitting up in an otherwise well infant is not uncommon.

Frequent spitting up, even in a baby with no other symptoms, can indicate that there is an underlying problem such as gastroesophageal reflux.

IMPORTANT CONDITIONS TO REPORT

Signs that the baby is unwell in combination with spitting up.

Decrease in stools and urinations.

Poor feeding behavior.

Weight loss, failure to gain adequately.

See also Gastroesophageal (GE) reflux; Let-down; Milk ejection reflex; Pyloric stenosis and breastfeeding

▶ Stooling patterns

DEFINITION   Stools (bowel movements) can be an important indication of how well the baby is doing at breastfeeding.

Baby's first stools (meconium) are greenish-black and tarry. The stool is sticky. By the second or third day, the stool becomes less black and more green (transitional stool), and when the large milk volume is available (around day three) the stool changes to yellow.

After day three, some babies stool a small stain in the diaper at every nursing. Others stool once or twice a day. If the baby is stooling only once or twice a day, the amount should be more substantial. After the early months of life, breastfed babies may stool less frequently, going days between large, soft stools. However, other older breastfed babies may continue to stool frequently.

Ask about

Age of baby.
Number of stools per day.
Number of feedings per day.
Weight gain pattern of baby.

ASSESSMENT

PROMPT CARE NEEDED?

Are any of the following present?

No stool in 24 hours in the newborn period.

Gray or white stool.

Bloody stool.

Lethargy (sleepy, difficult to rouse).

Hard to latch-on.

Subtle feeding cues.

Weak suck.

IF YES, *Seek pediatric care now and call lactation care provider now.*

ROUTINE CARE NEEDED?

Are any of the following present?

One or two small stools a day in newborn period.

Poor weight gain (less than 0.5 oz a day on average).

Fussy, unsatisfied baby.

IF YES, *Report to pediatric care provider and call lactation care provider today.*

SELF CARE INFORMATION

Improving the number of feedings and the quality of the feedings will increase the number of stools and the stool volume.

Keeping a feeding and diaper diary for a few days can help to describe what is happening to the lactation care provider or health care provider.

IMPORTANT CONDITIONS TO REPORT

Decreased stooling.

Increased sleepiness.

See also Bowel movements, infant; Constipation

▶ # Storage of breastmilk

DEFINITION   Safely preserving expressed milk.

Notes

Glass and hard plastic containers with tight lids are recommended for breastmilk storage. All containers should be food-grade. Plastic bags designed for milk storage may be used, but it may be difficult to prevent spillage and puncture of these bags.

When expressed for the healthy, full term infant, milk can be safely stored:[174]

Up to four hours at room temperature (lower than 75° F), but should be refrigerated immediately if possible (with frozen gel pack in an insulated lunch bag or cooler if refrigerator is not available).

Up to 72 hours in the refrigerator.

Up to three months in the built-in freezer section of a refrigerator.

Up to six months in a deep freezer.

Milk that will not be used fresh within 72 hours should be frozen as soon as possible.

When milk is being expressed for the premature or sick infant, it should be handled and stored according to the NICU/SCU guidelines.

See also Collection and storage of breastmilk; Milk storage bags

Footnotes

[174]Arnold, L.D.W. (2004). *Safe storage of expressed breastmilk for the healthy infant and child.* East Sandwich, MA: Health Education Associates.

▶ # STS care

See also Kangaroo care; Skin-to-skin (STS) care

Sudden Infant Death Syndrome (SIDS)

DEFINITION   Sudden Infant Death Syndrome (SIDS) is the unexpected death of a healthy appearing baby under the age of 1.

SIDS is rare in the first month of life and most cases of SIDS occur before 6 months of age.

In the United States there are more SIDS cases in the fall and winter seasons as compared to the spring and summer months.

The National "Back to Sleep" Campaign encourages parents to put their babies to sleep on their backs. Since the initiation of this campaign, the number of babies to die from SIDS per year has been reduced by 50%.

About 2200 babies die per year from SIDS in the United States.

SIDS is sudden and silent. The baby shows no signs of suffering.

The risk of SIDS increases if babies are not put to sleep on their backs, if they are overheated, if they are exposed to secondhand smoke, and if they have unsafe bedding.

Babies who are using pacifiers to help regulate their breathing should not be put to bed without their pacifiers until the physician gives the okay.

SELF CARE INFORMATION

Learn about safe sleeping practices for babies.

Protect the baby from secondhand smoke.

See also Co-sleeping; Crib death; Smoking and lactation

Supernumerary nipple tissue

DEFINITION   Accessory mammary glands and additional (supernumerary) nipples are usually found along the milk line that extends from the underarms to the thighs. They may be found outside of the line as well.

Breast tissue may produce milk, but without a nipple pore, it cannot be released.

During pregnancy and lactation, extra nipple tissue may enlarge and become prominent. A mother may find that what she thought was a mole is actually a supernumerary nipple.

Age of baby.

Onset of symptoms.

ASSESSMENT

PROMPT CARE NEEDED?

Are any of the following present?

Enlarged, painful areas along the milk line coupled with maternal fever higher than 101° F (38.5° C).

IF YES, *Call obstetric care provider within 2 to 4 hours.*

ROUTINE CARE NEEDED?

Are any of the following present?

Enlarged, painful areas along the milk line.

IF YES, *Call lactation care provider today.*

SELF CARE INFORMATION

Comfort measures such as ice packs or moist heat may ease the pain.

The areas will return to normal and become comfortable in a few days.

IMPORTANT CONDITIONS TO REPORT

Fever.

Reddened areas of the body.

Extreme pain in the area of the extra nipple tissue.

See also Accessory breast tissue; Hyperadenia; Hyperthelia

▶ Supplemental feeding

DEFINITION   Feedings that replace breastfeedings are considered supplemental feedings.

Age of baby.

Age of baby when supplemental feedings started.

Type of supplements.

How supplements are fed.

Amount of supplement per 24 hours.

Reactions from supplement.

ASSESSMENT

EMERGENT CARE NEEDED?

Are any of the following present?

Difficulty breathing.

IF YES, *Seek emergency care now.*

PROMPT CARE NEEDED?

Are any of the following present?

Meconium bowel movements after 5 days of life.

Fewer than three bowel movements daily in breastfed newborn after the first 2 days of life.

No urine in six hours.

Brick dust urine (uric acid crystals) after 2 days of life.

Dark colored urine.

Fewer than four urinations daily in the breastfed newborn after day 5 of life.

Noticeably sunken fontanelles (soft spot on top of head).

Decreased activity.

Baby below birthweight at 10 to 14 days of life.

Cessation of weight gain.

Eczema.

Hives.

Vomiting.

Diarrhea.

Blood in the stools.

IF YES, *Seek pediatric care now.*

ROUTINE CARE NEEDED?

Are any of the following present?

Education needed about supplemental feeding.

Education wanted about decreasing amount of supplement.

Education wanted about increasing milk volume.

IF YES, *Call lactation care provider.*

SELF CARE INFORMATION

Complementary feedings are those that are added to breastfeeding.

IMPORTANT CONDITIONS TO REPORT

Signs of dehydration (scanty, dark urine).

Lethargy.

Difficulty breathing.

Eczema.

Hives.

Vomiting.

Diarrhea.

Blood in the stools.

Irritability and excessive crying.

See also At-breast supplementation; Formula, infant; Mixed feeds

▶ Surgery and breastfeeding

DEFINITION   Mothers and babies can have surgery and continue breastfeeding. Decisions (even in an emergency) must be made about:

How the baby will be fed during the separation.

How the mother's breasts will be kept comfortable during the separation.

If the separation will be prolonged, how the mother's milk supply will be stimulated and maintained.

When and where the mother and baby can be reunited.

Medications or anesthesia used.

Restrictions after discharge.

SELF CARE INFORMATION

It's important to ensure that all health care providers are informed that the mother and baby are breastfeeding.

See also Breast surgery; Hospitalization and breastfeeding

▶ Swaddling

DEFINITION   Wrapping babies is traditional in some societies. Wrapping a young baby is called swaddling. Many babies are happier with the tight feeling of swaddling to remind them of the womb. When wrapping a baby who is going to breastfeed, there are two important considerations:

Babies nurse best when their hips and knees are flexed. Swaddle the baby in a flexed position.

Babies help to stimulate the mother's lactation hormones with their hands. Do not swaddle the hands. Leave the hands free to embrace the breast during the nursing.

▶ Switch nursing

DEFINITION   With switch nursing the mother moves the baby from one breast to the other and back again during the feeding. This is thought to stimulate the milk supply.

The baby would nurse on one breast for five minutes. The mother breaks suction and moves the baby to the other breast. She does this several times during the course of one feeding. The feeding should continue until the baby indicates fullness.

See also Cluster feeding; Increasing milk supply

► Tail of Spence

DEFINITION   The Tail of Spence is the part of the mammary gland tissue that extends into the underarm (axillary region). Sometimes the Tail of Spence is visible and enlarged during lactation.

Because this is part of the mammary gland, lumps, plugs, and other problems can develop in the Tail of Spence.

SELF CARE INFORMATION
Examine the Tail of Spence for lumps as you would the breast.
Position the baby to move any milk out of the Tail of Spence if milk is not draining efficiently from that area.

IMPORTANT CONDITIONS TO REPORT
Lumps in the armpit that do not move with nursing.
Pain in the armpit.
Reddened areas in the armpit.
Fever and flulike feelings.

See also Breast structure; Engorgement; Mastitis

► Taking the baby off the breast

DEFINITION   Babies make a seal at the breast with their lips and tongue. In addition, the breast is drawn into the mouth and held there firmly during suckling. To take the baby off of the breast the mother needs to break the seal. She can do this by inserting her clean finger into the corner of the baby's mouth or by pressing down onto her breast to break the seal.

SELF CARE INFORMATION
Ideally, babies should end the feeding themselves.

IMPORTANT CONDITIONS TO REPORT
Nipple pain.
Baby does not end feeding.
Deep breast pain.

See also Latch-on; Sore nipples; Weaning

▶ Tandem nursing

DEFINITION Nursing two babies not from the same pregnancy.

Usually, the mother has nursed the older baby through the pregnancy, but that is not always the case. Some mothers invite a weaned baby to nurse along with the newborn.

Ask about

Age of babies.

ASSESSMENT
ROUTINE CARE NEEDED?
Are any of the following present?
Need for nutrition evaluation.
IF YES, *Seek dietary consultation.*
Are any of the following present?
Mixed feelings about tandem nursing.
Need for practical help or strategies.
Nipple pain in pregnancy.
Help required with weaning.
IF YES, *Call lactation care provider.*

SELF CARE INFORMATION

Be open to adjusting expectations to meet reality.
Nurse the younger baby first and frequently.
Find time for non-nursing interactions with the older baby.

See also Breastfeeding during pregnancy

▶ Taste of milk

DEFINITION   Human milk does not look or taste like cow's milk. At first, during the colostral phase, milk is creamy or yellow in color. Mature milk is more bluish.

Human milk tastes very sweet to the adult palate.

Flavors in the mother's diet do flavor her milk and amniotic fluid. This is probably how babies learn the tastes of their family foods.

In research, babies nursed longer after their mothers had eaten garlic.[175] They seemed to prefer the flavored milk.

ASSESSMENT

ROUTINE CARE NEEDED?
   Are any of the following present?
   Fussy baby.
   Concerns about the effect of food(s) the mother is eating.

IF YES,   *Call lactation care provider.*

SELF CARE INFORMATION

Eat the foods that your family likes when you are breastfeeding.

Mothers whose babies may be allergic (family history of allergies) should avoid eating peanuts.

IMPORTANT CONDITIONS TO REPORT

Allergic symptoms in baby.

See also Cabbage; Maternal diet

Footnotes
   [175]Mennella, J.A., & Beauchamp, G.K. (1993). The effects of repeated exposure to garlic-flavored milk on the nursling's behavior. *Pediatric Research, 34*(6), 805–808.

▶ TB and breastfeeding

See also Tuberculosis (TB) and breastfeeding

▶ Teenaged mothers

DEFINITION   Adolescent mothers can breastfeed. They have similar issues, problems, and concerns as non-teen mothers.

Ask about

Age of baby.
Age of mother.

ASSESSMENT

ROUTINE CARE NEEDED?

Are any of the following present?
Poor dietary habits.

IF YES,   *Seek dietary consultation.*

Are any of the following present?
Need for support.
Need for practical breastfeeding management strategies.

IF YES,   *Call lactation care provider.*

SELF CARE INFORMATION

Teenagers who breastfeed have higher bone density later in life, compared to teens who have babies but do not breastfeed.

Teens should be encouraged to eat well to support the needs of their own bodies. Eating well helps provide energy and maintain optimal health. Eating well does not help women make more milk; only more frequent feeding or milk removal can do that.

See also Adolescent breastfeeding; Maternal diet; Milk production

▶ Teething

DEFINITION   Babies do not need to be weaned because they are teething or because they have teeth, although mothers may be told this by friends or family.

Because their gums are uncomfortable, teething babies may try chewing at the breast.

Mothers may have sore nipples when the baby is teething.

Ask about

Age of baby.
Presence of teeth.

ASSESSMENT

ROUTINE CARE NEEDED?

Are any of the following present?

Difficulty nursing during teething period.
Sore nipples during teething period.
Biting at the breast during feeding.
Questions about soothing a breastfeeding, teething baby.

IF YES,   *Call lactation care provider.*

Are any of the following present?

Questions about infant tooth care.

IF YES,   *Call pediatric care provider or dentist.*

SELF CARE INFORMATION

Teething is a temporary (but reoccurring) stage that can be difficult for some babies and families.

IMPORTANT CONDITIONS TO REPORT

Persistent refusal to feed in a teething infant.

See also Biting; Clenching or clamping onto the nipple/areola; Sore nipples

► TE fistula

See also Tracheoesophageal (TE) fistula

► Ten Steps to Successful Breastfeeding

DEFINITION   Optimal steps created by the World Health Organization (WHO) and United Nations Children's Fund (UNICEF) to be practiced in all maternity units worldwide. These steps form the basis of Baby-Friendly Hospital Initiative.

Baby-Friendly USA is the agency responsible for implementing the Baby-Friendly Hospital Initiative in the United States.

"The steps for the United States are:

1. Have a written breastfeeding policy that is routinely communicated to all health care staff.
2. Train all health care staff in skills necessary to implement this policy.
3. Inform all pregnant women about the benefits and management of breastfeeding.
4. Help mothers initiate breastfeeding within one hour of birth.
5. Show mothers how to breastfeed and how to maintain lactation even if they should be separated from their infants.
6. Give infants no food or drink other than breastmilk, unless medically indicated.
7. Practice rooming-in—allow mothers and infants to remain together 24 hours a day.
8. Encourage unrestricted breastfeeding.
9. Give no pacifiers or artificial nipples to breastfeeding infants.
10. Foster the establishment of breastfeeding support groups and refer mothers to them on discharge from the hospital or clinic."[176]

Notes

Baby-Friendly USA
327 Quaker Meeting House Road
East Sandwich, MA 02537
Phone: 508-888-8092
Web site: www.babyfriendlyusa.org

Footnotes

[176]Baby-Friendly Hospital Initiative. (n.d.). *The ten steps to successful breastfeeding*. Retrieved August 4, 2005, from http://www.babyfriendlyusa.org/eng/10steps.html.

▶ Test weighing

DEFINITION Weighing a baby before and after a feeding to estimate the amount of milk transferred is called test weighing.

Test weighing with digital scales, accurate to 1 g or 2 g, has been shown in research to be fairly accurate. Test weighing with other types of scales has not been shown to reflect an approximate intake.

Ask about

Age of baby.
Reason for test weighing.

ASSESSMENT

PROMPT CARE NEEDED?

Are any of the following present?

Pediatric referral for evaluation of milk supply.

Infrequent feeding (less than eight breastfeedings daily).

Insufficient urination or stooling.

Perception of milk supply problem.

IF YES, *Seek lactation care today.*

ROUTINE CARE NEEDED?

Are any of the following present?

Concern about the amount of milk baby is getting while breastfeeding.

Fear of inadequate milk supply.

IF YES, *Call lactation care provider today.*

SELF CARE INFORMATION

The test weight reflects only an estimate of the feeding that was test weighed.

Babies do not seem to transfer the same amount at each breastfeeding.

IMPORTANT CONDITIONS TO REPORT

Baby is difficult to rouse.

Baby has difficulty breathing or observer has difficulty determining whether baby is breathing.

Baby has inadequate urinations or stools.

Baby becomes lethargic.

See also Electronic scales; Milk transfer, estimating; Slow weight gain, baby

▶ # Thawing and warming frozen milk

DEFINITION   Techniques used to safely prepare frozen milk for consumption by baby.

> **Notes**
>
> Thaw milk in its container.
>   Milk can be safely thawed by:
>   Placing frozen containers in the refrigerator.
>   Holding frozen containers under lukewarm running tap water.
>   Placing frozen containers in lukewarm water. Hot water is not recommended
>   due to potential nutrient loss.
>   Milk should never be boiled or microwaved.
>   Milk does not need to be overly warm before being fed to infant.[177]

See also Collection and storage of breastmilk; Storage of breastmilk

Footnotes

[177] Arnold, L.D.W. (2004). *Safe storage of expressed breastmilk for the healthy infant and child.* East Sandwich, MA: Health Education Associates.

▶ Thrush

DEFINITION   Overgrowth of *Candida albicans* or other common fungi.

Symptoms of yeast infection of the breast include red, shiny looking skin on the nipple or areola, flaky skin, and sharp, itching pain that persists between feedings. Infant symptoms of yeast overgrowth or "thrush" include white patches of growth on the inner buccal surface (cheek) or tongue, and occasionally pain on latch. Infants may also have diaper area yeast overgrowth.

Ask about

Onset.
Medications taken in past month.

ASSESSMENT

PROMPT CARE NEEDED?

Are any of the following present?

Sharp, itching, persistent nipple pain (during as well as between feedings).
Flaky, shiny, or itchy skin on the nipple surface.
Presence of white patches in infant's mouth.

IF YES,   *Call medical care provider today.*

ROUTINE CARE NEEDED?

Are any of the following present?

Nipple pain during feeding.

IF YES,   *Call lactation care provider today.*

SELF CARE INFORMATION

Finish all medications prescribed.

If administering nystatin suspension to the infant, pour a dose into a clean cup or spoon. Half of the dose should be used for each side of the mouth. Suspension may be applied with a cotton swab. A clean swab should be used for each application. Take care not to introduce used swabs into the bottle of suspension.

IMPORTANT CONDITIONS TO REPORT

Persistent symptoms after completion of a course of treatment.
Recurrent symptoms.

Candida overgrowth may follow or increase after antibiotic treatment.

Recommended treatment for candidiasis is topical antifungal (nystatin).

If symptoms are not relieved by topical treatment, feeding evaluation should occur to rule out positioning or attachment problems contributing to pain.

Medical evaluation should rule out other conditions resulting in redness and pain, including **eczema**, reaction to surface allergens, trauma, **Raynaud's phenomenon**, concomitant bacteria, and infection.

Subsequent treatment with oral antifungals such as ketaconazole or fluconazole may resolve symptoms.

Lactation evaluation should rule out contributing problems with latch or distortion of nipple in baby's mouth.

See also Nipple pain

▶ Thyroid disease

DEFINITION   Breastfeeding is not contraindicated for women who have had thyroid disease—either hypothyroidism (low levels of the thyroid hormones) or hyperthyroidism (high levels of the thyroid hormones)—and now have normal thyroid levels.

Women with hypothyroidism are prescribed thyroid replacement therapy and can breastfeed. The medications for this condition are compatible with breastfeeding.

A woman whose hyperthyroid problem (thyroiditis) is suspected during pregnancy or lactation presents a special problem in the diagnosis and treatment. The mother should tell all health care providers that she is breastfeeding.

Many of the signs and symptoms of thyroid disease can seem "normal" to a postpartum woman. The symptom that is unique to breastfeeding is difficulty initiating and maintaining an adequate milk supply.

Both high and low levels of thyroid hormones can affect the milk supply.

Ask about

Age of baby.
Weight gain pattern of baby.

EMERGENT CARE NEEDED?

Are any of the following present?

About baby

Extreme lethargy or irritability.

Sudden change in baby's muscle tone (extremely floppy or stiff) or repetitive jerking movements (e.g., seizure activity).

Baby shows sudden disinterest in feeding.

Unable to wake baby.

Baby does not calm, even with cuddles.

Meconium bowel movements after 5 days of life.

Fewer than three bowel movements daily in breastfed newborn after the first 2 days of life.

No urine in six hours.

Brick dust urine (uric acid crystals) after 2 days of life.

Dark colored urine.

Fewer than four urinations daily in the breastfed newborn after day 5 of life.

Noticeably sunken fontanelles (soft spot on top of head).

Decreased activity.

Baby below birthweight at 10 to 14 days of life.

Cessation of weight gain.

Lethargy.

Hard to latch-on.

Weak suck.

Sleepy, difficult to rouse.

IF YES, *Seek pediatric care now.*

PROMPT CARE NEEDED?

Are any of the following present?

About mother

Signs and symptoms of hypothyroidism, including:

Persistent fatigue.

Weakness.

Weight gain or difficulty losing weight (difficult to ascertain in postpartum).

Coarse, dry hair.

Dry, rough skin.

Hair loss (difficult to notice in pregnant and postpartum women unless it is severe).

Inability to tolerate cold as well as others in the same environment.

Muscle cramps and aches.

Constipation.

Depression (may be assumed to be "baby blues").

Irritability.

Memory loss.

Abnormal menstrual periods (it is normal for breastfeeding women to not menstruate in the first several months postpartum).

Decreased sexual desire (normal in postpartum women).

Signs and symptoms of hyperthyroidism, including:

Palpitations.

Heat intolerance.

Nervousness.

Insomnia.

Breathlessness.

Increased bowel movements.

Light or absent menstrual periods.

Fatigue.

Weight loss.

Fast heart rate.

Trembling hands.

Muscle weakness.

Warm, moist skin.

Hair loss.

IF YES,   *Report to maternal medical care provider today.*

ROUTINE CARE NEEDED?

Are any of the following present?

Questions about building up milk supply after diagnosis of thyroid problem.

Questions about drug compatibility.

IF YES,   *Call lactation care provider today and consult up-to-date drug references.*

SELF CARE INFORMATION

Postpartum thyroid problems can initially present as postpartum depression or just normal tiredness or fatigue. Mothers who struggle with milk supply should have a thorough medical evaluation if the supply does not improve with increased frequency and expression.

IMPORTANT CONDITIONS TO REPORT

Increasing sleepiness in baby.
Increasing fatigue and inability to cope in the mother.
Feelings of hopelessness or depression.
Symptoms of thyroid disease.

See also Hyperthyroidism; Hypothyroidism; Lactational Amenorrhea Method (LAM); Maternal fatigue; Postpartum depression; Slow weight gain, baby

▶ Toddler and young child nursing

DEFINITION Nursing is different as the baby grows through new ages and stages. Each stage is a new experience for mother and child. Breastfeeding is still a valuable experience for toddlers and young children, and breastmilk continues to provide nourishment and immune factors.

Ask about

Age of baby.

ASSESSMENT

ROUTINE CARE NEEDED?
Are any of the following present?
Strategies needed for breastfeeding toddlers and young children.
Strategies needed for weaning toddlers and young children.

IF YES,   *Call lactation care provider.*

Nursing is different at different ages; do not expect the experience to always be the same.

See also Closet nursing; Milk production; Tandem nursing; Weaning

▶ # Tongue exercises

DEFINITION   Because the tongue is a muscle, it can be exercised. If a baby is having a problem nursing because of the tongue, occupational therapists, speech and language therapists, and physical therapists can help babies' tongues become more fit for suckling through specific exercises.

Ask about

Age of baby.
Weight gain pattern of baby.

ASSESSMENT

PROMPT CARE NEEDED?
Are any of the following present?
About baby
Lethargy (sleepy, difficult to rouse).
Hard to latch-on.
Weak suck.
Extreme irritability in baby.
Sudden change in baby's muscle tone (extremely floppy or stiff) or repetitive jerking movements (e.g., seizure activity).
Baby shows sudden disinterest in feeding.
Baby does not calm, even with cuddles.
Meconium bowel movements after 5 days of life.
Fewer than three bowel movements daily in breastfed newborn after the first 2 days of life.
No urine in six hours.

Brick dust urine (uric acid crystals) after 2 days of life.

Dark colored urine.

Fewer than four urinations daily in the breastfed newborn after day 5 of life.

Noticeably sunken fontanelles (soft spot on top of head).

Decreased activity.

Baby below birthweight at 10 to 14 days of life.

Cessation of weight gain.

IF YES, *Seek pediatric care now.*

ROUTINE CARE NEEDED?

Are any of the following present?

Baby appears not to be using tongue correctly during feeding, resulting in difficulty latching baby onto breast or sustaining feedings.

Nipple pain for mother.

Clicking sounds heard during feeding.

IF YES, *Call lactation care provider today and refer to occupational therapist, speech and language therapist, or physical therapist as needed.*

SELF CARE INFORMATION

A baby's tongue can be trained to suckle more effectively by doing specific exercises.

See also Down syndrome; Occupational therapy; Pierre Robin sequence

▶ Tongue-tie

DEFINITION A tight lingual frenulum (the membrane attaching the tongue to the bottom of the mouth). This condition is also called ankyloglossia.

When the frenulum is tight, it can restrict the movement of the tongue, resulting in breastfeeding problems for some mothers and babies.

Ask about

Age of baby.

Appearance of tongue.

PROMPT CARE NEEDED?

Are any of the following present?

Tight lingual frenulum in baby.

Nipple or breast pain.

Difficulty latching baby to breast and/or sustaining latch.

History of recurrent breast infection.

Milk supply problems.

Poor growth of breastfed infant.

IF YES, *Call lactation care provider today.*

Are any of the following present?

Presence of tight lingual frenulum in baby in conjunction with feeding problems and/or breast/nipple problems in breastfeeding mother.

IF YES, *Report to pediatrician.*

SELF CARE INFORMATION

Practice skin-to-skin contact frequently.

Feed baby at first sign of hunger cues (signs that say "feed me" include hand-to-face or hand-to-mouth movements, lip smacking, seeking with lips, rooting, and head bobbing).

Practice good attachment:

Watch for feeding cues and offer the breast as soon as it is seen.

Wait for baby to open mouth wide (greater than a 100° angle).

Pull baby in so that chin touches the breast first, and nipple enters the mouth along the top of the tongue; this should result in a wide open mouth on breast.

Lips should be flanged outward.

Baby's lips should look off center when compared with the areola; the bottom lip should be farther away from the nipple than the top lip.

IMPORTANT CONDITIONS TO REPORT

Unresolved symptoms.

Ongoing concerns.

See also Nipple pain

Footnotes

[178]Ballard, J.L., Auer, C.E., & Khoury, J.C. (2002). Ankyloglossia: Assessment, incidence, and effect of frenuloplasty on the breastfeeding dyad. *Pediatrics, 110*(5), e63.

▶ Torticollis

DEFINITION   Injury and spasms of the muscles of the neck cause the head to fall to one side, often with the chin pointing to the other side. Womb position and birth injury may contribute to the development of this condition, which develops gradually over the first days of life. Nursing mothers of babies with torticollis may need help finding comfortable positions for nursing.

See also Birth injury

▶ Tracheoesophageal (TE) fistula

DEFINITION   A tracheoesophageal (TE) fistula is a small opening between the trachea, which leads from the mouth to the lungs, and the esophagus, which leads from the mouth to the stomach. The two passageways are right next to each other in the throat.

When a baby is born with a TE fistula there is a chance that food (breastmilk or formula) can easily get into the lungs and cause chemical pneumonia. Therefore, the baby is usually not fed right away.

TE fistulas are considered a surgical emergency.

The mother should begin expressing milk as soon as possible in order to initiate and maintain her milk supply. Her milk may be given to the baby through a feeding tube until the baby is able to go to the breast.

Ask about

Age of baby.
Surgical history.

ASSESSMENT

ROUTINE CARE NEEDED?
Are any of the following present?
Problems with milk supply with baby with TE fistula.
Baby has difficulty breastfeeding after surgery.

IF YES, *Call lactation care provider today.*

SELF CARE INFORMATION
The mother should begin expressing milk as soon as possible in order to initiate and maintain her milk supply. Her milk may be given to the baby through a feeding tube until the baby is able to go to the breast.

IMPORTANT CONDITIONS TO REPORT
Complications as described by the hospital discharge team.

See also Breathing, sucking, swallowing; Hospitalization and breastfeeding; Tube feeding

▶ Transitional milk

DEFINITION The stages of human milk are: (1) colostrum, (2) transitional milk, and (3) mature milk. Milk content changes gradually from colostrum to mature milk in the first two weeks after the baby is born. From about seven days to two weeks postpartum the milk is called transitional milk.

See also Colostrum; Mature milk

▶ Transition to breastfeeding

DEFINITION   Babies may be fed away from the breast for some time and then transition to breastfeeding. For example, a premature baby may be tube fed at first and then need to learn how to suckle at the breast and effectively transfer milk.

Ask about

Age of baby.
How the baby is currently being fed (away from the breast).
What the baby is currently being fed.

ASSESSMENT

ROUTINE CARE NEEDED?
Are any of the following present?
Strategies needed to transition baby to breastfeeding.
Desire to feed the baby at the breast.

IF YES, *Call lactation care provider.*

SELF CARE INFORMATION
Babies can be successfully breastfed, even after a substantial time being fed away from the breast.

See also At-breast supplementation; Milk production; Premature infant; Relactation; Skin-to-skin (STS) contact

▶ Triplets

DEFINITION   Three babies from the same pregnancy are called triplets.

Mothers can make enough milk to support triplets, usually with a combination of expressing and nursing.

SELF CARE INFORMATION

Pumping should start as soon as possible after the babies are born.

Many mothers of multiples have found it helpful to keep a journal of "who nursed when," number of wet and dirty diapers, and weight gain for each baby, to ensure that none of the babies is being overlooked.

Mothers of triplets may have been on bed rest during their pregnancies and can become easily fatigued. Advise them to ask for help.

Suggest easy ways for mothers to snack and drink while caring for triplets.

IMPORTANT CONDITIONS TO REPORT

Lethargy.

Decrease in urine and stools.

Change in breastfeeding behavior.

Problems with feeding.

See also **Higher order multiples (HOM); Multiple infants (twins, triplets, and higher order multiples); Premature infant**

▶ Tubal ligation

DEFINITION   Tubal ligation is a surgical procedure that is commonly referred to as "tying the tubes."

The fallopian tubes transport mature eggs from the ovary to the uterus about one time a month. Sperm travels from the uterus up the fallopian tube. If the sperm encounters a mature egg, fertilization may occur.

Tubal ligation is a form of permanent sterilization. To stop fertilization, the egg is prevented from traveling down the tube and the sperm is prevented from traveling up.

Ask about

Mothers often make a plan to have a tubal ligation before leaving the hospital after the birth of a baby.

ASSESSMENT

ROUTINE CARE NEEDED?
Are any of the following present?
Nursing after surgery.

IF YES, *Ask the surgeon about the course of the surgery and recovery and how long separation from baby will be.*

ROUTINE CARE NEEDED?
Are any of the following present?
Possibility of drugs and anesthesia passing into the milk.

IF YES, *Consult up-to-date drug references.*

SELF CARE INFORMATION
Always tell your health care providers that you intend to breastfeed or that you are breastfeeding.
Ask your health care providers if there are choices in drugs and anesthesia that would make the separation from the baby shorter.
When you are reunited with the baby, start with skin-to-skin care.

See also Hospitalization and breastfeeding; Skin-to-skin (STS) care

Drug References

American Academy of Pediatrics Committee on Drugs. (2001). Transfer of drugs and other chemicals into human milk. *Pediatrics, 108*, 776–789.

Briggs, G.G., Freeman, R.K., & Yaffee, S.J. (Eds.). (2002). *Drugs in pregnancy and lactation* (6th ed.). Philadelphia: Lippincott, Williams, and Wilkins.

Hale, T.W. (2004). *Medications and mothers milk.* Amarillo, TX: Pharmasoft Publishing.

Lawrence, R.A., & Lawrence, R.M. (2005). *Breastfeeding: A guide for the medical profession* (6th ed.). St. Louis: Mosby.

▶ Tube feeding

DEFINITION   A baby can be fed through tubing threaded through its nose or mouth and ending in the stomach or small intestine. Sometimes the tube is attached to a pump that feeds the baby continuously. Other times babies are fed a "bolus" feed through a syringe attached to the tubing.

Premature babies are often tube fed before they can coordinate their suck-swallow-breathe reflex or have the cardio-respiratory stability to feed orally.

Term babies may be tube fed for a variety of medical and surgical reasons. Colostrum and breastmilk can be fed to the baby through the tube.

Babies who are tube fed are usually given pacifiers to suck on.

Ask about

Age of baby.
Baby's feeding history.

ASSESSMENT

ROUTINE CARE NEEDED?

Are any of the following present?

Questions about obtaining a breast pump.
Transition to breastfeeding.
Questions about milk supply.
Questions about expressing milk.
Questions about collecting and storing milk.

IF YES,   *Call lactation care provider.*

Even though the baby can only be given a small amount of milk now, mothers whose babies are being tube fed should maximize their milk production.

Skin-to-skin care offers a way to feel close to the baby, even when breastfeeding is not possible.

IMPORTANT CONDITIONS TO REPORT

Decreasing milk supply.

See also At-breast supplementation; Gavage feeding; Premature infant; Skin-to-skin (STS) care; Transition to breastfeeding

▶ Tubercles of Montgomery (Montgomery glands)

DEFINITION   A group of 12–20 tubercles scattered around the areola of the breast that enlarge during pregnancy and lactation. These tubercles are connected to a combination of lactiferous glands and sebaceous glands. The substance secreted is both lubricating and antimicrobial.

SELF CARE INFORMATION

Excessive cleaning of the breast and areola is not necessary or recommended.

IMPORTANT CONDITIONS TO REPORT

Blocked or infected Montgomery glands (these can be difficult to distinguish from herpes lesions and should be reported to obstetrician for differential diagnosis).

See also Blisters on nipple or breast; Breast structure

▶ Tuberculosis (TB) and breastfeeding

DEFINITION   Tuberculosis (TB) is a disease that is primarily spread through the air. The disease is spread when a person with active TB coughs, sneezes, speaks, sings, or laughs. Tiny droplets fly through the air.

It usually takes lengthy contact with someone who has active TB before a person can become infected.

People who have been treated with appropriate drugs for at least two weeks are no longer contagious and do not spread the germ to others.

A mother with newly diagnosed active TB is separated from her baby during the initial two weeks of treatment. She can express her milk and it can be fed to her baby. The baby will be tested and may also be treated.

TB can be responsible for mastitis. This is called tuberculosis mastitis. If the mother has this form of TB, the organism can be transmitted in her milk.

Except for women with tubercular mastitis, TB has not been found to pass through the milk.

Ask about

Age of baby.
Diagnosis of TB.

ASSESSMENT

PROMPT CARE NEEDED?
Are any of the following present?
Plan for feeding baby during separation needed.

IF YES, *Call pediatric care provider today and seek lactation care today.*

ROUTINE CARE NEEDED?
Are any of the following present?
Plan for expressing milk needed.
TB drug regime compatibility with breastmilk and breastfeeding.
Transition to breastfeeding.

IF YES, *Seek lactation care today.*

SELF CARE INFORMATION
Treatment for TB can save your life. Take all the medications as prescribed. If you cannot take the drug for some reason, tell your doctor right away.

IMPORTANT CONDITIONS TO REPORT
Declining milk supply.

See also Contraindicated conditions; Expression of mothers' milk;
Hospitalization and breastfeeding; Transition to breastfeeding

▶ Twins

DEFINITION   Two babies from the same pregnancy are called twins. Twins may be
identical or fraternal.

Mothers can make enough milk to support twins. Nursing two babies at the
same time boosts milk production.

ASSESSMENT

ROUTINE CARE NEEDED?

Are any of the following present?

Strategies needed for managing the nursing of twins.

Strategies needed for managing milk supply for twins.

IF YES,   *Call lactation care provider today.*

SELF CARE INFORMATION

Pumping should start as soon as possible after the babies are born.

Many mothers of multiples have found it helpful to keep a journal of "who nursed
when," number of wet and dirty diapers, and weight gain for each baby, to ensure
that none of the babies is being overlooked.

Mothers of twins may have been on bed rest during their pregnancies and can
become easily fatigued. Advise them to ask for help.

Suggest easy ways for mothers to snack and drink while caring for twins.

IMPORTANT CONDITIONS TO REPORT

Lethargy.

Decrease in urine and stools.

Change in breastfeeding behavior.

Problems with feeding.

See also Multiple infants (twins, triplets, and higher order multiples); Premature infant

▶ Type 1 diabetes (IDDM)

DEFINITION   A chronic disease causing high levels of sugar in the blood, diabetes is caused by too little insulin or resistance to insulin. Also known as insulin dependent diabetes mellitus (IDDM).

Type 1 diabetes is usually diagnosed in childhood. The pancreas makes little or no insulin, requiring daily injections of this hormone that regulates sugar metabolism.

Women with this condition can breastfeed their babies.

Ask about

Onset.

ASSESSMENT

EMERGENT CARE NEEDED?

Are any of the following present?

Insulin shock (**hypoglycemia**) in the breastfeeding woman. (Symptoms of insulin shock include rapid pulse, rapid breathing, dizziness or altered consciousness, weakness, blurred vision, headache, sweating, and numbness of hands or feet.)

IF YES,   *Seek emergency care now.*

PROMPT CARE NEEDED?

Are any of the following present?

Difficulty maintaining blood glucose levels during breastfeeding.

IF YES,   *Report to medical care provider and seek dietary consultation.*

SELF CARE INFORMATION

Women with diabetes are more prone to infection. Monitor breasts and nipples daily for any red, infected, or painful areas.

If insulin dependent, be aware that less insulin may be required during breastfeeding—watch for signs of low blood sugar.

IMPORTANT CONDITIONS TO REPORT

Any symptoms of infection.

Difficulty regulating blood sugar.

Notes

Women with diabetes should be encouraged to breastfeed.

Research suggests that women who have experienced gestational diabetes are less likely to develop diabetes if they breastfeed their babies.[179]

See also Autoimmune diseases

Footnotes

[179]Kjos, S.L., Henry, O., Lee, R.M., Buchanan, T.A., & Mishell, D.R., Jr. (1993). The effect of lactation on glucose metabolism in women with recent gestational diabetes. *Obstetrics & Gynecology, 82*(3), 451–455.

▶ Typhoid fever

DEFINITION   A life-threatening illness caused by the organism *Salmonella typhi* (*S. typhi*). Although typhoid fever affects about 12.5 million people per year worldwide, there are only about 400 cases per year in the United States.

The *S. typhi* organism lives only in humans. People with typhoid fever carry the organism in their bloodstream and intestinal tract. They will become ill and shed the organism in their stool. A few people carry the illness but do not become ill. They also shed the organism in their stool.

You can contract typhoid fever if you eat food or drink beverages that have been handled by a person who is shedding *S. typhi*. Sewage contaminated by *S. typhi* can get into the drinking water and be used for washing food. The food or drink will pass along the organism.

People with typhoid fever usually have a sustained fever as high as 103° F to 104° F (39° C to 40° C). Among other symptoms, they may have stomach pains, feel weak, and lose their appetites.

Vaccines are available. They are advisable for people who are traveling to parts of the world where typhoid fever is common. Travelers should determine whether drinking water in their intended destination is safe.

There is no evidence that *S. typhi* is passed through mothers' milk.

Ask about

Age of baby.
Onset of typhoid fever.

ASSESSMENT

EMERGENT CARE NEEDED?

Are any of the following present?

Mother unable to care for baby.

Mother too ill to breastfeed or express milk on her own.

IF YES, *Seek medical and lactation care now.*

PROMPT CARE NEEDED?

Are any of the following present?

Compatibility of prescribed drugs with breastfeeding.

IF YES, *Consult up-to-date drug references.*

ROUTINE CARE NEEDED?

Are any of the following present?

Transitioning baby back to breastfeeding.

Lowered milk supply.

IF YES, *Call lactation care provider today.*

SELF CARE INFORMATION

Take all medications as prescribed, even after you feel better.

Follow all of the self care instructions (drink extra fluids, rest, etc.).

Practice good hygiene through regular hand washing.

Follow eating and drinking guidelines when traveling to areas of the world with poor sanitation.

IMPORTANT CONDITIONS TO REPORT

Declining milk supply.

See also Expression of mothers' milk; Hospitalization and breastfeeding; Medications

Drug References

American Academy of Pediatrics Committee on Drugs. (2001). Transfer of drugs and other chemicals into human milk. *Pediatrics, 108,* 776–789.

Briggs, G.G., Freeman, R.K., & Yaffee, S.J. (Eds.). (2002). *Drugs in pregnancy and lactation* (6th ed.). Philadelphia: Lippincott, Williams, and Wilkins.

Hale, T.W. (2004). *Medications and mothers milk.* Amarillo, TX: Pharmasoft Publishing.

Lawrence, R.A., & Lawrence, R.M. (2005). *Breastfeeding: A guide for the medical profession* (6th ed.). St. Louis: Mosby.

▶ Uncoordinated suckling

DEFINITION Efficient milk transfer at the breast depends on a coordinated suck and swallow.

Babies more likely to have an uncoordinated suck at first include:

Babies who are born prematurely.

Babies who have been exposed to certain drugs.

Babies who have neurological impairment.

Age of baby.
Feeding history.
Weight gain history.

ASSESSMENT

EMERGENT CARE NEEDED?

Are any of the following present?

Difficulty breathing even when not feeding.
Difficullty breathing after feeding.
Baby pulls off of the breast to breathe.
Extreme **lethargy or irritability** in baby.
Sudden change in baby's muscle tone (extremely floppy or stiff) or repetitive jerking movements (e.g., seizure activity).
Baby shows sudden disinterest in feeding.
Unable to wake baby.
Baby does not calm, even with cuddles.
Meconium bowel movements after 5 days of life.
Fewer than three bowel movements daily in breastfed newborn after the first 2 days of life.
No urine in six hours.
Brick dust urine (uric acid crystals) after 2 days of life.
Dark colored urine.
Fewer than four urinations daily in the breastfed newborn after day 5 of life.
Noticeably sunken fontanelles (soft spot on top of head).
Baby below birthweight at 10 to 14 days of life.
Cessation of weight gain.

IF YES, *Seek pediatric care now.*

PROMPT CARE NEEDED?

Are any of the following present?

Diagnosis of neuromuscular problem in a breastfeeding baby.

IF YES, *Refer for consultation with occupational, physical, or speech therapist experienced with breastfeeding babies.*

> **Are any of the following present?**
>> Baby does not stay on the breast.
>> Baby is not gaining adequately.
>> Baby does not seem to transfer milk.
>
> **IF YES,** *Call lactation care provider now.*

ROUTINE CARE NEEDED?
> **Are any of the following present?**
>> Difficulty maintaining milk supply.
>
> **IF YES,** *Call lactation care provider today.*

SELF CARE INFORMATION

As soon as it is determined that the infant has an uncoordinated suck, mother should express her milk regularly in order to maintain her supply and to collect milk to feed the baby.

Increased opportunities to practice breastfeeding can be helpful to promote coordinated sucking.

Skin-to-skin holding may improve motor organization of babies.

IMPORTANT CONDITIONS TO REPORT

Inadequate stooling or urinations.

Lethargy.

Difficult to rouse.

Lower milk volume.

See also **Alternate breast massage; Botulism, infantile; Breast pump; Lethargy; Sleepy baby; Weak suck; Weight gain, baby–low**

▶ UNICEF

See also **United Nations Children's Fund (UNICEF)**

▶ Unilateral

DEFINITION   One sided.

▶ United Nations Children's Fund (UNICEF)

DEFINITION   "UNICEF is the driving force that helps build a world where the rights of every child are realized. We have the global authority to influence decision-makers, and the variety of partners at grassroots level to turn the most innovative ideas into reality. That makes us unique among world organizations, and unique among those working with the young."[180]

Notes

UNICEF International: UNICEF House
3 United Nations Plaza
New York, NY 10017
Phone: 212-326-7000
Web site: www.unicef.org

UNICEF USA
338 East 38th Street
New York, NY 10016
Phone: 212-686-5522
Web site: www.unicefusa.org

See also Baby-Friendly Hospital Initiative (BFHI); Baby-Friendly USA; Ten Steps to Successful Breastfeeding

Footnotes

[180]United Nations Children's Fund. (n.d.). *About UNICEF: Who we are.* Retrieved August 4, 2005, from http://www.unicef.org/about/who/index.html.

▶ United States Breastfeeding Committee (USBC)

DEFINITION   "The USBC is a collaborative partnership of organizations. The mission of the committee is to protect, promote and support breastfeeding in the U.S. The USBC exists to assure the rightful place of breastfeeding in society."[181]

> **Notes**
>
> United States Breastfeeding Committee (USBC)
> 2025 M Street NW
> Suite 800
> Washington, DC 20036
> Phone: 202-367-1132
> E-mail: info@usbreastfeeding.org
> Web site: www.usbreastfeeding.org

Footnotes

[181]United States Breastfeeding Committee. (n.d.). *A brief history of the United States Breastfeeding Committee.* Retrieved August 24, 2005 from http://www.usbreastfeeding.org/History.html.

▶ United States Department of Agriculture (USDA), WIC program

DEFINITION   WIC is a supplemental food program for women, infants, and children that is administered through the United States Department of Agriculture (USDA).
"The mission of WIC is to safeguard the health of low-income women, infants, and children up to age 5 who are at nutritional risk by providing nutritional foods to supplement diets, information on healthy eating, and referrals to health care."[182]

Breastfeeding rates among WIC participants are rising. The percentage of WIC participants who initiated breastfeeding increased by 69% over a 10-year period. The percentage of women who breastfed at 6 months increased by 145% during the same time period.[183]

Notes

WIC at FNS Headquarters:
Supplemental Food Programs Division
Food and Nutrition Service - USDA
3101 Park Center Drive
Alexandria, VA 22302
Phone: 703-305-2746
Fax: 703-305-2196
Web site: www.fns.usda.gov/wic

Footnotes

[182]The Special Supplemental Nutrition Program for Women, Infants, and Children. (2003). *WIC's mission*. Retrieved August 4, 2005, from http://www.fns.usda.gov/wic/aboutwic/mission.htm.

[183]United States Department of Agriculture. (2003). *WIC and breastfeeding rates* (Food and Nutrition Research Report, Number 34-2). Washington, DC.

▶ Universal precautions

DEFINITION   Universal precautions are infection control guidelines designed to protect workers from exposure to diseases and certain body fluids. Universal precautions do not apply to breastmilk, except for workers in a milk bank setting.

Wearing gloves when handling breastmilk (thawing, heating, and preparing feedings) helps to ensure that the milk will not be contaminated.

▶ Urinary tract infection (UTI)

DEFINITION   A urinary tract infection (UTI) is an infection anywhere in the urinary tract. This includes the kidneys, ureter, bladder, and urethra.

Usually, a UTI is caused by bacteria that can also live in the intestines, in the vagina, or around the urethra, which is at the entrance to the urinary tract. The body typically removes the bacteria.

Signs and symptoms of UTI include:

  Burning sensation during urination.

  Frequent urge to urinate, even with scanty amount of urine.

  Pain in the back or in the lower abdomen.

  Cloudy, dark, bloody, or unusual smelling urine.

  Fever or chills.

Breastfeeding is not contraindicated when the mother has a UTI. Breastfeeding confers some protection against urinary tract infections in infants.[184]

Ask about

Age of baby.

Onset of UTI.

ASSESSMENT

ROUTINE CARE NEEDED?

Are any of the following present?

Prescribed medication compatibility with breastfeeding.

IF YES,   *Consult up-to-date drug references.*

SELF CARE INFORMATION

Follow medical advice and take medication as prescribed.

See also Acute infection

Footnotes

  [184]Pisacane, A., Graziano, L., Mazzarella, G., Scarpellino, B., & Zona, G. (1992). Breastfeeding and urinary tract infection. *Journal of Pediatrics, 120*(1), 87–89.

► **USBC**

  See also United States Breastfeeding Committee (USBC)

► ## USDA

See also Special Supplemental Food Program for Women, Infants, and Children (WIC)

► ## Uterine bleeding

DEFINITION Flow of blood from the healing wall of the uterus. Vaginal blood flow is expected after delivery. This blood is also called lochia.

Three types of lochia are recognized, including lochia rubra (red), lochia serosa (pink), and lochia alba (white). Lochia rubra, a red discharge, begins after delivery and continues for two to three days. Lochia serosa, a paler, pinkish discharge continues for the next week or so. Lochia alba, a whitish discharge, starts around the tenth day postpartum and should be resolved within a month.[185]

Ask about

Onset.
Date of delivery.

ASSESSMENT

EMERGENT CARE NEEDED?

Are any of the following present?

Soaking a sanitary napkin with bright red blood at a rate of one napkin or more per hour.

Clots in the bloody discharge.

Foul odor to the discharge (even if occasional).

Dizziness.

Fever.

Abdominal pain.

IF YES, *Call obstetric care provider now or seek emergency care now.*

PROMPT MEDICAL CARE NEEDED?

Are any of the following present?

Soaking a sanitary napkin with bright red blood at a rate of one napkin every two to three hours.

Abdominal tenderness.

Low-grade fever.

Lightheadedness.

IF YES,   *Call obstetric care provider within 2 to 4 hours.*

PROMPT LACTATION CARE NEEDED?

Are any of the following present?

Problems with milk supply in a woman diagnosed with retained placental fragments.

IF YES,   *Call lactation care provider today.*

ROUTINE CARE NEEDED?

Are any of the following present?

Soaking a sanitary napkin with bright red blood at a rate of one napkin every three or more hours.

Abdominal tenderness.

IF YES,   *Call obstetric care provider today.*

SELF CARE INFORMATION

Monitor blood flow.

IMPORTANT CONDITIONS TO REPORT

Continuation of symptoms.

Sudden gushing of blood.

Multiple blood clots passed.

Concerns about milk supply.

As time progresses, the volume of lochia should also decrease. Sudden return of bright red bleeding is of concern and should be evaluated medically. Retained placental fragments can be indicated by ongoing lochia rubra. In this event, mature milk production may not occur until placental fragments are expelled or removed.

See also Lochia; Postpartum hemorrhage; Retained placental fragments

Footnotes

[185]Varney, H., Kriebs, J.M., & Gegor, C.L. (Eds.). (2004). *Varney's midwifery* (4th ed., p. 1043). Sudbury, MA: Jones & Bartlett Publishers.

▶ # UTI

See also Urinary tract infection (UTI)

▶ # Vaccinations and immunizations

DEFINITION   Breastfeeding provides baby's first immunization (vaccination). After that, breastfed babies should be immunized on the same schedule as babies who are not breastfed.

Mothers who are breastfeeding can receive most immunizations except smallpox vaccination. Mothers should not receive the smallpox vaccine even if they are pumping their milk and feeding their babies breastmilk in a bottle.

ASSESSMENT

ROUTINE CARE NEEDED?
Are any of the following present?
Vaccination or immunizations for mother or baby.

IF YES,   *Consult up-to-date drug references.*

SELF CARE INFORMATION

Follow medical recommendations for after immunization care.

Babies are comforted by nursing during and after painful procedures.

IMPORTANT CONDITIONS TO REPORT

The health care provider will provide a list of important conditions to report after vaccinations and immunizations.

See also Immunization

Drug References

American Academy of Pediatrics Committee on Drugs. (2001). Transfer of drugs and other chemicals into human milk. *Pediatrics, 108,* 776–789.

Briggs, G.G., Freeman, R.K., & Yaffee, S.J. (Eds.). (2002). *Drugs in pregnancy and lactation* (6th ed.). Philadelphia: Lippincott, Williams, and Wilkins.

Hale, T.W. (2004). *Medications and mothers milk.* Amarillo, TX: Pharmasoft Publishing.

Lawrence, R.A., & Lawrence, R.M. (2005). *Breastfeeding: A guide for the medical profession* (6th ed.). St. Louis: Mosby.

► Varicella zoster virus

DEFINITION   Refers to the characteristic lesions, "chicken pox," resulting from infection with *Varicella zoster,* a virus of the herpes family. This highly infectious virus is passed via droplet and direct contact with lesions. Exposure can be serious for the newborn. If mother is judged safe to be with her infant, and she has no lesions on the breast area, breastfeeding is considered safe.

Ask about

Onset.

Age of baby.

Infection of any household members.

EMERGENT CARE NEEDED?

Are any of the following present?

Eruption of chicken pox in a newborn infant.

Presence of chicken pox lesions on the breast and nipple area.

IF YES, *Report to medical care provider immediately.*

Notes

Mothers who are infected in the early perinatal period may infect their infants by passing droplets and allowing infant contact with lesions. Infection risk may be decreased by administering varicella zoster immunoglobulin (VZIG) to the infant.

If a breastfeeding mother is separated from her baby, she should be encouraged to express or pump her milk eight or more times daily to maintain her milk supply. If she has no lesions on the breast or nipple area, her milk may be given to the baby. Careful handwashing should be practiced to avoid involving the breast or collected milk.

If only siblings are infected, baby and mother should be isolated and continue breastfeeding.

See Lawrence & Lawrence for an excellent protocol for *Varicella zoster* in the peripartum.[186]

See also Acute infection

Footnotes

[186]Lawrence, R.A., & Lawrence, R.M. (2005). *Breastfeeding: A guide for the medical profession* (6th ed., p. 655). St. Louis: Mosby.

▶ Vasospasm of breast and nipple

DEFINITION   Nipple pain may happen because of Raynaud's phenomenon/syndrome. This is a condition in which blood flow to the extremities is temporarily reduced. The condition has also been called nipple vasospasm. The affected extremity becomes cold and numb and turns white. As the blood flow returns, it may quickly turn blue and then reddish pink. This is the tri-color sign of Raynaud's. There is also a bi-color sign (white and pink). As the color returns the pain increases. The pain can be brief, lasting for just a few minutes, or prolonged, lasting up to an hour.

The reaction occurs in response to cold, wetness, stress, and certain medications.

Usually the fingers and toes are affected, but the nipples are also extremities and can therefore be affected.

Ask about

Age of baby.
History of nipple pain.

ASSESSMENT

ROUTINE CARE NEEDED?
Are any of the following present?
Persistent nipple pain.
Breast pain in reaction to cold, wet, and nursing.
Tri-color sign (white, blue, pink) or bi-color sign (white, pink) of the nipple when cold or wet.

IF YES, *Call obstetric care provider today and call lactation care provider today.*

IMPORTANT CONDITIONS TO REPORT
If Nifedipine is prescribed, seek medical help in the case of adverse reactions described in the package insert.

SELF CARE INFORMATION
Nifedipine (Adalat, Procardia) is a prescription medication (calcium channel blocker) that has been used to treat Raynaud's Phenomenon/Syndrome in nursing mothers.
Mothers with Raynaud's syndrome are usually advised to avoid caffeine and nicotine.

See also Nifedipine; Painful breastfeeding; Sore nipples

▶ Vegetarians

DEFINITION   Although many vegetarian diets are compatible with breastfeeding, some vegetarian diets (such as macrobiotic and vegan) may not be nutritionally adequate and can put the breastfed infant at risk of malnutrition. The major concerns of vegetarian diets are deficiencies of vitamins B_{12}, B_2, and D, and also the mineral zinc.

Ask about

Type of diet.
Age of baby.
Nutritional supplements taken.

ASSESSMENT

EMERGENT CARE NEEDED?

Are any of the following present?

Infant tetany (a condition characterized by painful muscle spasms and tremors).

Infant seizures.

IF YES,   *Seek emergency care now.*

PROMPT CARE NEEDED?

Are any of the following present?

Infant lethargy.

Change in infant feeding behavior.

Infant weight loss after the first week of life.

Slow growth in the breastfed infant of a macrobiotic mother.

IF YES,   *Seek pediatric care within 2 to 4 hours.*

SELF CARE INFORMATION

Nutritional risks of vegetarian diets are especially associated with protein, vitamins B_{12} and B_2, vitamin D, and zinc deficiencies.

IMPORTANT CONDITIONS TO REPORT

Lethargy and poor feeding behavior can be early signs of nutritional inadequacies.

Notes

Many people who are vegetarians are knowledgeable about including foods and supplements that balance their diets.

See also Macrobiotic diet of the mother; Maternal diet

▶ Vitamin supplements

DEFINITION　The American Academy of Pediatrics recommends that all babies receive a vitamin D supplement. This vitamin is ordinarily made in the skin when babies are exposed to sunlight. Today, babies may not be outside enough and when they are, they may be coated in sunscreen which prevents vitamin D from being formed in the skin.

When formula is manufactured, vitamin D is added. Mothers of breastfed babies give it separately as a liquid.

Mothers eating vegan diets are usually advised to supplement their diets with B vitamins, especially vitamin B_{12}. Vitamin D might also be advised for vegans.

Mothers who are eating a variety of foods are usually encouraged to continue taking their prenatal vitamins during lactation.

Age of baby.

ROUTINE CARE NEEDED?
Are any of the following present?
Questions about vitamin supplements for baby.
Questions about vitamin supplements for mother.

IF YES, *Call medical care provider and seek dietary consultation.*

See also Macrobiotic diet of the mother; Vegetarians

▶ Vomiting

DEFINITION Spitting up or vomiting in the infant can be differentiated from projectile vomiting by the distance it travels. Projectile vomit clears the chin of the infant. It may travel several feet. Spitting up does not clear the chin on its way out.

Spitting up, even after every feeding, may not be an indication that there is anything wrong with the baby. The mother may have a very powerful let-down reflex, for example.

SELF CARE INFORMATION
Occasional spitting up in an otherwise well infant is not uncommon.
Frequent spitting up, even in a baby with no other symptoms, can indicate that there is an underlying problem, such as gastroesophageal reflux.

IMPORTANT CONDITIONS TO REPORT
Projectile vomiting.
Bilious (green) vomit in a newborn (considered a surgical emergency unless proven otherwise).
Signs that the baby is unwell in combination with spitting up.
Decrease in stools and urinations.
Poor feeding behavior.
Weight loss, failure to gain adequately.

See also Gastroesophageal (GE) reflux; Let-down; Milk ejection; Projectile vomiting; Pyloric stenosis and breastfeeding

▶ WABA

See also World Alliance for Breastfeeding Action (WABA)

▶ Waking a sleepy baby

DEFINITION   Babies cycle between sleep and wakefulness more rapidly than adults. They have twice as many light sleep cycles as adults.

Newborn babies sleep about 18 hours a day on average, but their sleep is more interrupted than that of adults.

When babies cycle into lighter sleep (about every 20 minutes) their eyeballs move under their closed lids. They can nurse well at this stage of sleep, which is called REM (rapid eye movement) sleep.

Some babies are sleepy at first, making it difficult to get in 10–12 effective nursings a day.

There can be many reasons for this temporary condition, such as jaundice, drug effects from labor analgesia, and a difficult labor and birth.

Babies who are underfed are lethargic and sleepy. The more underfed they are, the more lethargic they become.

Sleepy babies should have a breastfeeding evaluation to determine whether or not they are being adequately fed.

Ask about

Age of baby.
Weight gain pattern.
History of sleepiness.

EMERGENT CARE NEEDED?

Are any of the following present?

Cannot rouse baby.

Baby sleeps more than 3 hours between feedings consistently.

Shallow breathing or breathing difficult to observe. (Observe the newborn's breathing for at least 1–2 minutes. Sleeping newborns often exhibit periodic breathing which may include rapid shallow breaths interspersed with brief pauses in breathing.)

Meconium bowel movements after 5 days of life.

Fewer than three bowel movements daily in breastfed newborn after the first 2 days of life.

No urine in six hours.

Brick dust urine (uric acid crystals) after 2 days of life.

Dark colored urine.

Fewer than four urinations daily in the breastfed newborn after day 5 of life.

Low muscle tone/floppiness.

IF YES, *Seek pediatric care now.*

PROMPT CARE NEEDED?

Are any of the following present?

Baby nurses fewer than 10 times in 24 hours.

Baby consistently falls asleep after sucking briefly at the breast.

Baby is not gaining at least 0.5 oz a day in the newborn period.

Baby does not sustain active suckling or feeding at the breast.

IF YES, *Seek lactation care today.*

SELF CARE INFORMATION

Babies need to be fed in order to sleep well, but sleepy babies are not necessarily well fed.

Parents who observe the baby for feeding cues—hand-to-face or hand-to-mouth movements, lip smacking, seeking with lips, rooting, and head bobbing—may find it easier to feed the baby at the baby's best time.

Young babies tend to cluster their feedings. Nurse the baby again when baby gives the next feeding cue (i.e., watch the baby, not the clock to determine the timing of the next feeding). The baby never completely empties the breast.

IMPORTANT CONDITIONS TO REPORT

Babies that are hard to rouse and sleep longer than three hours between nursings should be evaluated.

Babies who fall asleep after a minute or two at the breast should be evaluated.

See also Co-sleeping; Feeding cues; Feeding patterns; Hyperbilirubinemia; Hypotonia; Infant behavior; Lethargy; Milk production

▶ Water for the nursing baby (Water supplementation)

DEFINITION   Water is not needed for the nursing baby, even in hot, dry climates. Because babies have immature kidneys and a different body composition than adults, they are more vulnerable to water imbalance before 6 months of age.

Ask about

Age of baby.

Amount of water being supplemented.

ASSESSMENT

EMERGENT CARE NEEDED?

Are any of the following present in a baby being given extra water?

Seizures or convulsions, particularly facial movements and jerking of a body part.

Baby stops breathing and turns blue.

IF YES,   *Seek emergency care now.*

SELF CARE INFORMATION

Water is not needed for the nursing baby, even in hot, dry climates.

Because babies have a different body composition than adults, they are more vulnerable to water imbalance.

IMPORTANT CONDITIONS TO REPORT

More than eight wet diapers a day.

Giving baby extra water.

Seizures or convulsions, particularly facial movements and jerking of a body part.

Baby stops breathing and turns blue.

See also Components of breastmilk; Dehydration and breastfeeding; Jaundice

▶ WDWN (Well developed, well nourished)

DEFINITION An acronym used to indicate that an individual appears to be adequately fed.

▶ Weak suck

DEFINITION Milk production stimulation and milk transfer depend on an effective suck.

Babies more likely to have a weak suck at first include:

Babies who are born prematurely.

Babies who have been exposed to certain drugs.

Babies who have neurological impairment.

Ask about

Age of baby.

Feeding history.

Weight gain history.

ASSESSMENT

EMERGENT CARE NEEDED?

Are any of the following present?

Difficulty breathing even when not feeding.

Difficulty breathing after feeding.

Baby pulls off of the breast to breathe.

Extreme lethargy or irritability in baby.

Sudden change in baby's muscle tone (extremely floppy or stiff) or repetitive jerking movements (e.g., seizure activity).

Baby shows sudden disinterest in feeding.

Unable to wake baby.

Baby does not calm, even with cuddles.

Meconium bowel movements after 5 days of life.

Fewer than three bowel movements daily in breastfed newborn after the first 2 days of life.

No urine in six hours.

Brick dust urine (uric acid crystals) after 2 days of life.

Dark colored urine.

Fewer than four urinations daily in the breastfed newborn after day 5 of life.

Noticeably sunken fontanelles (soft spot on top of head).

Baby below birthweight at 10 to 14 days of life.

Cessation of weight gain.

IF YES, *Seek pediatric care now.*

PROMPT CARE NEEDED?

Are any of the following present?

Diagnosis of neuromuscular problem in a breastfeeding baby.

IF YES, *Refer for consultation with occupational, physical, or speech therapist experienced with breastfeeding babies.*

Are any of the following present?

Baby does not stay on the breast.

Baby is not gaining adequately.

Baby does not seem to transfer milk.

IF YES, *Call lactation care provider now.*

ROUTINE CARE NEEDED?

Are any of the following present?

Difficulty maintaining milk supply.

IF YES, *Call lactation care provider today.*

SELF CARE INFORMATION

As soon as it is determined that the infant has an uncoordinated suck, mother should express her milk regularly in order to maintain her supply and to collect milk to feed the baby.

Increased opportunities to practice breastfeeding can be helpful to promote coordinated sucking.

IMPORTANT CONDITIONS TO REPORT

Inadequate stooling or urinations.

Lethargy.

Baby difficult to rouse.

Lower milk volume.

See also Botulism, infantile; Breast pump; Lethargy; Sleepy baby; Uncoordinated suckling; Weight gain, baby–low

▶ Weaning

DEFINITION   Weaning is a process that begins when the baby is fed anything except breastmilk and continues until the baby is no longer receiving mother's milk.

Ask about

Age of baby.
Feeding history.

ASSESSMENT

ROUTINE CARE NEEDED?
Are any of the following present?
Weaning information required because of prescribed drug.

IF YES,   *Consult up-to-date drug references.*

ROUTINE CARE NEEDED?
Are any of the following present?
Questions about how long breastfeeding should last.
Need for weaning strategy or management.

IF YES,   *Call lactation care provider.*

SELF CARE INFORMATION

Every mother has unique feelings about her breastfeeding experience, including how and when it should end.
Mothers are sometimes instructed to wean for reasons that are not legitimate, such as the onset of baby's teething.

IMPORTANT CONDITIONS TO REPORT

Breast discomfort.
Fever.
Red streaks on breast.
Concerns about weaning.

See also Abrupt weaning; Closet nursing; Nursing strike

Drug References

American Academy of Pediatrics Committee on Drugs. (2001). Transfer of drugs and other chemicals into human milk. *Pediatrics, 108,* 776–789.

Briggs, G.G., Freeman, R.K., & Yaffee, S.J. (Eds.). (2002). *Drugs in pregnancy and lactation* (6th ed.). Philadelphia: Lippincott, Williams, and Wilkins.

Hale, T.W. (2004). *Medications and mothers milk.* Amarillo, TX: Pharmasoft Publishing.

Lawrence, R.A., & Lawrence, R.M. (2005). *Breastfeeding: A guide for the medical profession* (6th ed.). St. Louis: Mosby.

▶ Weight gain, baby—high

DEFINITION Well fed breastfed babies gain more rapidly in the early months compared to standard growth charts and to formula fed babies. It is not thought possible for women to overfeed babies at the breast.

Ask about

Age of baby.
Weight gain pattern of baby.

ASSESSMENT

PROMPT CARE NEEDED?

Are any of the following present?

About mother

Reddened areas of the breast.

Fever higher than 101° F (38.5° C).

Extreme breast discomfort.

Flu-like aching throughout body.

Recurrent mastitis.

IF YES, *Call obstetric care provider within 2 to 4 hours and seek lactation care today.*

SELF CARE INFORMATION

Oversupply can cause discomfort for mother and baby. Careful management of the mother's milk supply can increase the baby's comfort.

IMPORTANT CONDITIONS TO REPORT

Recurrent symptoms.

Unresolved symptoms.

See also Milk flow, too fast; Overactive let-down reflex

▶ Weight gain, baby—low

DEFINITION Breastfed babies should gain a minimum of 0.5 oz to 1 oz a day on average in the early weeks. New studies indicate that breastfed babies gain even faster than was previously believed, probably because in the past, breastfeeding was done on a schedule and not as frequently as we now know is ideal.

Ask about

Age of baby.

Weight gain pattern.

PROMPT CARE NEEDED?

Are any of the following present?

Extreme lethargy or irritability in baby.

Sudden change in baby's muscle tone (extremely floppy or stiff) or repetitive jerking movements (e.g., seizure activity).

Baby shows sudden disinterest in feeding.

Unable to wake baby.

Baby does not calm, even with cuddles.

Meconium bowel movements after 5 days of life.

Fewer than three bowel movements daily in breastfed newborn after the first 2 days of life.

No urine in six hours.

Brick dust urine (uric acid crystals) after 2 days of life.

Dark colored urine.

Fewer than four urinations daily in the breastfed newborn after day 5 of life.

Noticeably sunken fontanelles (soft spot on top of head).

Decreased activity.

Baby below birthweight at 10 to 14 days of life.

Cessation of weight gain.

Sleeping at the breast.

IF YES, *Seek pediatric care now.*

ROUTINE CARE NEEDED?

Are any of the following present?

Sleeps at the breast after a few sucks.

Hard to latch-on.

No audible swallows.

Pediatric referral for consultation.

IF YES, *Seek lactation care today.*

IMPORTANT CONDITIONS TO REPORT
Decrease in number of urinations or stools.
Increased sleepiness, hours spent sleeping.
Baby is harder to rouse.

See also Hypotonia; Jaundice

▶ Weight loss, baby

DEFINITION   Weight loss is not expected after the first few days postpartum.

See also Insufficient milk supply; Weight gain, baby–low

▶ Weight loss, mother

DEFINITION   Weight loss of up to 5 lb a month in the first months postpartum has not been associated with poorer growth of the nursing baby.

Exclusively breastfeeding mothers are more likely to be closer to their pre-pregnancy weight at six months postpartum when compared to mixed feeding or formula feeding mothers.

ASSESSMENT

ROUTINE CARE NEEDED?

Are any of the following present?

Desire to exercise while breastfeeding.
Desire to lose weight while breastfeeding.

IF YES,   *Call lactation care provider.*

SELF CARE INFORMATION
Weight loss of up to 5 lb a month in the first months postpartum has not been associated with poorer growth of the nursing baby.

Exclusive breastfeeding is the best route to weight loss in the first six months post-partum. Continued breastfeeding after six months contributes to additional weight loss.

IMPORTANT CONDITIONS TO REPORT
Rapid weight loss of more than 3 lb per week after the first six weeks postpartum.

See also Exclusive breastfeeding; Exercise and breastfeeding

▶ Wellstart International

DEFINITION "Wellstart International's mission is to advance the knowledge, skills, and ability of health care providers regarding the promotion, protection, and support of optimal infant and maternal health and nutrition from conception through the completion of weaning."[187]

> **Notes**
>
> Wellstart International
> P.O. Box 80877
> San Diego, CA 92138-0877
> Phone: 619-295-5192
> Web site: www.wellstart.org
> Wellstart offers professional education and support materials, as well as local breast-feeding services.

Footnotes
[187]Wellstart International. (2003). *Mission.* Retrieved August 4, 2005, from http://www.wellstart.org/about.html.

▶ Wet diapers

DEFINITION Wet diapers, in addition to stooling patterns, can be an important indication of breastfeeding success.

Age of baby.

History of urination.

ASSESSMENT

EMERGENT CARE NEEDED?

Are any of the following present?

No wet diaper or stool in 6–8 hours after the first 2 days of life.

Red dusty urine in diaper after the first 2 days of life.

Urine crystals in diaper after the first 2 days of life.

Lethargy/difficulty rousing baby.

Baby sleeps at the breast consistently.

IF YES, *Seek pediatric care now.*

PROMPT CARE NEEDED?

Are any of the following present?

No wet diaper or stool in 4–6 hours after the first 2 days of life.

Baby falls asleep after a few sucks.

Poor latch.

IF YES, *Seek lactation care now and report to pediatric care provider.*

ROUTINE CARE NEEDED?

Are any of the following present?

Need for reassurance that baby is getting enough nourishment with no other symptoms.

IF YES, *Call lactation care provider today.*

SELF CARE INFORMATION

Wet diapers, in addition to stooling patterns, can be an important indication of breastfeeding success.

IMPORTANT CONDITIONS TO REPORT

No wet diaper or stool in 6 hours after the first 2 days of life.

Red, dusty urine in diaper after the first 2 days of life.

Urine crystals in diaper after the first 2 days of life.
Lethargy.

See also Bowel movements, infant; Stooling patterns; Water for the nursing baby (Water supplementation)

▶ Wet-nursing

DEFINITION   Historically, women who nursed babies who were not their own were called wet-nurses. Wet-nurses usually were not nursing their own babies at the same time and may have been paid for their service.

Because of concerns about transmission of HIV, hepatitis, herpes, and other organisms, wet-nursing is discouraged in the United States today.

See also Cross nursing; Donor milk

▶ WHO

See also Baby-Friendly Hospital Initiative (BFHI); Ten Steps to Successful Breastfeeding; World Health Organization (WHO)

▶ WHO Code (International Code of Marketing of Breast-milk Substitutes)

DEFINITION   A document adopted by the World Health Assembly in 1981 and amended by several subsequent resolutions as a minimum requirement to protect infant health. The International Code sets forth a series of expectations about the behavior of the infant formula industry, health care systems, health care providers, governments, and other parties regarding the protection of breastfeeding and ethical marketing of breastmilk substitutes.

▶ WIC program

DEFINITION   WIC is a supplemental food program for women, infants, and children that is administered through the United States Department of Agriculture (USDA).

"The mission of WIC is to safeguard the health of low-income women, infants, and children up to age 5 who are at nutritional risk by providing nutritional foods to supplement diets, information on healthy eating, and referrals to health care."[188]

Breastfeeding rates among WIC participants are rising. The percentage of WIC participants who initiated breastfeeding increased by 69% over a 10-year period. The percentage of women who breastfed at 6 months increased by 145% during the same time period.[189]

> ### Notes
>
> WIC at FNS Headquarters:
> Supplemental Food Programs Division
> Food and Nutrition Service - USDA
> 3101 Park Center Drive
> Alexandria, VA 22302
> Phone: 703-305-2746
> Fax: 703-305-2196
> Web site: www.fns.usda.gov/wic

Footnotes

[188]The Special Supplemental Nutrition Program for Women, Infants, and Children. (2003). *WIC's mission*. Retrieved August 4, 2005, from http://www.fns.usda.gov/wic/aboutwic/mission.htm.

[189]United States Department of Agriculture. (2003). *WIC and breastfeeding rates* (Food and Nutrition Research Report, Number 34-2). Washington, DC.

See also Special Supplemental Food Program for Women, Infants, and Children (WIC)

▶ Witches' milk

DEFINITION Both boy and girl babies have enlarged breasts when they are born. The swelling lasts for a few days, whether or not the baby is being breastfed. If the breast is squeezed, witches' milk will come out. The milk is actually very similar to mother's milk, and is created in response to maternal hormones that have crossed the placenta.

SELF CARE INFORMATION
Over time the baby's breasts will get smaller and this newborn milk will disappear.

IMPORTANT CONDITIONS TO REPORT
Milk continuing beyond the early weeks.
Bloody discharge from the baby's nipples.

▶ WNL (Within normal limits)

DEFINITION An acronym used to indicate that an individual's growth and development is typical.

▶ Working mothers

DEFINITION Mothers who work for pay may do so away from home or in the home. They may be separated from their babies or have their babies nearby. In the United States, more than half of the mothers with babies under the age of 1 are employed.

Ask about

Amount of separation—hours per day, days per week.
Start date of work.
Age of baby.
Mother's plans to continue breastfeeding.
Mother's plans to express milk.
Accommodations at work for expressing and saving milk.
How the baby will be fed away from the mother.

ROUTINE CARE NEEDED?

Are any of the following present?

Information needed about managing work and breastfeeding.

IF YES, *Call lactation care provider today.*

SELF CARE INFORMATION

Stress does not seem to affect milk supply, but frequent milk removal is needed to maintain or improve the milk supply.

Milk can be collected and frozen in the early weeks to supplement milk collected after mother's return to work.

Milk supply is best maintained by using a pump that is intended for that purpose (i.e., electric rental grade pump for longer separation; casual use pump for occasional expression).

Select child care facilities carefully.

Expressed milk is a raw food and should be refrigerated as soon as possible after expression.

The timing of return to work and the number of hours spent away from the baby affect the duration of breastfeeding more than the type of work a woman does.

IMPORTANT CONDITIONS TO REPORT

Problems with expressing milk (check that the equipment is working properly).

Breast problems.

Problems with the infant accepting expressed milk.

Notes

Ongoing support and help with problem solving may be needed after returning to work.

See also Collection and storage of breastmilk; Day care; Decrease in milk supply; Pump; Reverse cycle nursing

▶ World Alliance for Breastfeeding Action (WABA)

DEFINITION   The World Alliance for Breastfeeding Action (WABA) protects, promotes, and supports breastfeeding worldwide.

"WABA is a global network of individuals and [organizations] concerned with the protection, promotion and support of breastfeeding worldwide. WABA action is based on the Innocenti Declaration, the Ten Links for Nurturing the Future and the Global Strategy for Infant & Young Child Feeding."[190]

WABA coordinates World Breastfeeding Week.

Notes

World Alliance for Breastfeeding Action (WABA)
P.O. Box 1200
10850 Penang, Malaysia
Web site: www.waba.org.my

Footnotes

[190]World Alliance for Breastfeeding Action. (n.d.) *Untitled*. Retrieved August 4, 2005, from http://www.waba.org.my/.

▶ World Health Organization (WHO)

DEFINITION   The World Health Organization (WHO) is a specialized agency of the United Nations that directs and coordinates international health work.

WHO's main functions are to give world guidance in the field of health, to set global standards for health to cooperate with governments in strengthening national health programs, and to develop and transfer appropriate health technology, information, and standards.

See also Baby-Friendly Hospital Initiative (BFHI); Ten Steps to Successful Breastfeeding

▶ X-ray, diagnostic

DEFINITION X-ray is a type of high energy radiation. In low doses, x-rays are used to diagnose diseases by making pictures of the inside of the body.
  Diagnostic x-rays have no effect on lactation.

ASSESSMENT
ROUTINE CARE NEEDED? *Are any of the following present?*   Mother requires diagnostic x-ray.
IF YES, *Inform mother that diagnostic x-rays have no effect on lactation.*

See also Radioactive agents

▶ Yeast infection

DEFINITION Overgrowth of *Candida albicans* or other common fungi.
  Symptoms of yeast infection of the breast include red, shiny looking skin on the nipple or areola, flaky skin, and sharp, itching pain that persists between feedings. Infant symptoms of yeast overgrowth or "thrush" include white patches of growth

on the inner buccal surface (cheek) or tongue, and occasionally pain on latch. Infants may also have diaper area yeast overgrowth.

Ask about

Onset.
Medications taken in past month.

ASSESSMENT

PROMPT CARE NEEDED?

Are any of the following present?

Sharp, itching, persistent nipple pain (not just during feedings).
Presence of white patches in infant's mouth.
Baby with yeast infection in the diaper area.

IF YES, *Call obstetric and pediatric care providers today.*

ROUTINE CARE NEEDED?

Are any of the following present?

Nipple pain during feeding.

IF YES, *Seek lactation care today.*

SELF CARE INFORMATION

Finish all medications prescribed.
If administering nystatin suspension to the infant, pour a dose into a clean cup or spoon. Half of the dose should be used for each side of the mouth. Suspension may be applied with a cotton swab. A clean swab should be used for each application. Take care not to introduce used swabs into the bottle of suspension.

IMPORTANT CONDITIONS TO REPORT

Persistent symptoms.
Recurrent symptoms.

Candida overgrowth may follow, or increase after antibiotic treatment.

Recommended treatment for candidiasis is topical antifungal (nystatin).

If symptoms are not relieved by topical treatment, feeding evaluation should occur to rule out positioning or attachment problems contributing to pain.

Medical evaluation should rule out other conditions resulting in redness and pain, including **eczema**, reaction to surface allergens, trauma, **Raynaud's phenomenon**, concomitant bacteria, and infection.

Subsequent treatment with oral antifungals such as ketaconazole and fluconazole may resolve symptoms.

When yeast is diagnosed in the nursing mother or child, both should be treated. In addition, any artificial nipples or pacifiers used should be discarded and replaced after treatment.

Lactation evaluation should rule out contributing problems with latch or distortion of nipple in baby's mouth.

See also Candidiasis; Nipple pain; Thrush

Appendix A

Sample Triage Documentation Form

SAMPLE INTAKE FORM

DATE ___/___/___   TIME: _____   LC: _____

MOTHER:

Name _____

Telephone _____

Address _____

_____

Referred by _____

Significant Hx _____

OB/CNM _____

INFANT(S):

Name(s) _____

DOB _____ Birthweight _____

Age today _____

Recent weight_____ on _____

Significant Hx _____

_____

Ped/FP _____

Delivered at _____ Hospital _____ Home

_____ Birth Center

CALLED CONCERNING:

_____

_____

_____

SUGGESTIONS GIVEN:

_____

_____

_____

DISPOSITION RECOMMENDED:

☐ **Emergent Medical:** Referred to _____

☐ **Prompt Medical:** Referred to ____Pediatrician ____Obstetrician
____Family Practitioner ____Other (indicate) _____

☐ **Emergent/Prompt Lactation Care:** ___Consult Appt Sched for __/__ @ ___
☐ Referral to other LC _____

☐ **Routine:** ☐ Mother to call back as needed ☐ Consult Appt Suggested
☐ Referred to _____

Follow-up call planned for __/__ @ ___
Who will call? ☐ Call Center Staff or ☐ Mother ☐ Information pack sent

Follow-up completed on __/___ by _____

| Length of call: _____ min. |

Appendix B

Sample Disposition Form for Telephone Answering

In this agency...

"Seek emergency care now" means refer to

_____

_____

"Seek medical care now" means refer to

_____

_____

_____

"Seek medical care in 2 to 4 hours" means refer to

_____

_____

_____

"Seek medical care today" means refer to

_____

_____

"Call pediatric care provider today" means refer to

_____

_____

"Call obstetric care provider today" means refer to

_____

_____

"Call lactation care provider now" means refer to

_____

_____

"Call or seek lactation care today" means refer to

_____

_____

"Seek dietary consultation" means refer to

_____

_____

Referral numbers:

WIC_____   _____

Social Services_____   _____

Pump and other equipment phone numbers

_____

_____

Drug references may be located

_____

_____

Contraindications Protocol

_____

_____

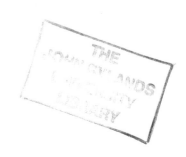